A Series of Textbooks for Public Health

PREVENTIVE MEDICINE

预防医学

主　编 / 赵进顺　倪春辉　孟晓静

副主编 / 孙桂菊　李煌元

秘　书 / 严玮文

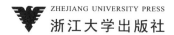

ZHEJIANG UNIVERSITY PRESS
浙江大学出版社

Contributors

叶海亚·阿布卡里亚/Abqariyah，Yahya（马来亚大学医学院社会和预防医学系/Department of Social and Preventive Medicine，Faculty of Medicine，University of Malaya）

艾自胜/Ai，Zisheng（同济大学医学院医学统计学教研室/Department of Medical Statistics，School of Medicine，Tongji University）

柏建岭/Bai，Jianling（南京医科大学公共卫生学院生物统计学系/Department of Biostatistics，School of Public Health，Nanjing Medical University）

珍妮·鲍曼/Bowman，Jenny（自由撰稿人和编者 freelance writer and editor）

岑晗/Cen，Han（宁波大学医学院公共卫生学院/School of Public Health，Medical School of Ningbo University）

戴悦/Dai，Yue（福建医科大学公共卫生学院卫生管理学系/Department of Health Management，Public Health School，Fujian Medical University）

黄民耀/Derry，Minyao Ng（宁波大学医学院/Medical School of Ningbo University）

丁玉松/Ding，Yusong（石河子大学医学院预防医学系/Department of Preventive Medicine，School of Medicine，Shihezi University）.

董长征/Dong，Changzheng（宁波大学医学院公共卫生学院/School of Public Health，Medical School of Ningbo University）

范引光/Fan，Yinguang（安徽医科大学公共卫生学院流行病与卫生统计学系/Department of Epidemiology and Health Statistics，School of Public Health，Anhui Medical University）

冯丹/Feng，Dan（中山大学公共卫生学院营养学系/Department of Nutrition，School of Public Health，Sun Yat-sen University）

冯晴/Feng，Qing（南京医科大学公共卫生学院营养与食品卫生学系/Department of Nutrition and Food Hygiene，School of Public Health，Nanjing Medical University）

凤志慧/Feng，Zhihui（山东大学公共卫生学院职业与环境健康学系/Department of Occupational and Environmental Health，School of Public Health，Shandong University）

郭欣/Guo，Xin（山东大学公共卫生学院卫生毒理与营养学系/Department of Toxicology and Nutrition，School of Public Health，Shandong University）

玛丽亚·哈莱姆/Haleem，Maria（宁波大学医学院/Medical School of Ningbo University）

韩丽媛/Han，Liyuan（中国科学院大学华美医院，中国科学院大学宁波生命与健康产业研究院/Hwa Mei Hospital，Ningbo Institute of Life and Health Industry，University of Chinese Academy of Sciences）

何灿霞/He，Canxia（宁波大学医学院公共卫生学院/School of Public Health，Medical School of Ningbo University）

何斐/He，Fei（福建医科大学公共卫生学院流行病与卫生统计学系/Department of Epidemiology and Health Statistics，Public Health School，Fujian Medical University）

胡付兰/Hu，Fulan（深圳大学医学部公共卫生学院流行病与卫生统计学教研室/Department of Epidemiology and Biostatistics，School of Public Health，Health Science Center，Shenzhen University）

华启航/Hua，Qihang（宁波大学医学院公共卫生学院/School of Public Health，Medical School of Ningbo University）

荆春霞/Jing，Chunxia（暨南大学基础医学院公共卫生与预防医学系/Department of Public Health and Preventive Medicine，School of Medicine，Jinan University）

敬媛媛/Jing，Yuanyuan（川北医学院预防医学系/Department of Preventive Medicine，North Sichuan Medical College）

孔璐/Kong，Lu（东南大学公共卫生学院劳动卫生与环境卫生学系/Department of Occupational and Environmental Health，School of Public Health，Southeast University）

冷瑞雪/Leng，Ruixue（安徽医科大学公共卫生学院流行病与卫生统计学系/Department of Epidemiology and Health Statistics，School of Public Health，Anhui Medical University）

李煌元/Li，Huangyuan（福建医科大学公共卫生学院预防医学系/Department of Preventive Medicine，Public Health School，Fujian Medical University）

李京/Li，Jing（潍坊医学院公共卫生学院预防医学系环境卫生教研室/Division of Environmental Health，Department of Preventive Medicine，School of Public Health，Weifang Medical University）

李静/Li，Jing（徐州医科大学公共卫生学院卫生学系/Department of Hygiene，School of Public Health，Xuzhou Medical University）

李举双/Li，Jushuang（温州医科大学公共卫生与管理学院预防医学系/Department of Preventive Medicine，School of Public Health and Management，Wenzhou Medical University）

李晓枫/Li，Xiaofeng（大连医科大学公共卫生学院流行病学教研室/Department of Epidemiology，School of Public Health，Dalian Medical University）

李永华/Li，Yonghua（济宁医学院公共卫生学院食品安全与健康教研室/Department of Food Safety and Health，School of Public Health，Jining Medical University）

李育平/Li，Yuping（扬州大学临床医学院，江苏省苏北人民医院/Clinical Medical School of Yangzhou University，Northern Jiangsu People's Hospital）

李真/Li，Zhen（宁波大学医学院公共卫生学院/School of Public Health，Medical School of Ningbo University）

廖奇/Liao，Qi（宁波大学医学院公共卫生学院/School of Public Health，Medical School of Ningbo University）

林玉兰/Lin，Yulan（福建医科大学公共卫生学院流行病与卫生统计学系/Department of Epidemiology and Health Statistics，Public Health School，Fujian Medical University）

刘丽亚/Liu，Liya（宁波大学医学院公共卫生学院/School of Public Health，Medical School of Ningbo University）

卢光玉/Lu，Guangyu（扬州大学医学院预防医学系/Department of Preventive Medicine，Medical College of Yangzhou University）

马俊香/Ma，Junxiang（首都医科大学公卫学院劳动卫生与环境卫生学系/Department of Occupational and Environmental Health，School of Public Health，Capital Medical University）

马儒林/Ma，Rulin（石河子大学医学院预防医学系/Department of Preventive Medicine，School of Medicine，Shihezi University）

安妮·马穆沙什维利/Mamuchashvili，Anny（宁波大学医学院/Medical School of Ningbo University）

毛广运/Mao，Guangyun（温州医科大学公共卫生与管理学院预防医学系，温州医科大学附属眼视光医院临床研究中心/Department of Preventive Medicine，School of Public Health and Management，and Center on Clinical Research of the Eye Hospital，Wenzhou Medical University）

毛盈颖/Mao，Yingying（浙江中医药大学公共卫生学院流行病与卫生统计学教研室/Department of Epidemiology and Health Statistics，School of Public Health，Zhejiang Chinese Medical University）

孟琼/Meng，Qiong（昆明医科大学公共卫生学院流行病与卫生统计学系/Department of Epidemiology and Health Statistics，School of Public Health，Kunming Medical University）

孟晓静/Meng，Xiaojing（南方医科大学公共卫生学院职业卫生与职业医学系/Department of Occupational Health and Occupational Medicine，School of Public Health，Southern Medical University）

倪春辉/Ni，Chunhui（南京医科大学公共卫生学院实验教学中心/Experimental Teaching Center，School of Public Health，Nanjing Medical University）

潘红梅/Pan，Hongmei（昆明医科大学公共卫生学院营养与食品科学系/Department of Nutrition and Food Science，School of Public Health，Kunming Medical University）

庞道华/Pang，Daohua（济宁医学院公共卫生学院营养与食品卫生学教研室/Department of Nutrition and Food Hygiene，School of Public Health，Jining Medical University）

培尔顿·米吉提/Peierdun，Mijiti（新疆医科大学公共卫生学院流行病学教研室/Department of Epidemiology，School of Public Health，Xinjiang Medical University）

仇梁林/Qiu，Lianglin（南通大学公共卫生学院营养与食品卫生学系/Department of Nutrition and Food Hygiene，School of Public Health，Nantong University）

曲泉颖/Qu，Quanying（锦州医科大学公共卫生学院流行病学教研室/Department of Epidemiology，School of Public Health，Jinzhou Medical University）

邵方/Shao，Fang（南京医科大学公共卫生学院生物统计学系/Department of Biostatistics，School of Public Health，Nanjing Medical University）

沈冲/Shen，Chong（南京医科大学公共卫生学院流行病学系/Department of Epidemiology，

School of Public Health，Nanjing Medical University）

施红英/Shi，Hongying（温州医科大学公共卫生与管理学院预防医学系/Department of Preventive Medicine，School of Public Health and Management，Wenzhou Medical University）

孙桂菊/Sun，Guiju（东南大学公共卫生学院营养与食品卫生学系/Department of Nutrition and Food Hygiene，School of Public Health，Southeast University）

孙桂香/Sun，Guixiang（徐州医科大学公共卫生学院流行病与卫生统计学系/Department of Epidemiology and Health Statistics，School of Public Health，Xuzhou Medical University）

孙宏鹏/Sun，Hongpeng（苏州大学医学部公共卫生学院少儿卫生与社会医学系/Department of Child Health and Social Medicine，School of Public Health，Medical College of Soochow University）

孙鲜策/Sun，Xiance（大连医科大学公共卫生学院劳动卫生与环境卫生教研室/Department of Occupational and Environmental Health，School of Public Health，Dalian Medical University）

唐春兰/Tang，Chunlan（宁波大学医学院公共卫生学院/School of Public Health，Medical School of Ningbo University）

唐少文/Tang，Shaowen（南京医科大学公共卫生学院流行病学系/Department of Epidemiology，School of Public Health，Nanjing Medical University）

童智敏/Tong，Zhimin（昆山疾病预防控制中心/Kunshan Municipal Center for Disease Control and Prevention）

王春平/Wang，Chunping（潍坊医学院公共卫生学院预防医学系/Department of Preventive Medicine，School of Public Health，Weifang Medical University）

王辉/Wang，Hui（北京大学医学部公共卫生学院妇幼卫生系/Department of Maternal and Children Health，School of Public Health，Peking University Health Science Center）

王建明/Wang，Jianming（南京医科大学公共卫生学院流行病学系/Department of Epidemiology，School of Public Health，Nanjing Medical University）

王津涛/Wang，Jintao（四川大学华西公共卫生学院环境卫生与职业医学系/Department of Environmental Health and Occupational Medicine，West China School of Public Health，Sichuan University）

王乐三/Wang，Lesan（中南大学湘雅公共卫生学院流行病与卫生统计学系/Department of Epidemiology and Health Statistics，Xiangya School of Public Health，Central South University）

王丽君/Wang，Lijun（暨南大学医学院公共卫生与预防医学系/Department of Public Health and Preventive Medicine，School of Medicine，Jinan University）

王强/Wang，Qiang（江苏大学医学院预防医学与卫生检验系/Department of Preventive Medicine and Public Health Laboratory Science，School of Medicine，Jiangsu University）

王少康/Wang，Shaokang（东南大学公共卫生学院营养与食品卫生学系/Department of

Nutrition and Food Hygiene，School of Public Health，Southeast University）

王涛/Wang，Tao（温州医科大学公共卫生与管理学院预防医学系/Department of Preventive Medicine，School of Public Health and Management，Wenzhou Medical University）

王晓珂/Wang，Xiaoke（南通大学公共卫生学院职业医学与环境毒理学系/Department of Occupational Medicine and Environmental Toxicology，School of Public Health，Nantong University）

王子云/Wang，Ziyun（贵州医科大学公共卫生学院流行病与卫生统计学系/Department of Epidemiology and Health Statistics，School of Public Health，Guizhou Medical University）

黄丽冰/Wong，Li Ping（马来亚大学医学院社会和预防医学系/Department of Social and Preventive Medicine，Faculty of Medicine，University of Malaya）

吴冬梅/Wu，Dongmei（南京医科大学公共卫生学院职业医学与环境卫生学系/Department of Occupational Medicine and Environmental Health，School of Public Health，Nanjing Medical University）

吴继国/Wu，Jiguo（南方医科大学公共卫生学院环境卫生学系/Department of Environmental Health，School of Public Health，Southern Medical University）

吴秋云/Wu，Qiuyun（徐州医科大学公共卫生学院卫生学系/Department of Hygiene，School of Public Health，Xuzhou Medical University）

吴思英/Wu，Siying（福建医科大学公共卫生学院流行病与卫生统计学系/Department of Epidemiology and Health Statistics，School of Public Health，Fujian Medical University）

吴莹/Wu，Ying（南方医科大学生物统计教研室/Department of Biostatistics，Southern Medical University）

肖艳杰/Xiao，Yanjie（锦州医科大学公共卫生学院流行病学系/Department of Epidemiology，School of Public Health，Jinzhou Medical University）

徐进/Xu，Jin（宁波大学医学院公共卫生学院/School of Public Health，Medical School of Ningbo University）

许望东/Xu，Wangdong（西南医科大学公共卫生学院循证医学中心/Department of Evidence-Based Medicine，School of Public Health，Southwest Medical University）

严玮文/Yan，Weiwen（南京医科大学公共卫生学院预防医学实验教学中心/Experimental Teaching Center of Preventive Medicine，School of Public Health，Nanjing Medical University）

杨丹婷/Yang，Danting（宁波大学医学院公共卫生学院/School of Public Health，Medical School of Ningbo University）

杨艳/Yang，Yan（西南医科大学公共卫生学院营养与食品卫生教研室/Department of Nutrition and Food Hygiene，School of Public Health，Southwest Medical University）

姚美雪/Yao，Meixue（徐州医科大学公共卫生学院流行病与卫生统计学系/Department of Epidemiology and Health Statistics，School of Public Health，Xuzhou Medical University）

叶洋/Ye，Yang（江苏大学医学院预防医学与卫生检验系/Department of Preventive Medicine and Public Health Laboratory Science，School of Medicine，Jiangsu University）

易洪刚/Yi，Honggang（南京医科大学公共卫生学院生物统计学系/Department of Biostatistics，School of Public Health，Nanjing Medical University）

尹洁云/Yin，Jieyun（苏州大学医学部公共卫生学院流行病与卫生统计学教研室/Department of Epidemiology and Health Statistics，School of Public Health，Medical College of Soochow University）

于广霞/Yu，Guangxia（福建医科大学公共卫生学院预防医学系/Department of Preventive Medicine，School of Public Health，Fujian Medical University）

俞琼/Yu，Qiong，（吉林大学公共卫生学院流行病与卫生统计学教研室/Department of Epidemiology and Health Statistics，School of Public Health，Jilin University）

袁芝琼/Yuan，Zhiqiong（大理大学公共卫生学院营养与食品卫生学教研室/Department of Nutrition and Food Hygiene，School of Public Health，Dali University）

曾芳芳/Zeng，Fangfang（暨南大学医学院公共卫生与预防医学系/Department of Public Health and Preventive Medicine，School of Medicine，Jinan University）

查龙应/Zha，Longying（南方医科大学公共卫生学院营养与食品卫生学系/Department of Nutrition and Food Hygiene，School of Public Health，Southern Medical University）

张丹丹/Zhang，Dandan（浙江大学基础医学院病理学与病理生理学系/Department of Pathology and Pathophysiology，School of Basic Medical Sciences，Zhejiang University）

张俊辉/Zhang，Junhui（西南医科大学公共卫生学院流行病与卫生统计学教研室/Department of Epidemiology and Health Statistics，School of Public Health，Southwest Medical University）

张莉娜/Zhang，Lina（宁波大学医学院公共卫生学院/School of Public Health，Medical School of Ningbo University）

张利平/Zhang，Liping（潍坊医学院公共卫生学院预防医学系环境卫生教研室/Division of Environmental Health，Department of Preventive Medicine，School of Public Health，Weifang Medical University）

张巧/Zhang，Qiao（郑州大学公共卫生学院卫生毒理学教研室/Department of Toxicology，School of Public Health，Zhengzhou University）

张思懋/Zhang，Simin（南京医科大学公共卫生学院社会医学和健康教育系/Department of Social Medicine and Health Education，School of Public Health，Nanjing Medical University）

张晓宏/Zhang，Xiaohong（宁波大学医学院公共卫生学院/School of Public Health，Medical School of Ningbo University）

赵进顺/Zhao，Jinshun（宁波大学医学院公共卫生学院/School of Public Health，Medical School of Ningbo University）

赵苒/Zhao，Ran（厦门大学公共卫生学院预防医学系/Department of Preventive Medicine，School of Public Health，Xiamen University）

赵秀兰/Zhao，Xiulan（山东大学公共卫生学院营养与毒理学系/Department of Nutrition and Toxicology，School of Public Health，Shandong University）

赵研/Zhao，Yan（匹兹堡大学医学中心/University of Pittsburgh Medical Center）

郑馥荔/Zheng，Fuli（福建医科大学公共卫生学院预防医学系/Department of Preventive Medicine，School of Public Health，Fujian Medical University）

仲崇科/Zhong，Chongke（苏州大学医学部公共卫生学院流行病与卫生统计学教研室/Department of Epidemiology and Health Statistics，School of Public Health，Medical College of Soochow University）

周舫/Zhou，Fang（郑州大学公共卫生学院劳动卫生教研室/Department of Occupational Health，School of Public Health，Zhengzhou University）

周志衡/Zhou，Zhiheng（广州市华立科技职业学院健康学院/Health College of Guangzhou Huali Science and Technology Vocational College；深圳市福田区第二人民医院/ The Second People's Hospital of Futian District，Shenzhen）

邹祖全/Zou，Zuquan（宁波大学医学院公共卫生学院/School of Public Health，Medical School of Ningbo University）

Preface

Public health is the science and art of disease prevention. It targets many facets necessary to the well-being of society, including prolonging life, the promotion of physical health through organized community efforts directed at environmental sanitation, the control of community infections, the education of the individual in the principles of personal hygiene, the development of the social machinery to ensure that every individual in the community has an adequate standard of living for the maintenance of health, and the organization of medical and nursing services to aid early diagnosis and enable preventive treatment of diseases. Public health includes many sub-branches, among which the most importantones are preventive medicine, medical statistics, epidemiology, and health services. Preventive medicine is an important part of medical science, which, when integrated with basic medicine and clinical medicine, forms the entire frame of modern medicine. Because preventive medicine, medical statistics, and epidemiology are three important compulsory subjects for international students majoring in clinical medicine, Zhejiang University Press organized public health experts from five universities in China and the University of Texas in the United States of America to compile an English textbook entitled *Preventive Medicine*, *Medical Statistics and Epidemiology*, which was published in 2014. In recent years, this textbook has played an important role in teaching preventive medicine, medical statistics, and epidemiology to international students majoring in clinical medicine in China.

With the continuous expansion and internationalization of higher education in China and many developments in preventive medicine, medical statistics, and epidemiology, a revised edition of this important textbook was required. In 2018, Zhejiang University Press organized experts to reprint the textbook. For the revised edition, the quality was raised significantly to meet global demands. The authors endeavor to improve the quality of this textbook and reflect the latest developments in the fields of preventive medicine, medical statistics, and epidemiology. In addition, the authors present a resource to standardize and unify the quality of teaching and materials for international students majoring in clinical medicine in China.

The new edition is a series of textbooks for public health including *Preventive Medicine*, *Medical Statistics*, and *Epidemiology*.

This book, *Preventive Medicine*, consists of six chapters. The first chapter introduces the concept of preventive medicine and its tasks, health determinants, disease prevention strategies and clinical and community prevention services. Chapter 2 introduces the relationship between environment and health, the source, classification, environmental fate of pollutants, the impact of the environment on health, and the toxicology of chemical pollutants. Chapter 3 describes the living environment and health, including air, water, soil environment, and health, focusing on the sources of pollutants in the environment, health hazards and control measures. Chapter 4 is about occupational health. It introduces the classification of occupational harmful factors and the types of health damage; the principles of diagnosis, treatment, and prevention of occupational diseases; the exposure risk of common occupational toxicants, dust and physical factors; the resulting health damage; and relevant preventative and control measures. Chapter 5 is about food nutrition and health, focusing on the basics of nutrients, life cycle nutrition, public nutrition, nutrition and diseases, and foodborne diseases. Chapter 6 introduces the social, psychological, and behavioral factors associated with health. Social factors focus on the role of economic, cultural and health services on health, and psychological factors focus on the impact of stress on health and related interventions. Compared with the previous edition, this new edition is more comprehensive and is easier for learners to understand the relationship between environment and health, which is conducive to the prevention and control of environmentally related diseases.

In addition to this textbook, a concise bilingual manual with *pinyin* has been compiled. The authors envision this manual to be useful in bridging the language barrier faced by international students studying clinical medicine in China, especially those starting internships in Chinese hospitals, or by Chinese doctors who intend to practice in a foreign country and hope to have a convenient guide to refer to while practicing. This manual consists of the following parts: Part 1 includes a translation of all laboratory reports used in Chinese hospitals, which are categorized by department for ease of use, how to interpret each report, and the normal values; Part 2 consists of questions to ask during history taking in both English and Chinese with *pinyin*, to allow a doctor or an intern to obtain information despite the language barrier; Part 3 includes various tips and checklists of the most common physical examination; Part 4 lists the common communication skills necessary for various patient scenarios, including but not limited to "Breaking Bad News" and "Explaining Medication"; Part 5 consists of case report forms (discharge summary for hospitalized patients and medical records for outpatient department); Part 6 is a guide on the use of the basic Chinese hospital software; Part 7 shows clinical formulae needed in the clinical practice. This manual will be easy and convenient to use and ensures that any student or doctor have quick and easy access to topics of interest.

In addition, courseware presented in MS PowerPoint is available to supplement this book. And a question bank can be accessed by scanning the QR code at the end of each chapter. Institutions that use this book as teaching material can contact Zhejiang University Press.

More than 40 institutions of higher education both in China and abroad participated in the compilation of this series of textbooks. This series of textbooks is the crystallization of the knowledge and experience of experts in the field of public health from countries such as China, the United States of America, and Malaysia. All editorial committees pooled their best efforts together to ensure that this series of textbooks is not only innovative but also practical and reflects the latest developments in the related fields.

Finally, a special thanks goes to Mrs. Linda Bowman for her wonderful help in the process of reviewing the manuscript.

However, due to limited time, mistakes and omissions in the books are inevitable; therefore we sincerely seek the readers' feedback. For comments and suggestions, please email us at zhaojinshun@nbu. edu. cn

Zhao Jinshun, Ni Chunhui, Meng Xiaojing

Contents

Chapter 1　Introduction to Preventive Medicine

1. 1　Concept of Preventive Medicine

Modern medicine encompasses basic medicine, clinical medicine, and preventive medicine. What is preventive medicine? Stated simply, preventive medicine is a medical science aiming to prevent sickness before it happens or to avert resulting complications when a sickness or disease is already underway. Preventive medicine focuses on the health of individuals, communities, and defined populations. This important interdisciplinary branch of medicine focuses on the health of whole populations and all the factors influencing their health, encompassing elements of socioeconomics, the role of legislation, health equity, and the disparities found in communities and certain populations.

Preventive medicine can be practiced by governmental agencies, such as the Centers for Disease Control and Prevention (CDC), primary care physicians, and the individual. All physicians can promote preventative medicine, and some choose to specialize in it. Physicians who specialize in preventive medicine use health or medical statistics and epidemiology as well as a mix of medical, biological, social, economic, and behavioral sciences to study the causes of diseases and injuries. All doctors can incorporate some degree of preventive medicine into their practice, but primary care physicians are especially able to help people stay healthy and avoid illness. Most areas of clinical medicine focus narrowly on a single age group, ailment, or body part, but preventive medicine is not limited by these boundaries. It focuses on all populations, including patients and healthy people. Practicing preventive medicine can lower medical costs and reduce the productivity drain associated with preventable illness.

1. 2　Contents and Objectives of Preventive Medicine

Preventive medicine includes various speciality areas, such as the living environment and health, the occupational environment and health, food nutrition and health, social, psychological, and behavioral factors and health, public health, and public health promotion, emphasizing the relationship of health with different environments or factors. The objectives of preventive medicine are to protect, promote, and maintain health and well-being, and to prevent disease, disability, and death in all populations, prolonging life and enhancing the quality of life.

Preventive medicine is a very important part of public health. When we fall ill, we rely on doctors and health care professionals to help us recover—this refers to clinical medicine, which helps to treat a sickness or disease already underway, but what if we could avoid illness in the first place? We name this concept preventive medicine. Preventive medicine consists of measures taken to prevent diseases or injuries rather than curing them or treating their symptoms. This method contrasts with curative medicine in clinical practice. Preventive medicine very frequently works at the level of population health rather than individual health.

1.3   A Brief History of Preventive Medicine

Preventive medicine dates back to the 18th century. It was developed as a branch of medicine distinct from public health. Curiously, it came into existence even before the causative agents of disease were known. China has recognized the value of preventative care for millennia. The Hemudu culture (5000 B. C. —3300 B. C.) was a Neolithic culture that flourished just south to the Hangzhou Bay in Ningbo, China. In the remains of the Hemudu culture, a number of plants have been found that are effective in preventing and curing some kinds of diseases. Ancient wells, which ensured good-quality drinking water, have also been discovered in the ruins. Archaeological findings from the Indus Valley of northern India, dating from about 2000 B. C. , provide evidence of bathrooms and drains below street level in homes and sewers. Drainage systems have also been discovered among the ruins of the Middle Kingdom of ancient Egypt (2000 B. C. —1700 B. C.). *The Book of Leviticus*, written about 1500 B. C. , is believed to contain the first written health code in the world. The book dealt with personal and community responsibilities and included guidance regarding the cleanliness of the body, sexual health behaviors, protection against contagious diseases, and the isolation of diseased individuals. In ancient China, physicians suggested " treatment before a sickness is underway", which can be considered as the earliest evidence of preventive medicine. An ancient Chinese medical book (475 B. C. —221 B. C.) entitled *Huangdi Neijing* (*Yellow Emperor's Classic Canon*) (Figure 1. 1) stated that the superior-grade doctor prevents illness, the middle-grade doctor attends to impending sickness, and the low-grade doctor only focuses

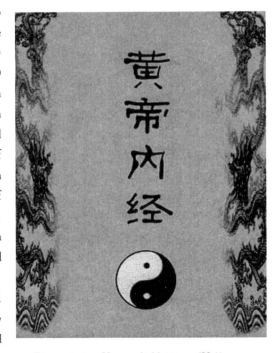

Figure 1. 1   *Huangdi Neijing* (*Yellow Emperor's Classic Canon*)—an Ancient Chinese Medical Book

on actual disease treatment. This is entirely consistent with the primary, secondary, and tertiary prevention strategies advocated today.

To prevent diseases due to nutritional deficiency, James Lind (1716—1794), a naval surgeon, advocated the intake of fresh fruits and vegetables for the prevention of scurvy (a disease resulting from a deficiency of vitamin C) in 1753. To prevent communicable diseases, Edward Jenner (1749—1823), a British physician, developed a vaccination against smallpox in 1796 (Figure 1.2). These two discoveries marked the new era of preventive medicine.

Preventive medicine is a medical discipline that focuses on preventing diseases and promoting a general state of health and well-being. When applied to a whole population, preventive medicine includes aspects such as extensive work in public health, pest and insect control, vaccinations, food safety, and improvements in hygiene, safe water supplies, homes, and individuals. This wide range of topics shows that many specialities are incorporated into successful preventive

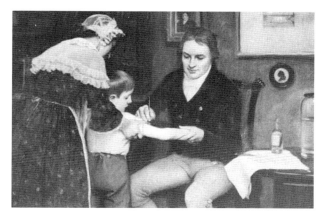

Figure 1.2   Edward Jenner Giving a Smallpox Vaccine to a Child

programmes. In developing nations, doctors who specialize in this field focus on improving hygiene and living conditions to prevent disease outbreaks and on vaccinating and educating the population. In developed nations, preventive medicine focuses more on extensive research, monitoring of food supplies, and well-trained epidemiology teams to track down the source of an outbreak when one emerges.

When practiced on an individual basis, preventive medicine involves looking at the body as a whole rather than at the individual parts. Many Eastern disciplines already view the body in this way, and practitioners of traditional Chinese and Indian medicine and other similar disciplines work with their patients to keep the body balanced, happy, and healthy. Measures to treat the body as a whole include herbal regimens, massage, psychotherapy, and dietary changes. The West has slowly accepted the value of this view for individuals, especially for treating rising obesity rates, and many doctors are starting to incorporate whole-body therapy into their practice.

In addition to medicine and biology, preventive medicine considers economic and social issues, as some populations are clearly more at risk of contracting dangerous diseases than others. Many sociologists, psychologists, and economists work in the preventive medicine field to assist people of low income, education, and social status all over the world. Organizations that promote preventive medicine work closely with these individuals in the hope that all people on Earth can enjoy healthy, disease-free lives, which is also the global goal of the World Health Organization (WHO).

After several centuries of development, preventive medicine has made great achievements in public health. However, at present, and maybe for a long time in the future, preventive medicine still faces many challenges. Globally, some examples of the most critical challenges are threats from new and traditional infectious diseases; rapidly increasing morbidity and mortality of chronic diseases; severe environmental pollution, especially in developing countries; and imbalance in public health services between developed and developing countries.

In the past two centuries, preventive medicine has witnessed enormous achievements in the control of infectious diseases, because the previous leading cause of death has largely been reduced due to improved sanitation and food safety, vaccines, the prevention and control of infectious diseases with antibiotics, and improved nutrition. New knowledge of the microbiological origins of cancers, such as that of the cervix, stomach, and liver, have strengthened primary prevention and brought hope that new cures will be found for other chronic diseases of infectious origin. However, new infectious viruses, such as HIV, new forms of influenza, and the Ebola have taken both professional and popular opinion by surprise and renewed the challenges facing the world public health community. Furthermore, the emergence of antibiotic-resistant strains of common organisms, due to the overuse of antibiotics, and the lack of vaccines for many dangerous microorganisms pose problems for humanity. This stresses the need for new vaccines, effective antibiotics, and strengthened environmental control measures. Though progress is being made to control many infectious diseases, tuberculosis and other diseases remain critical problems, especially for developing countries. Tragically long delays in adopting "new" and cost-effective vaccines cause hundreds of thousands of preventable deaths each year in developing and mid-level developed countries.

Chronic diseases have become the leading cause of morbidity and mortality in the world. The most common chronic diseases and leading causes of death are cardiovascular disease, cancer, chronic respiratory disease, and diabetes. It is estimated that these four major chronic diseases will be responsible for 75% of deaths worldwide by 2030. Research suggests that they will become an even greater burden in the future. Most chronic diseases are caused by preventable and lifestyle factors, such as smoking, excess alcohol, obesity, high cholesterol, or lack of physical exercise.

Global environmental pollution, including habitation environmental pollution and occupational environmental pollution, is also an important challenge for preventive medicine. Pollution is the release of chemical, physical, biological, or radioactive contaminants into the environment. Because it is sometimes not visible to the naked eyes, and it disperses through the media into which it is emitted (usually air, water, soil, food, and vegetables), pollution's direct effects can sometimes be hard to identify. Illnesses and conditions caused by factors in the environment are collectively called environmental diseases. Pesticides, chemicals, radiation, air pollution, water pollution, soil pollution, and food and vegetable pollution are all man-made hazards that are believed to contribute to human illnesses. Potential illness-causing agents are everywhere: at home and at work.

Globalization creates wealth but has no rules that guarantee its fair distribution. The huge gaps in health outcomes are growing wider, and these gaps divide rather precisely along the lines of poverty and wealth, resulting in an imbalance of the landscape of public health services. The health systems in most countries have proved to be inadequate for the task. Developing countries cannot manage chronic diseases alongside the continuing high mortality from infectious diseases.

During the 19th century and the first half of the 20th century, due to feudal society, foreign country invasion, and consequently backwardness in the industrial and economic sector, preventive medicine in China developed much slower than in some Western countries. Since 1979, preventive medicine in China has achieved rapid development.

1.4   Health and Determinants

1.4.1   Definition of Health

To study preventive medicine, one must understand what "health" is. Health, as a term, is not easy to define. Most people consider a healthy person to be one who has no apparent symptoms of illness, injury, or pain. Medical professionals consider health to be the general condition of a person's mind and body, usually meaning to be free from illness, injury, or pain. The WHO considers health to be a state of complete physical, mental, and social well-being and not merely the absence of disease or infirmity.

Generally, the context in which individuals live is of great importance for their health status and quality of life. Now, it is increasingly recognized that health is maintained and improved not only through the advancement and application of health care and medicine, but also through the efforts and intelligent lifestyle choices of individuals and society.

In May 1998, the WHO adopted a resolution to support the new global "Health for All" policy. The new policy, *Health 21: Health for All in the 21st Century*, succeeds the *Global Strategy for Health for All by the Year 2000* launched in 1978. It sets out global priorities for the first two decades of the 21st century and 10 targets that aimed to create the necessary conditions for people throughout the world to reach and maintain the highest attainable level of health. The policy is fundamentally a charter for social justice, providing a science-based guide to better health development and outlining a process that will lead to progressive improvement in people's health. All member countries are expected to set their own targets within this framework, based on their specific needs and priorities.

1.4.2 Determinants of Health

There are several basic types of determinants of health: human biological factors, environmental factors, health care services, behavior and lifestyles, and social factors. These determinants may affect human health alone or in combination.

1.4.2.1 Human Biological Factors

(1) Hereditary Factors

Most health problems are caused by interactions of genetic and environmental risk factors. A person may be healthy in every other way but have inherited conditions such as haemophilia, diabetes, mental retardation, various eye problems, lack of resistance to disease, or any number of other problems. Research now provides evidence that traits inherited from parents can influence people's likelihood of becoming addicted to alcohol or another drug. Genetic factors may play the following three roles in human health.

① Decisive role—For example Down's syndrome, a typical and rare genetic disease.

② Dominant role—Favism is a good example. An individual with G6PD deficiency may develop acute haemolytic anaemia when he or she eats broad beans. Some external environmental conditions are needed for this kind of genetic disease.

③ Co-operator role—Most health problems are caused by the interaction of genetic and environmental risk factors, such as type Ⅱ diabetes, cancer, and congenital heart disease. Under these conditions, genetic and environmental factors act together. As shown in Figure 1.3, heredity may be involved in various stages of disease development.

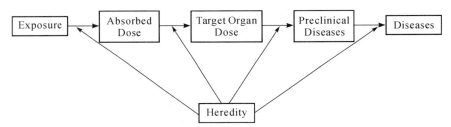

Figure 1.3   Heredity Plays a Co-operator Role in Disease Development

(2) Physiological and Biochemistry Factors

The physiological and biochemical system is a dynamic equilibrium system that maintains the normal functions of the body. However, the dynamic equilibrium may be disturbed by the exposure of harmful factors, aging, or genetic factors, initiating abnormal changes of physiology and biochemistry. These abnormalities could either be early pathological changes or important causes of diseases. For example, being overweight and obese raises the risks of metabolic diseases, cardiovascular diseases, and tumours. Being overweight and obese may result in abnormal changes of physiological indexes, such as the body mass index (B)MI, waist-to-hip ratio, blood pressure, and heart rate, while abnormal changes of biochemical indexes may occur in blood glucose, protein, lipid, vitamin and mineral, and hormone levels.

1.4.2.2 Environmental Factors

Considering the world population as a whole, the environment, which encompasses fresh water, food, and air, affects people's health more strongly than any other determinants. In the past, poor environmental management led to deaths from environment-related diseases, such as typhoid fever. Some estimates, based on morbidity and mortality statistics, indicate that the impact of the environment on people's health is as high as 80%.

Human evolution has been selective. People have adapted to their specific environments by producing biological defences against disease. People also have acquired intelligence, knowledge, and expertise that have allowed them to make significant changes in the environment, thereby creating conditions that lessen the likelihood of disease. This is accomplished mainly by controlling the causative agents of disease while they are still in the environment, before these agents reach human populations, so the body does not have to produce defences and therapeutic measures are not required. The crucial measures of defences against diseases in environmental health practice include:

① Water quality management—ensuring that potable water is available through treatment of water supplies;

② Water pollution control—reducing the effects of industrial and other waste on water supplies and recreational areas by the pretreatment of industrial and domestic waste;

③ Air pollution control—reducing the emissions of pollutants into the atmosphere;

④ Human waste disposal—disposing of human wastes in septic tank systems and sewage treatment plants;

⑤ Solid and hazardous waste management—treating and disposing of solid and hazardous wastes;

⑥ Food quality management—maintaining surveillance over food from the farm to the consumer to prevent contamination;

⑦ Occupational health practice—assuring a healthy and safe work environment;

⑧ Home and abroad travel sanitation—preventing the spread of communicable diseases between states and nations.

1.4.2.3 Health Care Services

Health care services ensure the maintenance or improvement of human health via the prevention, diagnosis, and treatment of disease, illness, injury, and other physical and mental impairments. Health care services are delivered by health professionals in allied health fields. Access to health care services may vary across communities or countries, and is largely influenced by social and economic conditions as well as health policies.

Health care services are the necessary services provided by health institutions and health professionals to individuals, groups, and society to prevent and control diseases and promote health by using health resources and means in a planned and purposeful manner.

Health care services are conventionally regarded as an important factor in promoting the general physical and mental health and well-being of people around the world. Health care service delivery systems are responsible for caring for patients as individuals, families, communities, and the population in general. Consideration should be given to providing integrated health care services from promotion and prevention to diagnostic, rehabilitation, and palliative care, as well as all levels of care, including self-care, home care, community care, primary care, long-term care, and hospital care.

1.4.2.4 Behavior and Lifestyles

Compared with other health determinants, behavior and lifestyle are likely to be the easiest to control.

People's behavior and lifestyles have a direct effect on their health. For instance, lack of sleep reduces the body's resistance to infections and leads to bodily degeneration. People who smoke or drink heavily might develop health problems rather quickly despite having good health previously. Many Americans follow a lifestyle that may lead to an early demise. They indulge in high-fat, high-sugar, high-salt, and low-fiber diets; meanwhile, they use moving sidewalks, escalators, elevators, cars, buses and other means of transportation that limit their exercise. Because all these behaviors and lifestyles are risk factors for heart disease, it is not difficult to understand why heart disease is the number-one killer in the United States.

In contrast to the overindulgence and sedentariness that characterize life in developed countries, the behavior and lifestyles in underdeveloped countries lead to their own health problems, dominated by malnutrition and other diseases, which are mainly caused by a lack of proper nutrition.

Healthy behaviors and lifestyles help maintain and improve people's health and well-being. Many governments and health organizations are now working on promoting healthy behavior and lifestyles, including healthy eating, physical activities, weight management, and stress management.

1.4.2.5 Social Factors

The social factors of health include the economic and social conditions that influence individual and group differences in health status. These factors are found in people's living and working conditions, such as wealth, the distribution of income, influence, and power, rather than individual risk factors, such as behavioral or genetic risk factors that influence the risk of a disease or vulnerability to a disease. The distributions of social determinants are often shaped by public policies. The social determinants of health are mostly responsible for health inequities—the unfair and avoidable differences in health status present within and among countries.

1.5　Four Levels of Prevention

Preventive medicine strategies are typically described as consisting of the following four levels: primary, secondary, tertiary, and quaternary prevention. In the 1940s, Hugh R. Leavell and E. Gurney Clark coined the term primary prevention. They later expanded the term to include secondary and tertiary prevention. In 1986, M. Jamoulle introduced the concept of quaternary prevention to avoid a patient's risk of overmedicalization.

1.5.1　Primary Prevention

Primary prevention, or "etiology prevention", means avoiding exposure to pathogens, microorganisms, and health risk factors. Primary prevention addresses the root cause of a disease or injury.

Primary prevention also consists of "health promotion" and "specific protection". Health promotional activities do not target a specific disease but rather promote health and well-being on a general level, for example, eating nutritious meals and exercising daily, both of which prevent disease and create a sense of overall well-being. Scientific advancements in hereditary diseases have facilitated great progress in specific protective measures for individuals who are carriers of a disease gene. Similarly, specific protective measures such as water purification, sewage treatment, and the development of personal hygienic routines have become mainstream for the prevention of infectious disease. The prevention of sexually transmitted infections is also considered as primary prevention.

In recent years, a new concept named "primal and primordial prevention" has also been ranked as primary prevention. Primal prevention refers to any measure aimed at helping future parents provide their upcoming child with adequate attention as well as secure physical and affective environments during the child's primal period of life. Primordial prevention refers to any measure designed to prevent the development of risk factors in the first place, early in life.

Methods to avoid the occurrence of a disease either through eliminating disease agents or increasing the human body's resistance to disease, such as immunization against disease, maintaining a healthy diet and exercise regimen, and avoiding smoking, all belong to this category.

1.5.2　Secondary Prevention

Secondary prevention, or "triple early prevention", refers to early detection, early diagnosis, and early treatment of a sickness or disease to prevent an asymptomatic disease from progressing to a symptomatic disease. Secondary prevention aims to detect and treat a disease at the early stage.

Methods to detect and address an existing disease prior to the appearance of symptoms, such as the treatment of hypertension (a risk factor for many cardiovascular diseases) and cancer screenings, belong to this category.

1.5.3　Tertiary Prevention

Tertiary prevention, or "clinical prevention", means reducing the negative impact of an extant disease by restoring function, reducing disease-related complications, improving the quality of life, and prolonging life.

Tertiary prevention attempts to reduce the damage caused by a symptomatic disease by focusing on mental, physical, and social rehabilitation. The goals of tertiary prevention include preventing pain and damage, halting the progression and complications from the disease, and restoring the health and functions of the individuals affected by the disease.

Methods to reduce the harm of a symptomatic disease, such as disability or death through rehabilitation and treatment, belong to this category.

1.5.4　Quaternary Prevention

Quaternary prevention, or "over intervention prevention", means avoiding unnecessary or excessive interventions of the medical, health care, or prevention processes. Quaternary prevention is the action taken to prevent overmedicalization or overprevention of sick or healthy people.

Methods to mitigate or avoid the results of unnecessary or excessive interventions in the health system belong to this category.

Based on the above preventive strategies, a whole life cycle prevention strategy has been gradually established to control common and serious diseases, such as HIV, diabetes, and cancer in the past 10 to 20 years.

The whole life cycle refers to the human life from the beginning of the combination of germ cells to the final end of life, which includes pregnancy, neonatal, infancy, preschool, school age, adolescence, middle age, menopausal, old age, and terminal stage. Different stages and periods have their own characteristics with certain internal relations.

A person's health status in the early stages of life has a great impact on his or her health in the later stages. The process of growth and development is also a process of accumulating risk factors of diseases. For example, the susceptibility of chronic diseases changes little throughout the whole life cycle, while the levels of hazard exposure—such as smoking and environmental pollution—are eventually leading to cancer, cardiovascular diseases, and so on. Therefore, prevention must be implemented from the perspective of the whole life cycle and special actions must be developed for controlling different diseases. Figure 1.4 shows the interventions for HIV prevention as an example of the whole life cycle prevention strategy.

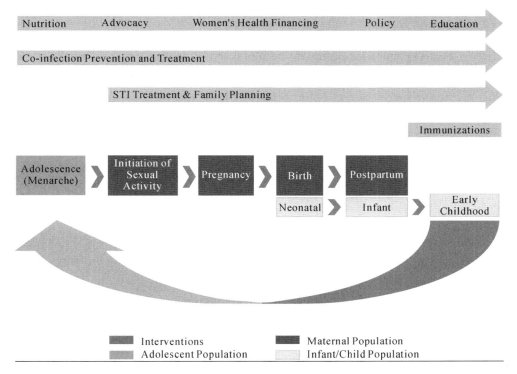

Figure 1. 4   The Maternal, Infant and Adolescent Life Cycle and Associated Health
Interventions for HIV Prevention

1.6   Clinical and Community Preventive Services

Preventive health services are most effective when provided to large groups, but health care professionals are often limited to providing them to individuals or small groups. To spread preventive health care services through clinical and community health care systems, *The Guide to Clinical Preventive Services* and *The Guide to Community Preventive Services* were released by the U. S. Preventive Services Task Force (USPSTF) in 1990 and 2000, respectively. These recommendations for clinical and community preventive services are intended to prevent or reduce the risk of heart disease, cancer, infectious diseases, and other conditions and events that affect the health of children, adolescents, adults, and pregnant women. The guides complement and illuminate each other to promote the development of public health and preventive medicine at the clinical and community levels.

1.6.1   Clinical Preventive Services

Clinical preventive services include medical screening tests, immunizations, health behavior counselling, and preventive medications and aim to save lives and promote well-being. Clinical preventive services also include the assessment of health risk factors for healthy people and asymptomatic "patients" in clinical settings. Individual preventive interventions are then implemented to prevent disease and promote health. The interventions mainly involve early screening, health education, immunization and preventive medications. Healthy and asymptomatic patients are the targets of interventions that are well known for primary and secondary prevention. A clinical preventive service is an individual-specific preventive service carried out under clinical conditions and provided by clinicians in their routine clinical work; it is a combination of health care and prevention.

Clinical doctors have a great advantage in practicing preventive services, as reflected in the following three aspects:

① Medical practitioners meet the "patients" face to face, which is very convenient and accurate in quantitatively evaluating the individual health risks of "patients" to determine the health intervention strategy for controlling the risk factors of the disease.

② Patients show good compliance with doctors' advice. Therefore, their enthusiasm and initiative for improving their behavior and lifestyle can be motivated effectively.

③ Medical practitioners can easily follow up on patients' health and behavior changes and then propose highly individualized recommendations for preventive health care over time, which will be beneficial to managing personal health, improving negative health behavior, and diagnosing and treating diseases early. These are all beneficial for improving the quality of life and prolonging the life span.

Clinical preventive services are mainly involved in health maintenance and health promotion and reduce the risk factors that lead to and exacerbate illness and injury and so on. There are six main services, as follows.

① Assessment and monitoring of individual risk factors. This is beneficial for detecting and controlling relevant health risks over time.

② Health counseling for healthy, sub-healthy, and preclinical patients and make disease prevention plans together.

③ Health screening. This aims to identify patients and sub-patients from the healthy population through a quick, simple physical examination, laboratory examination, and methods for assessing and monitoring risk factors to realize "early detection, early diagnosis, early treatment".

④ Vaccination (immunization). This is an efficient way to protect a susceptible population and prevent infectious diseases by injecting an antigen or antibody to enable the body to acquire specific resistance to certain diseases.

⑤ Chemoprophylaxis. Medicines, nutrients, and biological agents or natural substances are used to improve the ability to resist disease among asymptomatic patients or population with a high risk of illness. A typical example is the use of iodized salt to prevent iodine deficiency disorders. Chemoprophylaxis can also be classified as a kind of primary prevention.

⑥ Preventive treatment. Some treatment methods can be used to prevent a disease from an earlier stage to the later stage, such as surgical resection of intestinal polyps to prevent colorectal cancer.

1.6.2　Community Preventive Services

Community preventive services are health care services that focus on the maintenance, protection, and improvement of the health status of population groups and communities. They are community-oriented primary health care services; therefore, the types and forms of services are relatively stable. Community preventive services require a team of professionals for prevention, medicine, propaganda, and education to provide the best services for the community population.

Community preventive services are normally provided in the form of projects carried out among the community population. *The Guide to Community Preventive Services* is the gold standard of the evidence-based interventions for community health, public health practitioners, and decision makers. There are five consecutive basic steps in the implementation of community prevention services: community mobilization, community diagnosis, implementation, monitoring, and evaluation. Partners in the implementation of community prevention services may include governments, businesses, health care systems, schools, community organizations and individuals. Community participation is required throughout the entire community prevention service plan.

(Ni Chunhui, Zhao Jinshun, Wang Liping, Bowman Jenny)

Exercises

Chapter 2　Introduction to Environment and Health

2.1　Environment and Health

2.1.1　Introduction to Environment and Health

Environment is the sum total of all surroundings for human survival and reproduction. It encompasses air, food, and water for human survival, as well as the opportunity for intellectual, moral, social, and psychological development. Humans interact with their environment constantly. Human beings require materials from environment and places to carry on life's activities. As the most developed organisms on earth, humans generally understand the laws governing natural development and change their environment to improve their living conditions. Humans and the natural environment depend on and influence each other, following the law of unity of opposites. Some human activities, such as overconsumption, overexploitation, deforestation, and pollution, cause damage to the environment either directly or indirectly. In terms of disease prevention and health promotion, research on the relationship between human health and environment is needed to explore beneficial and adverse effects. The main goals are to control and eliminate adverse health effects while promoting beneficial health effects for the sustainable development of the environment and economy. Environmental health consists of preventing or controlling disease, injury, and disability related to the interactions between human beings and their environment.

2.1.2　Classification and Composition of Environment

The World Health Organization (WHO) defines environment, as it relates to health, as "all the physical, chemical, and biological factors external to a person, and all the related behaviors".

2.1.2.1　Classification of Environment

Environment is classified as natural environment and social environment. The natural environment encompasses all living and non-living things occurring naturally on earth, including air, water, soil, rock, and biological communities. It includes the primitive environment and secondary environment (Table 2.1). Social environment refers to the immediate physical and social setting where people live or events happen or develop. Social environment includes the culture in which individuals are educated or live, as well as the people and institutions with whom they interact.

Table 2. 1   Primitive and Secondary Environment

Item	Primitive Environment	Secondary Environment
Definition	Naturally formed, not or seldom affected by human activity	Formed or built by human activity
Examples of beneficial effects on health	Clean air, water, and soil, and appropriate sunlight and microclimate	Improved ecosystem attained by environment modification
Examples of adverse effects on health	Biogeochemical diseases caused by excess or deficiency of some micronutrients in water or soil, and acute or chronic adverse effects caused by natural disasters	Environmental pollution caused by industrial, agricultural, or life activities

2. 1. 2. 2 Composition of Environment

As an entity, environment is composed of media and factors. Environmental media refers to materials that surround organisms, such as air, water, soil, rock, and biological communities. Environmental factors include everything that shapes the environment: the identifiable elements in the chemical, physical, biological, social, economic, or political environment that affect the survival, operations, and growth of human beings. Environmental factors may affect living things either directly or indirectly.

(1) Chemical Factors

Chemical elements within the environment affect the types of organisms that can grow or thrive in the area. Some elements, like copper and zinc are important micronutrients for many organisms. However, chemical compositions, such as acidity level, can be detrimental to plant life in an area. Many herbicides have caused significant environmental damage. For example, the defoliant herbicide mixture known as Agent Orange was used by the U. S. military during the Vietnam War to destroy the foliage under which the Viet Cong took cover to hide the movement of their troops and set up ambushes. Agent Orange not only destroyed the plant life, it also caused extensive and long-term environmental damage. Air pollution, including vehicle exhaust and fossil fuel combustion from industrial sources (e. g. power stations), is another chemical factor that spreads quickly. Specific pollutants that may be found in these sources include nitrogen oxides, sulfur dioxide, carbon monoxide, lead, and particulate matter. Ozone is another important air pollutant. Indoor air pollution is mainly caused by carbon monoxide, tobacco smoke, solid fuels combustion and radon.

(2) Physical Factors

The physical factors that affect the environment are temperature, humidity, radiation, noise and vibration, and so forth. Normal physical factors, such as the moderate invisible, infrared, and ultraviolet light, are essential for human health and can promote growth and development. However, abnormal physical factors will damage human health. For example, high noise levels can contribute to cardiovascular effects in humans and an increased incidence of coronary artery disease. Noise poses a serious threat to physical and psychological health, and may negatively interfere with learning and behavior.

(3) Biological Factors

Biological factors include infectious pathogens, disease vectors, and biological toxins. Infectious pathogens, predominantly include microorganisms (bacteria, mycoplasma, viruses) and parasites (e. g. protozoan). Disease vectors include factors such as mosquitoes, which can carry and spread malaria. Biological toxins are produced by snakes, wasps, poisonous mushroom, and pufferfish, to name a few examples.

(4) Social, Psychological, and Behavioral Factors

Factors in the social environment include the political system, social and familial financial status, cultural traditions, and educational levels. Social participation and integration in the immediate social environment appear to be important to both mental and physical health. What also seems important is the stability of social connections, such as the composition and stability of households and the existence of stable and supportive local social environments or neighborhoods in which to live and work. A network of social relationships is an important source of support and presents an important influence on health behaviors. Social environments may also operate through effects on drug use, which also has consequences for violence and mental-health-related outcomes. Features of social environment that may operate as stressors (such as perceptions of safety and social disorder) have been linked to mental health, both in terms of negative stress and features that serve to buffer the adverse effects of stress.

2.1.3 The Interrelationship Between Environment and Human Health

2.1.3.1 Consistency of the Human Body to the Environment

The relationship between the human body and the environment is mainly material exchange, energy transfer, and information transmission by metabolism. Consistency exists between the human body and the environment. For example, the human body is mostly composed of water, about 62% by weight, and water must be replenished daily or the body functions will be affected. Similarly, about 75% of the Earth's surface is covered by water. The human body is composed of about 6% minerals: calcium, phosphorus, potassium, sulfur, sodium, chlorine, magnesium, and iron. Similarly, the Earth's crust contains about 100 chemical elements discovered thus far, and 8 of them make up more than 98% of the crust. These are, in order of abundance, oxygen, silicon, aluminum, iron, calcium, magnesium, sodium and potassium.

2.1.3.2 Adaptation of the Human Body to the Environment

Humans adapt to changes in the environment through genetic change, developmental adjustments, acclimatization, and cultural or technological advances. Genetic change in humans is slow but is known to occur. In Europe, during the last ice age, a species of hominid called Neanderthals developed a number of cold-weather adaptations that presumably helped them survive in the frigid climate. Among these were a stocky frame, large noses for efficient heat exchange and thick, robust bones that permitted the attachment of large muscles. Developmental adjustments are faster than genetic evolution, because they occur on a generational scale. After World War II, for example, the common diet of Japanese changed to include more animal protein. While this had no effect on Japanese adults, their children and grandchildren grew faster during childhood to an average of 7 inches taller. Acclimatization is even faster than developmental adjustments and can work within a single individual's lifetime. An example of this is the body's ability to add and shed fat in response to a changing diet. Cultural and technological changes are among the most complex adaptations humans use. Clothes, fire, and radio communications are all technologies humans have developed as insulation against the demands of the natural world. Bioconcentration and biomagnification reflect the adaptation of the human body to the environment. The former, which occurs within a trophic level, is the increase in concentration of a substance in certain tissues due to absorption from food and the environment. Biomagnification refers to the increasing concentration of a substance, such as a toxic chemical, in the tissues of tolerant organisms at successively higher levels in a food chain.

2. 1. 3. 3　Interaction Between the Environment and the Human Body

Human environment interaction refers to the dynamics between the environment and the human body, and it can also be used to predict the future of this interaction. Human environment interaction refers to the way people change their environment and how the environment changes them. In the recent past, concern for the environment has been widespread because environmental damage is worsening, and the climate is affected simultaneously. Various factors influence the human environment interaction. Some of these include population size and the practices of the different populations. It is important for policymakers to understand human environment interaction, because it affects the future of the human race. It is vital to try and modify this interaction to such a degree that both human life and the environment are preserved. Some of the ways in which humans directly influence the environment result from the need for food and clothing. Activities such as transportation also influence the environment. In addition, The National Institute of Environmental Health Sciences (NIEHS) Environmental Genome Project is examining the relationships between environmental exposures, inter-individual sequence variation in human genes, and disease risks. The NIEHS program targets the systematic identification and genotyping of single nucleotide polymorphisms (SNPs) in environmental response genes and has been expanded genome-wide. A better understanding of genetic influences on environmental response could lead to more accurate estimates of disease risks and provide a basis for disease prevention and early intervention programs directed at individuals and populations with increased risk.

2.2　Environmental Pollution and Health Effects

While exploiting and using natural environmental resources and creating new living environments, human beings discharge wastes from production and living activities into the environment, resulting in environmental pollution and deterioration of environmental quality. Various man-made or natural factors can cause significant changes in the composition of the environment, resulting in deterioration of environmental quality, destruction of ecological balance, and direct, indirect, or potential harmful effects on human health, which are called environmental pollution. Serious environmental pollution is called public nuisance.

2.2.1　Environmental Pollutants and Their Sources

Substances that enter the environment and can cause environmental pollution are called environmental pollutants. Pollutants discharged directly into the environment from pollution sources with no change to their physical and chemical properties are called primary pollutants. After primary pollutants enter the environment, they form new pollutants through physical, chemical, or biological effects in the environment that are completely different from the physical and chemical properties and toxicity of the original pollutants. These altered substances are called secondary pollutants. For example, mercury discharged directly from factory wastewater is a primary pollutant, and methyl mercury formed by microbial action in silt is a secondary pollutant. According to their properties, pollutants can be categorized as biological, physical, and chemical. At present, environmental pollution is dominated by chemical pollutants.

2.2.1.1　Productive Pollution

The "waste water, waste gas, and waste residue" produced during industrial and manufacturing processes are referred to as productive pollutants or "industrial three wastes". Industrial wastes contain a large number of substances that are harmful to human health. If untreated or improperly treated wastes are discharged into the environment in large quantities, they may cause air, water, soil, food, and other pollution, leading to deterioration of environmental quality. The main harmful substances found in industrial three wastes and their pollution sources are listed in Table 2.2.

Table 2. 2   The Main Harmful Substances and Pollution Sources of the Three Industrial Wastes

Items	Major Harmful Substances	Major Sources
Gas, fume, and dust.	Soot and dust. Toxic fume and dust: lead, arsenic, manganese, etc. The harmful gas: sulfur dioxide, nitrogen oxides, etc.	Thermal power stations, industrial boilers, etc. Machinery manufacturing, coal burning, etc. Chemical industry, etc.
Liquid waste	Inorganic chemicals: acids, bases, heavy metals, etc. Organic matter: phenols, organophosphorus compounds, oil, organic suspended matter, etc. Organisms: parasite, bacteria, etc.	Chemical industry, machinery, metallurgy, printing and dyeing, mining, papermaking industry, etc. Papermaking, leather, slaughtering, biological products, food processing, sugar, petrochemical, etc.
Waste residue	Inorganic waste residue: ore, slag, ash, etc. Organic waste residue: animal and plant carcasses, animal viscera and hair, skin, etc.	Mining, smelting, chemical industry, boiler, etc. Biological products, slaughtering, food processing, etc.

The long-term and extensive application of all kinds of pesticides (insecticides, fungicides, herbicides, plant growth regulators, etc.) in agricultural production can result in pesticide residues in crops, livestock products, and wildlife, and the air, water, and soil may also be polluted to varying degrees. The use of large amounts of pesticides and fertilizers affects not only soil structure and microbial shape, but also human health.

Human productive activities release a large number of synthetic chemicals into the environment, including chemical carcinogens, environmental endocrine disruptors (EEDs), and persistent organic pollutants (POPs). As a result, productive pollution including industrial or agricultural pollutants is the main source of environmental pollution at present. In 2010, the total amount of sulfur dioxide emissions in China was 21. 851 million tons, of which 18. 644 million tons (accounting for 85. 32%) came from industrial production and 8. 291 million tons from soot, of which 6. 032 million tons (accounting for 72. 75%) came from industrial production. Productive pollution generally belongs to organized emissions, which are relatively easy to control, even though the quantity of pollutants is large. But the pollutant composition is complex, and the toxicity is strong.

2. 2. 1. 2   Living Pollution

With the rapid growth of the population and the increased consumption level, the output of the "three wastes of life" (excrement, sewage, and garbage) is also on the rise. In some large and medium-sized cities, heavily polluted factories were relocated after urban reconstruction and living pollution has gradually become the main source of pollution. It is estimated that China produces more than 8 billion tons of municipal solid waste each year, including household garbage, sludge, livestock and poultry waste, and agricultural and forestry waste. As the government works to improve environmental protection, Chinese urban household garbage collection and transportation network is becoming increasingly efficient, and the number and capacity of household garbage treatment facilities are growing rapidly. By the end of 2010, Chinese cities and counties had disposed 22.1 million tons of household garbage annually, with a harmless disposal rate of 63.5%, including 77.9 percent in cities and 27.4% in the rural areas.

Domestic pollutants are typically large yield with complex compositions, containing a large amount of cellulose, sugar, fat, protein, and other substances, as well as a variety of pathogenic bacteria, viruses, parasites, and other pathogens. If the sanitary treatment of domestic pollutants is improper or inadequate, domestic pollutants will damage the air, water, soil, and food in the living environment, and could lead to the spread and prevalence of some infectious diseases. With modernization, great changes have taken place in the nature and composition of the "three wastes". For example, the amount of plastics, metals, and other macromolecular compounds in household garbage increases gradually, which not only increases the difficulty of harmless disposal of garbage and sewage, but also brings harm to human health through drinking water and food. Alkyl sulfonate-type synthetic detergents widely exist in domestic sewage, which can not only increase the surface tension of water, but also affect the sensory characteristics of water. In addition, phosphorus and other elements contained in alkyl sulfonate-type synthetic detergent can also act together with nitrogen and other elements in domestic sewage after entering water to enable proliferation of algae and other aquatic organisms, increase oxygen consumption, and rapidly deteriorate the sensory characteristics and chemical structure of water, leading to eutrophication. The biological toxins produced by the algae, such as microcystin, can cause acute and chronic poisoning to organisms.

It has been estimated that about 20% of air pollutants come from living pollution, mainly from soot, sulfur dioxide, carbon monoxide, carbon dioxide, and other harmful gases produced by coal burning and gas burning in domestic stoves and heating boilers.

The components of living pollutants are relatively complex compared with those of productive pollutants, but the treatment is relatively difficult because of the unorganized emissions.

2.2.1.3　Other Pollution

With the rapid development of the global economy, the number of automobiles is increasing rapidly and the aviation industry is developing day by day. The noise, vibration and exhaust gases produced during transportation have become the main sources of urban environmental pollutants, especially affecting the air quality of many large and medium-sized cities in China, which are facing the double burden of coal-burning pollution and traffic pollution.

The growing popularity and rapid growth of power equipment, wireless communications, radio and television, medical equipment, household appliances and so on can produce a variety of wavelengths including microwave electromagnetic waves. At present, electromagnetic radiation has become one of the most common environmental impact factors. Whether long-term exposure to electromagnetic fields is harmful to human health has been a topic of interest from both the public and multi-national governments. WHO established the international electromagnetic field project in 1996 and formally released its assessment of the possible adverse health consequences of electromagnetic fields in June 2007.

Medical and military atomic energy and radioisotope agencies discharge various types of radioactive wastes and drifting dust into the environment. In particular, the development and use of nuclear power poses a potential threat to the human environment. In recent years, due to natural disasters or accidents caused by negligence in management, radionuclide in nuclear power plants has leaked out, causing great harm to the ecological environment and people's health.

Electronic waste, also known as e-waste, refers to discarded electronic products that are no longer used, including various computers, household appliances, communication equipment, office equipment and other obsolete products used in daily life. E-waste contains a large number of toxic and harmful substances such as lead, cadmium, mercury, hexavalent chromium, polyvinyl chloride, and brominated flame retardants. In particular, in some areas where the dismantling of e-waste is the main industry, high-pollution exposure environments have been formed, with heavy metals and POPs as the main characteristics, causing serious health hazards to both employees and local residents. In February 2010 the United Nations environment program released the survey report "Recycling—From E-Waste to Resources" in Indonesia, pointing out that the increasing global e-waste is posing serious challenges to public health and the living environment in developing countries.

For a long time, the extensive use and abuse of antibiotics have led to antibiotic residue in soil, water and organisms, which is becoming an increasingly prominent environmental problem. Antibiotic pollution in the environment mainly comes from the use of medical drugs and agricultural veterinary drugs, and its health hazards are mainly manifested in broad-spectrum ecological toxicity and bacterial drug resistance. However, the increase and spread of drug-resistant environmental pathogens will pose a potential threat to human public health and clinical medication.

In addition, volcanic eruptions, forest fires, earthquakes and other natural disasters release a large amount of smoke and dust, waste gas, etc. These events can also affect the natural environment by varying degrees of pollution, causing damage to the ecosystem, which will affect human health, survival, and development.

2.2.2   Classification of Environmental Pollutants

There are many kinds of environmental pollutants, and they can be divided into three types according to their properties.

2.2.2.1   Physical Pollutants

Physical pollutants include noise, vibration, ionizing radiation, non-ionizing radiation, and thermal pollution to name a few examples. These pollutants can produce visual pollution, auditory pollution, and tactile pollution, and may even lead to long-term harm.

2.2.2.2   Chemical Pollutants

Chemical pollutants mainly come from human activities and man-made products, including inorganic substances such as mercury, cadmium, arsenic, chromium, lead, cyanide, fluoride, and organic compounds such as organophosphorus, organochlorine, polychlorinated biphenyls, phenols, polycyclic aromatic hydrocarbons. Persistent toxic substances are a typical class of special pollutants in the environment, the hazards of which include persistence, bioaccumulation, semi-volatility, migration, high toxicity, concealment, and hysteresis. These pollutants mainly include POPs and some heavy metals.

POPs refer to synthetic organic chemical pollutants that can persist in the environment and accumulate through the food chain, causing harmful effects on human health and the environment. These compounds have the characteristics of environmental persistence, bioaccumulation, long-distance migration, and high toxicity. They can cause disorder of the human endocrine system, destroy reproductive and immune systems, and induce cancer and neurological diseases.

2.2.2.3   Biological Pollutants

Biological pollutants include pathogens (microorganisms and parasites) and allergens (such as pollen, animal hair and dander, dust mites and molds, fish, eggs, and milk) that are harmful to humans and living things. Biological pollutants can be divided into animal (such as harmful insects, parasites, protozoa, aquatic animals), plant (such as weeds, seaweed) and microorganisms (such as viruses, bacteria, fungi). Biological pollution can be highly destructive and is characterized by unpredictability and long incubation periods.

2.2.3   Fate of Pollutants

The transformation of environmental pollutants refers to their spatial displacement and morphological changes. The former is the change of quantity, while the latter is a change in quality.

2.2.3.1   Migration of Pollutants

Migration of pollutants refers to their transfer from one place to another and from one medium to another, which is often accompanied by changes in the environment's pollutant concentration. The nature of pollutants and environmental factors affect pollutants' migration process.

① Physical migration—the mechanical movement of pollutants in the environment, such as the movement and diffusion of water flow and airflow, and settlement due to gravity.

② Chemical migration—dissolution, dissociation, oxidation-reduction, hydrolysis, complexation, integration, chemical precipitation, and biodegradation of pollutants.

③ Biological migration—the migration of pollutants through the body's physiological processes such as absorption, metabolism, reproduction, and death. After being absorbed by organisms, pollutants can be accumulated in the organism's bodies and further enriched through the food chain. The content of pollutants in the organism becomes significantly higher than their concentration in the environment, a phenomenon that is called bioenrichment.

2.2.3.2   Transformation of Pollutants

The process by which the morphological or molecular structures of environmental pollutants change under the influence of physical, chemical and biological factors. This process is achieved through the participation of environmental microorganisms or biological metabolism.

2.2.3.3   Self-Purification of Pollutants

Under the action of physical, chemical, or biological factors, the process of reducing the concentration or total amount of pollutants in a polluted environment varies with the environmental structure and state. According to its mechanism, self-purification can be divided into the following three categories.

① Physical purification—the process of reducing pollutant concentration and its degree of harm through dilution, diffusion, leaching, volatilization, and sedimentation. The physical purification capacity of a geographical environment mainly depends on the physical conditions of the geographical environment. For example, high temperature is conducive to the volatilization of pollutants, and high wind speed is conducive to the diffusion of pollutants. However, basin and valley form inversion layers, which weaken atmospheric diffusion and lead to atmospheric pollution.

② Chemical purification—chemical reactions such as peroxidation, reduction, chemical combination and decomposition, adsorption, condensation, exchange, and complexation in the geographical environment to reduce pollutants' degree of harm or convert them into harmless substances. The main environmental factors affecting environmental chemical purification are temperature, pH, and redox potential. For example, the higher the temperature is, the faster the chemical reaction rate is. Therefore, the self-purification effect of pollutants in a warm environment is stronger than in a cold environment. Harmful metal ions easily form hydroxide precipitation in alkaline environments, which is beneficial to purification.

③ Biological purification—the reduction or disappearance of the concentration of pollutants in the geographical environment through biological absorption and degradation. The capacity of biological purification is related to biological species, environmental temperature and humidity, and oxygen supply. In a warm, humid environment with sufficient nutrients and a good oxygen supply, plants have strong ability for absorption and purification, and aerobic microorganisms have strong ability for degradation and purification.

2.2.4   Health Effects of Environmental Pollutants

2.2.4.1   Spectrum of Health Effects of Environmental Pollutants

Environmental pollutants can cause different degrees of health effects in the population. This distribution is called the spectrum of health effects, which is an iceberg phenomenon. The diseased patients and deaths seen clinically are only the "top of the iceberg" and do not show the whole picture. Only by understanding all the factors of the crowd response and making a comprehensive quantitative assessment of its hazards, can we provide a reliable basis to formulate preventive measures and medical decision-making.

When environmental pollutants affect the population, individuals are exposed to different dose levels and exposure time. Individuals may have different responses due to age, gender, physical condition (health and disease) and genetic susceptibility to the environmental pollutants. The distribution pattern of a population's various responses to environmental pollutants is pyramidal and constitutes the pyramid-shaped health effect spectrum (Figure 2.1).

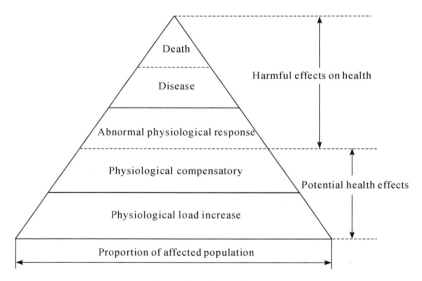

Figure 2. 1   Spectrum of Health Effects from Environmental Pollutants

Environmental pollutants can cause different degrees of health effects, which can be divided into five levels from weak to strong: ① Contaminant loading increases *in vivo* but does not cause changes in physiological function and biochemical metabolism; ② Some physiological and biochemical metabolic changes occur with the further increase of body load, but these changes are mostly physiologically compensatory and non-pathological; ③ Some abnormal changes of biochemical metabolism or physiological function have occurred, and they have adverse effects on health and pathological significance. The body is in a pathological compensatory and regulatory state without obvious clinical symptoms and can be regarded as quasi-sick (sub-clinical state); ④ Clinical symptoms and diseases caused by dysfunction of the body; ⑤ Deaths due to severe poisoning of environmental pollutants.

2.2.4.2　Health Effects of Environmental Pollutants

(1) Acute Health Effects

Acute health effects refer to contaminants entering the environment in a short period of time, resulting in harmful effects, acute poisoning, and even death of the exposed population in a relatively short period of time. Acute health effects are often caused by air pollution incidents. Many serious environmental pollution incidents have occurred throughout history, causing acute poisoning of large numbers of people and huge economic losses. For instance, the "Great Smog of London" in Britain, the "Chernobyl Disaster" in the Soviet Union, and the "Fukushima Daiichi Nuclear Accident" in Japan, to name a few examples.

(2) Chronic Health Effects

The harm caused by long-term and repeated effects of low concentration environmental pollutants on the human body is known as chronic health effects. Chronic health effects are caused by long-term accumulation of toxic substances in the body. Minamata disease in Japan from the 1950s to the 1960s is a typical incident of chronic poisoning caused by environmental pollution. This disease is caused by metal pollutants (mercury), which enter the human body as mercury (methyl mercury) through biological amplification of the food chain, and then accumulate in the body for several years.

(3) Genotoxicity

Genotoxicity refers to the changes of cellular genetic material (DNA) and genetic processes caused by chemical, physical, and biological factors in the environment. The genotoxicity of substances can be evaluated by measuring the interaction between genetic toxicants and DNA, and more by indirect detection of DNA repair or gene mutation and chromosome aberration.

(4) Carcinogenesis

According to statistics, $80\%—90\%$ of clinical cancer cases are closely related to long-term environmental exposure. Chemical factors in the environment play a major role in the process of tumorigenesis.

(5) Reproductive Toxicity and Developmental Toxicity

Reproductive toxicity refers to the damage of exogenous chemicals to male or female reproductive function or reproductive ability and the harmful effects on their offspring.

Developmental toxicity refers to any harmful effects on the development of the organism resulting from exposure to toxic agents before conception, during prenatal development, or post-natally until puberty. For instance, Thalidomide was widely used around the world in the late 1950s—1960s. It can effectively prevent vomiting during early pregnancy, but it also hinders the blood supply of pregnant women to their fetuses, resulting in a large number of babies born with phocomelia.

(6) Other Health Effects

Environmental toxicants can suppress immune function, cause allergic reaction, and initiate autoimmune response. The presence of some hormone-like pollutants in the environment can affect the production, release, transportation, metabolism, and function of natural hormones in the organism, they also interfere with the balance and stability of hormone levels and the development of the organism.

2.2.4.3　Determinants of Health Effects of Environmental Pollutants

(1) Chemical Structure and Physical Characteristics

The toxicity and reactivity of pollutants are related to their chemical structure. Furthermore, the physical characteristics of pollutants (solubility, volatility, etc.) can affect their absorption, distribution, accumulation, metabolism, excretion process and concentration in target organs, thus affecting the toxic effect of pollutants in the organism.

(2) Exposure Dose or Intensity

Exposure dose refers to the quantity of chemicals entering the body, often expressed in the quantity of chemicals exposed per unit weight (e. g. mg/kg). Exposure intensity refers to the number of physical factors acting on the body (e. g. noise in dB). Different doses of the same contaminant cause different levels of biological damage. The relationship between biological damage caused by environmental pollutants and dose can be expressed by dose-effect relationship or dose-response relationship. Dose-effect

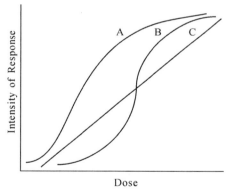

A: Parabolic curve; B: S-shaped curve; C: Straight curve

Figure 2.2　Types of Dose-Response Curves

relationship refers to biological changes in an organism, tissue, or organ caused by exposure to a certain dose of chemicals; dose effect can be expressed in units of measurement. Dose-response relationship is defined as the relationship between the dose of chemicals in the environment and the frequency of occurrence of the biological effect in a population, which is generally expressed in terms of incidence. Different chemicals in the environment have different dose-response relationships (Figure 2.2).

(3) Duration of Exposure

Under certain dose or intensity conditions, the duration or frequency of exposure to contaminants has an important impact on the consequences of pollutants. According to the time of exposure, exposure can be classified as acute (exposure in an accident or event), subchronic (repeated exposure for several weeks or months) and chronic (repeated exposure for several months or years). For many pollutants, different exposure times can result in completely different harmful effects.

(4) Combined Effect of Environmental Factors

Environmental pollutants are often not isolated, but act on the human body simultaneous with other chemical and physical factors. The toxic effects of two or more chemicals on the body at the same time or successively are called combined effects, which can be divided into non-interaction and interaction. The former includes addition joint action and independent action; the latter includes synergistic effect, potentiation joint action, and antagonistic joint action.

① Addition joint action: The toxic effects of various chemicals on the body are equal to the arithmetic sum of the effects of each chemical on the body alone.

② Independent action: Due to the different action modes and sites of various chemical substances, the toxic effects they cause do not affect each other, but rather show their own toxic effects respectively.

③ Synergistic effect: The total toxic effects of the chemicals on the body are greater than the sum of the toxic effects of each exogenous chemical on the body alone.

④ Potentiation joint action: A chemical is not toxic to the body itself, but its toxic effects are enhanced by simultaneous or subsequent exposure to another chemical.

⑤ Antagonistic joint action: The combined toxic effects of the chemicals on the body are lower than the sum of the individual toxic effects of each chemical.

(5) Individual Sensitivity

Under the same environmental exposure conditions, the human body has different response intensity and properties to environmental abnormal changes. People who are particularly sensitive to some pollutants comprise highly susceptible populations or sensitive populations. Many reasons might account for the differences in individual susceptibility, including individual health status, age, gender, nutritional status, and genetic factors.

2.3   Toxicology of Environmental Pollutants

2.3.1   Introduction to Toxicology

Historically, toxicology has been defined as the study of the adverse effects of xenobiotics on living organisms, which formed the basis of therapeutics and experimental medicine. Modern toxicology goes beyond the traditional definition, which has been expanded to study the effects of all exogenous harmful factors (chemical, physical, and biological factors) on living systems, the biologic mechanisms by which exogenous harmful factors modulate cells and their environment at the molecular level, as well as to evaluate and assess the possibility of exogenous harmful factors to endanger human health.

2.3.1.1　Different Areas of Toxicology

Toxicology has evolved rapidly during the last 100 years, especially after World War Ⅱ. Modern toxicology can be classified into three areas: descriptive toxicology, mechanistic toxicology, and regulatory toxicology. Descriptive toxicology deals with the toxicity of chemicals and provides important clues to mechanistic toxicology and information for safety evaluation and regulatory requirements. Mechanistic toxicology focuses on identifying and understanding the mechanisms by which chemicals exert toxic effects on living organisms. Regulatory toxicology examines the data provided by descriptive and mechanistic toxicology, to determine whether a chemical will be used at acceptable risk levels for a stated purpose. Each area has distinctive characteristics, but they all contribute to each other, and all are vitally important to chemical risk assessment.

In addition to the above categories, other specialized areas of toxicology include environmental toxicology, ecotoxicology, clinical toxicology, occupational toxicology, food toxicology, forensic toxicology, and radiotoxicology, according the field of application. According to the research objectives, toxicology can be classified into nanotoxicology, particulate matter toxicology, metal toxicology, pesticide toxicology, and receptor toxicology. Toxicology also includes cardiovascular toxicology, liver toxicology, kidney toxicology, and so on, according to target organs of toxic effects.

2.3.1.2　Some Important Toxicological Concepts

(1) Dose

Dose is an important factor for determining the toxic effect of exogenous toxicants to the body. Does generally refers to the amount of exogenous toxicants in contact with the body (exposure dose or external dose) or absorbed by the body (absorbed dose or internal dose) or directly leading to the damage of the body (biological effective dose or target dose) (Table 2.3). Dose is often expressed as a concentration of a substance in the body.

Table 2.3　Ways to Describe a Dose

Term	Definition
Exposure dose	The amount of a substance encountered in the environment
External dose	A dose acquired by contact with contaminated environmental sources
Absorbed dose	The amount of a substance available to the body's internal organs
Internal dose	The portion of a substance the body internalizes through ingestion, absorption, and other means
Administered dose	The quantity of a substance administered
Biologically effective dose	The portion of the internal dose required to cause a health outcome
Total dose	The dosage acquired by adding together all individual doses

(2) Lethal Dosage

A lethal dose (LD) is an indication of the lethality of a given substance or type of radiation. Because susceptibility varies from one individual to the other, the lethal dose represents a dose (usually recorded as dose per kilogram of the subject's body weight) at which a given percentage of subjects will die. LD may be based on the standard person concept, a theoretical individual who represents perfectly "average" characteristics, and thus might not apply to all sub-populations.

The most commonly used LD is the median lethal dose (LD_{50}), the point where 50% of the tested subjects died after exposure, and is expressed in the units of mg/kg body weight. Gases and aerosols are described in terms of lethal concentration (mg/m^3 or ppm), although this also depends on the duration of exposure, which must be included in the definition. Other variations of the term lethal dose are LD_{10} and LD_{90} (10% and 90% mortality, respectively).

(3) Dose-Response Relationship

Response refers to the proportion of individuals in a population who experience an effect when exposed to a certain toxicant. The relationship between the exposure characteristics and the spectrum of effects together are referred to as the dose-response relationship. Typically, the dose-response relationship for a toxicant is depicted by an S-shaped sigmoid curve (Figure 2.3). The lower portion of the curve shows no measurable response

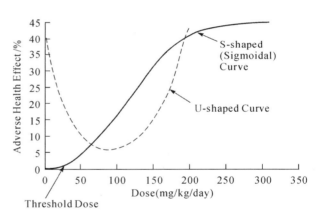

Figure 2. 3   Dose-Response Curves

until a threshold dose is reached. Once the threshold is reached, the dose-response curve becomes linear where each increase in dose is accompanied by an increase in response. As the dose increases further, a maximum response is reached, as indicated by the flattening of the sigmoid curve. Once the maximum response has been reached, any additional increase in dose may only prolong the effect. For essential nutrients, a U-shaped dose response curve is typical for an essential nutrient where too little or too much may result in adverse responses or death. Exposure to a toxicant can produce more than one toxic response, and the dose response relationship may be different for each response.

(4) Threshold

Threshold is the lowest dose of a toxicant that has a detectable effect. For any given toxicant, each cellular, biochemical, physiological, or clinical response may have a threshold. Some effects occur without a known threshold. Since susceptibility varies among animal species and among humans, the threshold is approximated. Thresholds are often used to categorize or rank chemical toxicity.

The threshold level refers to the amount of a substance necessary to elicit a response, below which there is no threshold. Some evidence indicates that effects increase as the dose increases, but sometimes the effects presented in response to the highest dose may have already been elicited in a lower dose. Carcinogens have no threshold, meaning that any amount of a carcinogenic chemical may elicit a response because it can damage the DNA, thus creating the conditions for cancerous proliferation.

(5) Latency

Latency refers to the time interval between toxic exposure and the occurrence of effects. The latency of toxicity varies greatly, from seconds to decades. When terminating fixed dose exposure, the length of latency depends mainly on the exposure dose.

2.3.2 Toxicokinetics

Two factors determine the toxic effects of environmental pollutants: the pollutant's toxicity and exposure dose, and the target dose and exposure duration. Once exposed to the human body, environmental toxicants undergo physiological processes, including absorption, distribution, metabolism, and excretion, which are known as toxicokinetics. Absorption, distribution, and excretion processes can also be termed biotransportation, because the structure and characteristics of the toxicants remain the same, and they can cross biological membranes. Metabolism is a form of biotransformation, consisting of metabolic processes that change the structure of an environmental toxicant. Biotransformation may increase (activate) or decrease (detoxify) the harmful properties of the toxicant.

As mentioned above, biotransportation involves crossing biological membranes with no alternations to a pollutant's characteristics. Biological membranes consist of cell membranes and membranes of organelles such as mitochondria, endoplasmic reticula, and nuclei. Biological membranes are dynamic structures composed of lipid bilayers, with hydrophobic lipids on both sides and a hydrophilic hydrocarbon chain in between. This structure allows hydrophobic pollutants to cross the membrane easily. There are several ways to cross biological membranes, including passive diffusion, active transport, and cytosis. Passive diffusion is the most common form of biotransportation, in which uncharged molecules of pollutants move along a concentration gradient. Active transport requires energy to move a substance through a membrane, against a concentration gradient with the aid of transporters. In the process of cytosis, a fluid membrane must be present. Cytosis usually involves pollutants wrapped by membrane-bound vessels and delivered in and out of organelles.

2.3.2.1 Absorption

Exposure dose is the amount of an environment pollutant that people encounter in the environment. Certain pollutants can only enter the human body through absorption, which is the transport of a chemical from the site of administration/exposure into plasma. There are various routes of absorption, including gastrointestinal absorption (injection), dermal absorption (through skin), and respiratory penetration (inhalation).

The primary site of gastrointestinal absorption is the small intestine. Its extensive surface area and voluminous perfusion help with passive diffusion. The rate of skin absorption depends largely on the pollutants' physical and chemical properties, such as the lipid-water partition coefficient, which is a measure of a molecule's relative solubility in the organic phase versus water. Inhalation is the primary route of exposure in areas with atmosphere pollution (e. g. PM_{10} and $PM_{2.5}$) or indoor air pollution (e. g. carbon monoxide). Through inhalation, large particles, such as dusts, are trapped by nasal hairs and could be removed in nose, while smaller particles could enter the tracheobronchial tree or even penetrate deeper into the alveoli depending on the size and physical characteristics (e. g. solubility) of the particles.

2.3.2.2　Distribution

Distribution is the transport of an environmental pollutant within the body, from plasma (systemic circulation) to cells and tissues. Pollutants are distributed unevenly depending on the blood flow volume and appetency to pollutants. Once distributed at the target tissue or organ where toxic effects are caused, the dose of the pollutant at that site is the target dose. When the absorption of a specific pollutant is faster than metabolism and excretion, the pollutant will accumulate in the tissue or organ, a process known as accumulation. The accumulation site is not necessarily the target site showing toxic effects; rather, the accumulation site is merely a storage vault, such as fat tissue and bone.

2.3.2.3　Metabolism

Metabolism is also known as biotransformation of environmental pollutants to metabolites. Metabolism mainly occurs in the liver, followed by the kidney, intestine and skin. There are two phases of metabolism, phase Ⅰ reactions and phase Ⅱ reactions, involving various enzymes and cofactors. Normally, environmental pollutants are detoxified or inactivated after biotransformation as solubility increases and hastens the excretion process. However, in some circumstances, biotransformation is an activation process. Benzopyrene (BP), for example, is not toxic in its original form, but once metabolized, it turns into cancer-causing carcinogens.

2.3.2.4　Excretion

Excretion is the removal of chemicals and their metabolites from the body. The major routes of excretion are renal elimination and biliary excretion, followed by intestine, lung, sweat, saliva and breastmilk.

2.3.3　Toxic Effects of Environmental Pollutants

2.3.3.1　General Toxic Effect

A general toxic effect is the body's non-specific toxic reaction to toxicants. The concept is comparable to special toxicity effects, such as carcinogenesis, mutagenesis, and teratogenesis. According to the duration of detoxification, general toxicity can be divided into acute toxicity, sub-acute toxicity, sub-chronic toxicity, and chronic toxicity. General toxic effects are important for safety evaluation and risk assessment of exogenous chemicals. The main purposes of general toxicity assessments include: confirming the toxicants' performances and characteristics; confirming the toxicants' dose-response relationship to obtain multiple toxicological parameters and LD_{50}; unveiling the toxicants' target organs; and confirming the reversibility of the damages toxicants cause.

2.3.3.2　Special Toxic Effect

(1) Mutagenesis

Mutagenesis refers to the process or state of mutation, which is the result of interactions between mutagens and genetic materials of organisms. It can be assessed directly by measuring the interaction of agents with DNA or more indirectly through the assessment of DNA repair or the production of gene mutations or chromosome alterations. Somatic cell mutations can cause tumors, teratogenesis, aging, and atherosclerosis, etc. Mutations occurring in any stage of germ cells can potentially affect offspring, leading to birth defects, miscarriages, or stillbirths.

(2) Carcinogenesis

Chemical carcinogenesis is a process in which chemicals induce malignant transformation of normal cells then develop into tumors. Chemicals that can cause such effects are called chemical carcinogens. Chemical carcinogenesis can be divided into three stages: initiation, promotion, and progression. According to the data from epidemiologic and animal studies, the International Agency for Research on Cancer has classified chemical carcinogens into five groups: ① Agent is carcinogenic; ② Agent is probably carcinogenic; ③ Agent is possibly carcinogenic; ④ Agent is not classifiable as to carcinogenicity; ⑤ Agent is probably not carcinogenic. Also, chemical carcinogens could be classified into three types according to their chemical carcinogenic mode: direct acting carcinogen, indirect acting carcinogen (metabolic activation is necessary for their carcinogenic activity), and tumor promoting agent.

(3) Teratogenesis

Teratogenesis is the process and characteristics of teratogenic agents causing defects in the morphology and structure of developing organisms. The results of teratogenesis include death of the developing organism, altered growth, structural abnormality, and functional deficiency.

(Zhao Jinshun, Ni Chunhui, Meng Xiaojing, Wang Chunping, Ma Rulin, Zheng Fuli, Zhou Fang, Wang Qiang)

Exercises

Chapter 3　Living Environment and Health

3.1　Introduction

Living environment refers to the totality of various conditions closely related to human life. It can be divided into natural environment and artificial environment according to whether it has been reconstructed artificially or not. Natural environment is the total of all kinds of natural factors, such as air, water, land, wildlife. Artificial environment refers to various conditions created artificially for human life, such as buildings, parks, service facilities for human life. There are various factors harmful to health in the living environment. These factors act on the body through environmental media such as air, water and soil, which endanger human health.

Pollution problems are not just problems of the air, water, or soil. Pollution affects all parts of the environment. The better we understand the earth, the better we can understand the problems that we are facing. An environmental viewpoint is one way of looking at the earth. This way of looking at problems goes beyond immediate questions and looks at how they affect the whole environment. A functioning and well-balanced environment is important to humans. We need clean air to breathe, clean water to drink, and healthy food to eat. All these are part of our environment and are interconnected. We now know that if we pollute the air, we may be affecting our food and water supply.

3.2　Air and Health

3.2.1　Composition and Structure of the Atmosphere

The atmosphere of Earth is the layer of gases, commonly known as air that surrounds the planet Earth and is retained by Earth's gravity. The atmosphere of Earth protects life on Earth by creating pressure allowing for liquid water to exist on the Earth's surface, absorbing ultraviolet solar radiation, warming the surface through heat retention (greenhouse effect), and reducing temperature extremes between day and night (the diurnal temperature variation). A person may survive for many days without food, or for a few days without water. Air is more immediately essential. Without air, a person can only survive for a few minutes.

The air that humans require is an odorless, colorless mixture of natural gases. It is composed of nitrogen (approximately 78%) and oxygen (21%). The remainder is mostly argon (0. 93%) and carbon dioxide (0. 032%) with traces of neon, helium, ozone, xenon, hydrogen, methane, and krypton. Air also contains a variable amount of water vapor, on average around 1% at sea level, and 0. 4% over the entire atmosphere. If anything else is added to the air, it becomes polluted.

In general, air pressure and density decrease with altitude in the atmosphere. However, temperature has a more complicated profile with altitude, and may remain relatively constant or even increase with altitude in some regions. Because the general pattern of the temperature/altitude profile is constant and measurable by means of instrumented balloon soundings, the temperature behavior provides a useful metric to distinguish atmospheric layers. The atmosphere is layered into four distinct zones of contrasting temperature due to differential absorption of solar energy (Figure 3.1). Understanding how these layers differ and what creates them helps us understand atmospheric functions.

The layer of air immediately adjacent to Earth's surface is called the troposphere. Ranging in depth from about 16 km (10 *mi*) over the equator to about 8 km (5 *mi*) over the poles, this zone is where most weather events occur. Due to the force of gravity and the compressibility of gases, the troposphere contains about 75% of the total mass of the atmosphere. The troposphere's composition is relatively uniform over the entire planet because this zone is strongly stirred by the wind. Air temperature drops rapidly with increasing altitude in this layer, reaching about -60℃ (-76℉) at the top of the troposphere. A sudden reversal of this temperature gradient creates a sharp boundary, the tropopause, which limits mixing between the troposphere and upper zones. This layer is most concerned by human.

The stratosphere extends from the tropopause up above 50 km (31 *mi*). Air temperature in this zone is stable or even increases with higher altitude. Although more dilute than the troposphere, the stratosphere has a very similar composition except for two important components: water and ozone (O_3). The fractional volume of water vapor is about one thousand times lower, and ozone is nearly one thousand times higher than in the troposphere. Ozone is produced by lighting and solar irradiation of oxygen molecules and would not be present if photosynthetic organisms were not releasing oxygen. Ozone protects life on Earth's surface by absorbing most incoming solar ultraviolet radiation.

Above the stratosphere, the temperature diminishes again, creating the mesosphere or middle layer. The lowest temperature in this region is about -80℃ (-120℉). At an altitude of 80 km (50 *mi*), another abrupt temperature change occurs. This is the beginning of the thermosphere, a region of highly ionized gases, extending out to about 1,600 km (1,000 *mi*). The temperature in the thermosphere is very high because molecules there are constantly bombarded by high-energy solar and cosmic radiations. There are so few molecules per unit area, thus, if a person were cruising through in a spaceship, the temperature increase would not be noticed.

The lower part of the thermosphere is called the ionosphere. This is where aurora borealis (northern lights) appears when showers of solar or cosmic energy cause ionized gases to emit visible light. There is no sharp boundary that marks the end of the atmosphere. Pressure and density decrease gradually as one travels away from Earth until they become indistinguishable from the near vacuum of intrastellar space. The composition of the thermosphere also gradually merges with that of intrastellar space, being made up mostly of helium and hydrogen.

3. 2. 2   Physical Properties of the Atmosphere

The Earth's atmosphere is the environment for most of its biological activity and exerts a considerable influence on the ocean and lake environments. Weather consists of the day-to-day fluctuations of environmental variables and includes the motion of wind and formation of weather systems such as hurricanes. Climate is the normal or long-term average state of the atmospheric environment. The atmosphere protects Earth's life forms from harmful radiations and cosmic debris.

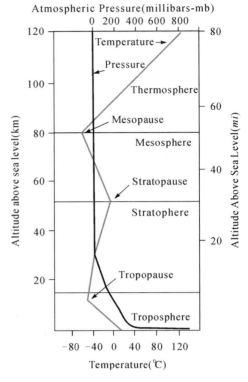

Figure 3. 1   Four Layers of the Earth's Atmosphere

3. 2. 2. 1   Solar Radiation

Solar radiation (or sunlight) is the energy that Earth receives from the Sun. Earth also emits radiation back into space, but at longer wavelengths that we cannot see. Part of the incoming and emitted radiation is absorbed or reflected by the atmosphere. Solar radiation is a central factor affecting a variety of human's life such as health, agriculture or the evolving transition process towards renewable energies. Solar radiation is more than the light and heat that we perceive from the sun. The sun is a star, after all, and it produces energy in many forms, from perceptible heat, visible and invisible spectrum of light, radiation, and more. Life on earth would be impossible without the sun, but our atmosphere also protects us from the more dangerous aspects of solar radiation.

Solar radiation is the total frequency spectrum of electromagnetic radiation produced by the sun. This spectrum covers visible light and near-visible radiation, such as x-rays, ultraviolet radiation, infrared radiation, and radio waves. Incoming solar radiation fluctuates from time to time and on average, about half of this radiation is reflected or absorbed by atmosphere. The absorption of solar radiation by the atmosphere is selective. Visible light passes through almost undiminished, whereas ultraviolet light is absorbed mostly by ozone in the stratosphere. Infrared radiation is absorbed mostly by carbon dioxide (CO_2) and water in the troposphere. On a cloudy day, as much as 90% of insolation is absorbed or reflected by clouds. Solar radiation is essential to life for two main reasons. First, the sun provides warmth; second, organisms are dependent on solar radiation for life-sustaining energy.

3.2.2.2 Ultraviolet Radiation

Ultraviolet (UV) radiation is electromagnetic radiation just like visible light, radar signals and radio broadcast signals (Figure 3.2). It has shorter wavelengths (higher frequencies) compared to visible light but has longer wavelengths (lower frequencies) compared to X-rays. UV radiation is divided into three wavelength ranges: UV-A (315—400 nm), UV-B (280—315 nm) and UV-C (100—280 nm). UV-A is less damaging to DNA, and hence is used in cosmetic artificial sun tanning (tanning booths and tanning beds) and psoralen and ultraviolet A radiation (PUVA) therapy for psoriasis. However, UV-A is now known to cause significant damage to DNA via indirect routes (formation of free radicalsand reactive oxygen species), and causes cancer. UV-B is also greatly absorbed by the Earth's atmosphere, and along with UV-C causes photochemical reaction leading to the production of the ozone layer. It may directly damages DNA and causes sunburn, however it is essential for vitamin D synthesis in the skin and fur of mammals. As one of the three types of invisible light rays (together with ultraviolet A and ultraviolet B) released by the sun, UV-C is the most dangerous type of ultraviolet light in terms of its potential threat to life on Earth. However, it cannot penetrate Earth's protective ozone layer. Due to absorption by the atmosphere, very little reaches Earth's surface. This spectrum of radiation has germicidal properties, as used in germicidal lamps.

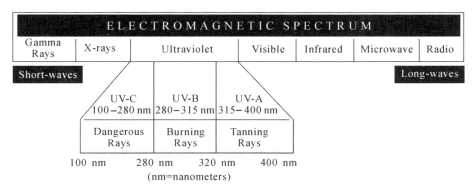

Figure 3.2 Electromagnetic Spectrum

Sunlight is the greatest source of UV radiation. Man-made ultraviolet sources include several types of UV lamps, arc welding, and mercury vapor lamps. Some UV exposure is essential for good health. It stimulates vitamin D production in the body. However, excessive exposure to ultraviolet radiation is associated with different types of skin cancer, sunburn, accelerated skin aging, as well as cataracts and other eye diseases. The severity of the effect depends on the wavelength, intensity, and duration of exposure.

We hear on the radio and read in the newspapers about the UV index as a part of the weather forecast. The UV index is a measure of the intensity of UV radiation in the sunlight that causes reddening of the skin (erythema). The UV index scale runs from 0 (when there is no sunlight) to 11+ (extreme). The UV index can increase the mid-teens at midday in the tropics. The implications of the UV index are summarized in Table 3.1.

Table 3.1   Implications of the UV Index and Grade

UV Index	Grade	Description	Protection Actions
0—2	1	Low	No sun protection. Wear a hat for going outside.
3—5	2	Moderate	Minimal sun protection (sun glasses and hat).
6—7	3	High	Protection required [sun glasses, hat and sun screen (SPF$\geqslant$15)].
8—10	4	Very High	Avoid the sun between 11 a.m. and 4 p.m. Take full precautions.
>10	5	Extreme High	Avoid the sun between 11 a.m. and 4 p.m. Take full precautions.

3.2.3   Types and Sources of Air Pollution

Air pollution worldwide is a growing threat to human health and the natural environment. Air pollution occurs when harmful or excessive quantities of substances including gases, particles, and biological molecules are introduced into Earth's atmosphere. It may cause diseases, allergies and even death to humans; it may also cause harm to other living organisms such as animals and food crops, and may damage the natural or artificial environment. Both human activity and natural processes can generate air pollution. Although some pollutants are released by natural sources such as volcanoes, coniferous forests, and hot springs, the effect of this pollution is very small compared to that caused by emissions from industrial sources, power and heat generation, waste disposal, and the operation of internal combustion engines. Fuel combustion is the largest contributor to air pollutant emissions, caused by humans, with stationary and mobile sources equally responsible. The air pollution problem is encountered outdoor as well as indoor.

An air pollutant is a material in the air that can have adverse effects on humans and the ecosystem. The substance can be solid particles, liquid droplets, or gases. A pollutant can be of natural origin or man-made. Pollutants are classified as primary or secondary. Primary pollutants are usually produced by processes such as ash from a volcanic eruption. Other examples include carbon monoxide gas from motor vehicle exhausts or sulphur dioxide released from the factories. The primary pollutants remain in the same chemical form as they are released from a source directly into the atmosphere. Secondary pollutants are not emitted directly. Rather, they form in the air when primary pollutants react or interact. The production of Peroxyacetyl Nitrate (PAN) during photochemical reactions is a typical example of secondary pollutant. Ground level ozone is a prominent example of secondary pollutants. Some pollutants may be both primary and secondary: They are both emitted directly and formed from other primary pollutants. The major pollutants which contribute to outdoor air pollution are sulfur dioxide, carbon monoxide, nitrogen oxides, ozone, total suspended particulate matter, lead, carbon dioxide, and toxic pollutants.

3. 2. 3. 1   Sources of Air Pollution

Sources of air pollution can be dichotomized into natural and anthropogenic sources. Natural sources include forest fires, dust storms, and volcanic eruptions. Plants such as ragweed contaminate the air with pollen. Decaying leaves and other forms of vegetation release gases that contribute to air pollution and cause haze. Anthropogenic air pollution, contamination produced by human activities (Table 3. 2), may also adversely affect human health. Some sources of anthropogenic air pollution include smoke from chimneys; gases from septic tanks and house sewer system vents; oily fumes and cooking odour; and fumes, gases, vapors and particles released from paint, household cleaners, hair sprays, and so forth.

Table 3. 2   Common Atmospheric Pollution Sources and Their Pollutants

Category	Source	Emitting pollutants
Agriculture	Open burning, spray pesticides	Suspended particulate matter, carbon monoxide, volatile organic compounds, pesticides
Mining and quarrying	Coal mining, crude oil and gas production, stone quarrying	Suspended particulate matter, sulphur dioxide, oxides of nitrogen, volatile organic compounds
Power generation	Electricity, gas, steam	Suspended particulate matter, sulphur dioxide, oxides of nitrogen, carbon monoxide, volatile organic compounds, sulphur trioxide, lead
Transport	Combustion engines	Suspended particulate matter, sulphur dioxide, oxides of nitrogen, carbon monoxide, volatile organic compounds, lead
Community service	Municipal incinerators	Suspended particulate matter, sulphur dioxide, oxides of nitrogen, carbon monoxide, volatile organic compounds, lead

Industrial pollution is created by the release of gases, vapors and fumes from industries that manufacture automobiles, clothing, cleaners, chemicals, plastics, furniture and other household products. Sources of air pollution may also be classified by the way they generate emissions: transportation, stationary combustion sources, industrial processes, solid waste disposal facilities and miscellaneous.

Transportation sources: This category includes most emissions produced from transportation sources during the combustion process. The internal combustion engines fueled by gasoline and diesel are the biggest sources in this category. The other sources include trains, ships, lawnmowers, farm tractors, planes, and construction machinery.

Stationary combustion sources: In this category the sources only produce energy and the emission is a result of fuel combustion. The sources include power plants as well as home heating furnaces. In developing countries, traditional biomass burning may be the major source of air pollutants.

Industrial processes: The sources which emit pollutants during manufacturing of products include petrochemical plants, petrochemical refining, food and agriculture industries, chemical processing, metallurgical and mineral product factories and wood processing industries are the major sources of air emissions. The smaller sources include dry-cleaning, painting and degreasing operations.

Solid waste disposal: This category includes facilities that dispose off unwanted trash. Refuse incineration and open burning are important sources.

Miscellaneous: These sources include forest fires, house fires, agriculture burning, asphalt road paving and coal mining.

3.2.3.2　Types of Air Pollution

There are two basic physical forms of air pollutants. The first is gaseous form. For example, sulfur dioxide, ozone and hydro-carbon vapors exist in the form of gas. Gases lack definite volume and shape and the molecules are widely separated. The second form is particulate matters. Particulate matter (PM) is a complex mixture of solids and liquids, including carbon, complex organic chemicals, sulphates, nitrates, mineral dust, and water suspended in the air. It varies in size. Some particles, such as dust, soot, dirt or smoke are large or dark enough to be seen with the naked eyes. But the most damaging particles are the smaller particles, known as PM10 or PM2.5. PM10 refers to particles with aerodynamic diameter that's smaller than 10 microns (10 μm). PM2.5 refers to particles with aerodynamic diameter smaller than 2.5 microns, and these are known as fine particles. The smallest fine particles, less than 0.1 micron in aerodynamic diameter, are called ultrafine particles.

The types of air pollution may be classified as point or area and natural (biogenic) sources. Point sources include stationary facilities that emit sufficient amounts of pollutants to be worth listing. Area sources are other point sources that individually emit small amount of pollutants. Dry cleaners in a city are an example of area sources. They contribute significantly to pollution as a group. Mobile sources include automobiles, trucks, air planes, ships, boats and lawnmowers. Natural sources are soil, water, vegetables, volcanic eruptions and lightning strikes.

3.2.4　Influences of Climate, Topography, and Atmosphere Processes

Climate, topography and physical processes in the atmosphere play an important role in transportation, concentration, dispersal, and removal of air pollutants. Wind speed is a fundamental atmospheric quantity caused by movement of air from high to low pressure, usually due to changes in temperature. Wind speed and wind direction are important in air quality monitoring. It can help identify the location of the pollution source, and provide a better overall picture of what's happening in the air. While wind rose give a succinct view of how wind speed and directions that typically distributed at a particular location over a period.

Temperature inversion affects air pollution levels. Temperature inversions occur when a stable layer of warmer air overlays cooler air, reversing the normal temperature decline with increasing height and preventing convection currents from dispersing pollutants. On most days, the temperature of air in the atmosphere is cooler at a higher altitude. This is because most of the Sun's energy is converted to sensible heat on the ground, which in turn warms the air at the surface. The warm air rises in the atmosphere, where it disperses and cools. However, sometimes the temperature of air actually increases

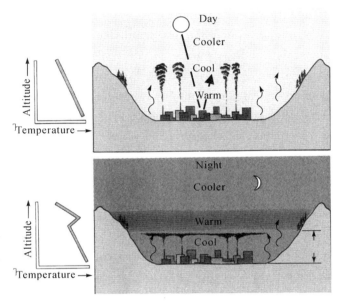

Figure 3.3 Temperature Inversion

with height. The situation of having warm air on top of cooler air is referred to as a temperature inversion, because the temperature profile of the atmosphere is "inverted" from its usual state (Figure 3.3). There are two types of temperature inversions: surface inversions that occur near the Earth's surface, and aloft inversions that occur above the ground. Surface inversions are most important in the study of air quality.

The Los Angeles Basin in the United States is a classic example of conditions that generate an atmospheric temperature inversion. During the day, the Sun heats the ground, warming the air near the surface and carrying dust and pollution aloft. Contaminated air is trapped by encircling mountains, forming a thick layer over the city. At night, the bare desert ground and paved streets radiate heat quickly into the cloudless sky. A layer of air immediately adjacent to the ground cools as well. This cooling is accelerated by cool, humid, on-shore breezes from the coast. The high particulate and pollutant levels in the upper air retain heat and form a cap that holds and concentrates contaminants.

The most common way surface inversions form is through the cooling of the air near the ground at night. Once the Sun goes down, the ground loses heat very quickly, and this cools the air that is in contact with the ground. However, since air is a very poor conductor of heat, the air just above the surface remains warm. Conditions that favor the development of a strong surface inversion are calm winds, clear skies, and long nights. Calm winds prevent warmer air above the surface from mixing down to the ground, and clear skies increase the rate of cooling at the Earth's surface. Long nights allow for the cooling of the ground to continue over a longer period of time, resulting in a greater temperature decrease at the surface. Since the nights in the wintertime are much longer than nights during the summertime, surface inversions are stronger and more common during the winter months. A strong inversion implies a substantial temperature difference exists between the cool surface air and the warmer air aloft. During the daylight hours, surface inversions normally weaken and disappear as the Sun warms the Earth's surface. However, under certain meteorological conditions, such as strong high pressure over the area, these inversions can persist for several days. In addition, local topographical features can enhance the formation of inversions, especially in the valleys.

Surface temperature inversions play a major role in air quality, especially during the winter when these inversions are the strongest. The warm air above cooler air acts like a lid, suppressing vertical mixing and trapping the cooler air at the surface. As pollutants from vehicles, fireplaces, and industry are emitted into the air, the inversion traps these pollutants near the ground, leading to poor air quality. The strength and duration of the inversion will control air pollution levels near the ground. A strong inversion will confine pollutants to a shallow vertical layer, leading to high air pollution levels, while a weak inversion will lead to the lower levels.

The effects of topography on the climate of any given region are powerful. Mountain ranges create barriers that alter wind and precipitation patterns. Topographical features such as narrow canyons channel and amplify winds, which affects the dilution and diffusion of air pollutants. Usually, the temperature in the urban always is higher than that in the suburbs, leading to the phenomenon of urban heat island. The temperature difference usually is larger at night than during the day, and is most apparent when winds are weak. Urban heat island is most noticeable during the summer and winter. The main cause of the urban heat island effect is from the modification of land surfaces. Waste heat generated by energy usage is a secondary contributor. As a population center grows, it tends to expand its area and increase its average temperature.

3.2.5   Effects of Air Pollution

3.2.5.1   Direct Health Effects

The health effects caused by air pollution may include difficulty in breathing, wheezing, coughing, asthma and worsening of existing respiratory and cardiac conditions. These effects can result in increased medication use, increased doctor or emergency department visits, more hospital admissions and premature death. The human health effects of poor air quality are far reaching, but mainly affect the body's respiratory and the cardiovascular system. Individual reactions to air pollutants depend on the type of pollutant a person is exposed to, the degree of exposure, and the individual's health status and genetics. The most common sources of air pollution include particulates, ozone, nitrogen dioxide, and sulphur dioxide. Children aged less than five years living in developing countries are the most vulnerable population in terms of total deaths attributable to indoor and outdoor air pollution. According to the responding time, the health effects can be divided into short-term and long-term effects.

Short-Term Health Effects(or Acute Health Effects):

Air pollution can cause irritation of the eyes, nose and throat, and it can lead to upper respiratory infections like bronchitis. It can also cause headaches and nausea. Air pollution can trigger asthma attacks as well.

Smog is air pollution that reduces visibility. Smog is unhealthy to humans and animals, and it can kill plants. Smog was common in industrial areas, and remains a familiar sight in cities today. Cities located in basins surrounded by mountains is more likely to have smog problems because the smog is trapped in the valley and cannot be carried away by wind. There are two types of smog: industrial smog and photochemical smog.

Events like the London smog of 1952 are often referred to as industrial smog because SO_2 emissions from burning coal play a key role. Typically, industrial smog—also called gray or black smog—develops under cold and humid conditions. Cold temperatures are often associated with inversions that trap the pollution near the surface. High humidity allows for rapid oxidation of SO_2 to form sulfuric acid and sulfate particles. Events similar to the 1952 London smog occurred in the industrial towns of Liege, Belgium, in 1930, killing more than 60 people, and Donora, Pennsylvania, the United States, in 1948, killing 20. Today coal combustion is a major contributor to urban air pollution in China, especially from emissions of SO_2 and aerosols.

Air pollution regulations in developed countries have reduced industrial smog events, but photochemical smog remains a persistent problem, largely driven by vehicle emissions. Photochemical smog is produced when sunlight reacts with nitrogen oxides and at least one volatile organic compound (VOC) in the atmosphere. Nitrogen oxides come from car exhaust, coal power plants, and factory emissions. VOCs are released from gasoline, paints, and many cleaning solvents. When sunlight hits these chemicals, they form airborne particles and ground-level ozone-or smog.

Photochemical smog is produced when pollutants from the combustion of fossil fuels react with sunlight. The energy in the sunlight converts the pollutants into other toxic chemicals. In order for photochemical smog to form, there must be other pollutants in the air, specifically nitrous oxides and other VOCs. When nitrous oxides and VOCs interact with sunlight, secondary pollutants are formed, such as ozone and peroxyacetyl nitrate. These secondary pollutants are known as photochemical smog. Ozone can be helpful or harmful. The ozone layer high up in the atmosphere protects us from the harmful effects of the ultraviolet radiation from the sun. But when ozone is close to the ground, it is bad for human health. Ozone can damage lung tissue, and it is especially dangerous to people with respiratory illnesses such as asthma. Ozone can also cause itchiness and burning eyes. Peroxyacetyl nitrate is one of the chemicals that are responsible for damaging lung tissue, and photochemical smog forms plenty of it. Photochemical smog typically develops in summer (when solar radiation is strongest) in stagnant conditions promoted by temperature inversions and weak winds.

In addition to London smog and photochemical smog, the world's worst short-term civilian pollution crisis was the 1984 Bhopal Disaster in India. Leaked industrial vapours from the Union Carbide factory, killed at least 3,787 people.

Long-Term Health Effects (or Chronic Health Effects):

Air pollution can lead to the chronic respiratory disease and lung cancer, one of the most common effects of being exposed to air pollution over long periods is difficulty in breathing, and in more serious cases, asthma. It is caused due to the swelling of the airway or the bronchioles, as they are called, because of the many pollutants in the air. Asthma causes major problems in an individual's daily life, and in extreme cases can lead to death, if not tended to promptly. Pneumonia is a very common disease, which seems to be on the rise, especially in the underdeveloped world because of the extreme high levels of pollution in these areas. It is caused by the inflammation of the lung tissue. If untreated, it can be quite deadly. The heart is the control center of the human body. The lungs constantly supply oxygen to the heart, which in turn pumps it through the blood to the entire the body. This perfect synergy of the heart and the other organs of the body ensure a healthy life. Over time, if we breathe in polluted air, it gets into our blood stream and causes many serious problems. These pollutants tend to accumulate in the coronary arteries and obstruct the flow of rich blood to the heart. This in turn affects the functioning of the heart, and can cause heart attacks.

Air pollution is also emerging as a risk factor for stroke, particularly in developing countries where pollutant levels are high. A 2007 study found that in women, air pollution is associated with ischemic stroke. Air pollution was also found to be associated with increased incidence and mortality from coronary stroke in a cohort study in 2011. Associations are believed to be causal and effects may be mediated by vasoconstriction, low-grade inflammation and atherosclerosis. Other mechanisms such as autonomic nervous system imbalance have also been suggested. Studies have shown that air pollution also affected short-term memory, learning ability, and impulsivity. It appears that inflammation had damaged those brain cells and prevented that region of the brain from developing, and the ventricles simply expanded to fill the space.

Ambient levels of air pollution have been associated with preterm birth and low birth weight. A 2014 WHO worldwide survey on maternal and perinatal health found a statistically significant association between low birth weights (LBW) and increased levels of exposure to PM2. 5. Women in regions with greater than average PM2. 5 levels had statistically significant higher odds of pregnancy resulting in a low-birth weight infant even when adjusted for country-related variables. The effect is thought to be from stimulating inflammation and increasing oxidative stress. A study by the University of York found that in 2010 exposure to PM2. 5 was strongly associated with 18% of preterm births globally, which was approximately 2. 7 million premature births. The countries with the highest air pollution associated preterm births were in South and East Asia, the Middle East, North Africa, and West sub-Saharan Africa. The WHO estimated in 2014 that air pollution causes the premature death of some 7 million people worldwide every year. Studies published in March 2019 indicated that the number may be around 8. 8 million. Urban outdoor air pollution is estimated to cause 1. 3 million deaths worldwide per year. Children are particularly at risk due to the immaturity of their respiratory organ systems.

3. 2. 5. 2   Indirect Health Effects

(1) Greenhouse Effects

The greenhouse effect happens when certain gases—known as greenhouse gases accumulate in Earth's atmosphere. A greenhouse gas (GHG) is a gas that absorbs and emits radiant energy within the thermal infrared range. These gases include carbon dioxide (CO_2), methane, nitrous oxide (N_2O), fluorinated gases, and ozone. Greenhouse gases let the Sun's light shine onto the Earth's surface, but they trap the heat that reflects up into the atmosphere. In this way, they act like the glass walls of a greenhouse. This greenhouse effect keeps the Earth warm enough to sustain life. Without the greenhouse effect, the average temperature of the Earth would drop from 14℃ (57℉) to as low as −18℃ (−0. 4℉). Some greenhouse gases come from natural sources. Evaporation adds water vapor to the atmosphere. Animals and plants release carbon dioxide when they respire or breathe. Methane is released naturally from some low-oxygen environments, such as swamps. Nitrous oxide is produced by certain processes in soil and water.

Since the Industrial Revolution of the late 1700s and early 1800s, people have been releasing large quantities of greenhouse gases into the atmosphere. That amount has skyrocketed in the past century. Greenhouse gas emissions increased 70% between 1970 and 2004. Emissions of CO_2, the most important greenhouse gas, rose by about 80% during that time. The amount of CO_2 in the atmosphere today far exceeds the natural range seen over the last 650,000 years.

Most of the CO_2 that people put into the atmosphere comes from burning fossil fuels. Cars, trucks, train, and plane are powered by fossil fuels, and likewise many electric power plants. Another way human release CO_2 into the atmosphere is by cutting down forests, because trees contain large amounts of carbon. Methane is added to the atmosphere through livestock farming, landfills, and fossil fuel production such as coalmining and natural gas processing. Nitrous oxide comes from agriculture and fossil fuel burning. Fluorinated gases include chlorofluorocarbons (CFCs), hydrochlorofluorocarbons (HCFCs), and hydrofluorocarbons (HFCs). These gases are used in aerosol cans and refrigeration. All these human activities add greenhouse gases to the atmosphere. As the level of these gases rises, so does the temperature of the Earth. The rise in Earth's average temperature contributed to human activity is known as global warming.

Action must be taken to reduce the amount of greenhouse gases released into the atmosphere. There are various ways of doing this, including driving less, using public transportation, reuse, recycle, using less electricity, eating less meat, or planting trees. Trees absorb carbon dioxide, keeping it out of the atmosphere. Ruminant animals such as cows are the main contributors to methane production.

(2) Acid Deposition

"Acid rain" is a broad term referring to a mixture of wet and dry deposition (deposited material) from the atmosphere containing higher than normal amounts of nitric and sulfuric acids. The precursors, or chemical forerunners, of acid rain formation result from both natural sources, such as volcanoes and decaying vegetation, and man-made sources, primarily emissions of sulfur dioxide (SO_2) and nitrogen oxides (NO_x) resulting from fossil fuel combustion. Acid rain occurs when these gases react in the atmosphere with water, oxygen, and other chemicals to form various acidic compounds. The result is a mild solution of sulfuric acid and nitric acid (Figure 3. 4).

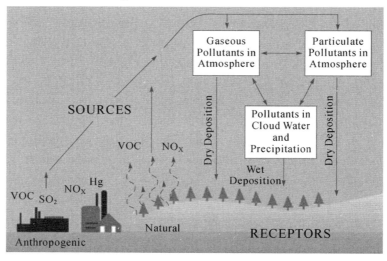

Figure 3. 4　Acid Deposition

Wet deposition refers to acidic rain, fog, and snow. If the acid chemicals in the air are blown into areas where the weather is wet, the acids can fall to the ground in the form of rain, snow, fog, or mist. As this acidic water flows over and through the ground, it affects a variety of plants and animals. The strength of the effects depends on several factors, including how acidic the water is; the chemistry and buffering capacity of the soils involved; and the types of fish, trees, and other living things that rely on the water. In areas where the weather is dry, the acid chemicals may become incorporated into dust or smoke and fall to the ground through dry deposition, sticking to the ground, buildings, homes, cars, and trees. Dry deposited gases and particles can be washed from these surfaces by rainstorms, leading to increased runoff. This runoff water makes the resulting mixture more acidic. About half of the acidity in the atmosphere falls back to earth through dry deposition.

Acid rain has been shown to have adverse effects on forests, freshwater, and soils, killing off insect and aquatic life forms (Figure 3.5). It also damages buildings and statues, and may adversely affect human health. The harm to people from acid rain is not direct. However, the pollutants that cause acid rain—sulfur dioxide (SO_2) and nitrogen oxides (NO_x)—do damage human health. These gases interact in the atmosphere to form fine sulfate and nitrate particles that can be transported long distances by winds and inhaled into human

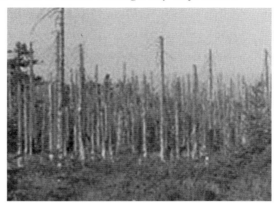

Figure 3.5   Effect of Acid Rain on a Forested Area of the Jizera Mountains, Czech Republic

lungs. Fine particles can also penetrate indoors. Many scientific studies have identified the relationships between elevated levels of fine particles and increased illness and premature death from heart and lung disorders, such as asthma, bronchitis, or lung cancer.

Acid rain causes acidification of lakes and streams and contributes to the damage of trees at high elevations and many sensitive forest soils. In addition, acid rain accelerates the decay of building materials and paints, including irreplaceable buildings, statues, and sculptures that are part of our nation's cultural heritage. Prior to falling to the Earth, SO_2 and NO_x gases and their particulate matter derivatives—sulfates and nitrates—contribute to visibility degradation and harm public health.

(3) Ozone Depletion

Ozone is present in the stratosphere. The stratosphere reaches 30 miles above the Earth, and at the very top it contains ozone. Ozone is a colorless gas. It is formed when oxygen molecules absorb ultraviolet photons, and undergo a chemical reaction known as photo dissociation or photolysis. In this process, a single molecule of oxygen breaks down into two oxygen atoms. The free oxygen atom (O), then combines with an oxygen molecule (O_2), and forms a molecule of ozone (O_3). The ozone molecules, in turn absorb ultraviolet rays between 310 to 200 nm (nanometers) wave length, and thereby prevent these harmful radiations from entering the Earth's atmosphere. The process of absorption of harmful radiation occurs when ozone molecules split up into a molecule of oxygen, and an oxygen atom. The oxygen atom (O), again combines with the oxygen molecule (O_2) to regenerate an ozone (O_3) molecule. Thus, the total amount of ozone is maintained by this continuous process of destruction, and regeneration.

Ultraviolet radiations (UVR), are high energy electromagnetic waves emitted from the Sun. UV radiation includes UV-A, the least dangerous form of UV radiation, UV-B, and UV-C, which is the most dangerous. UV-C is unable to reach the Earth's surface due to stratospheric ozone's ability to absorb it. The real threat comes from UV-B, which can enter the Earth's atmosphere, and has adverse effects.

Ozone layer depletion first captured the attention of the whole world in the latter half of 1970, and since then, a lot of research has been done to find its possible effects and causes. Various studies have also been undertaken to find out a possible solution. The production and emission of chlorofluorocarbons (CFCs), is the leading cause of ozone layer depletion (Figure 3.6). CFC's accounts for almost 80% of the total depletion of ozone. Other ozone-depleting substances (ODS), include hydrochlorofluorocarbons (HCFCs) and VOCs. These are often found in vehicle emissions, byproducts of industrial processes, refrigerants, and aerosols. ODS are relatively stable in the lower atmosphere of the Earth, but in the stratosphere, they are exposed to ultraviolet radiation and thus, they break down to release a free chlorine atom. This free chlorine atom reacts with an ozone molecule (O_3), and forms chlorine monoxide (ClO), and a molecule of oxygen. ClO reacts with an ozone molecule to form a chlorine atom, and two

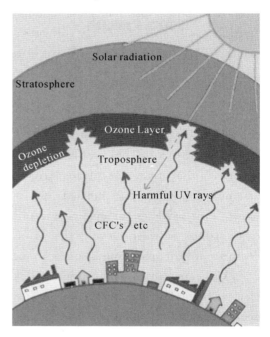

Figure 3.6 Ozone Depletion in the Stratosphere

molecules of oxygen. The free chlorine molecule again reacts with ozone to form chlorine monoxide. The process continues, and this results in the depletion of the ozone layer.

As ozone depletes in the stratosphere, it forms a "hole" in the layer. This hole enables harmful ultraviolet rays to enter the Earth's atmosphere. Every time 1% of the ozone layer is depleted, 2% more UV-B is able to reach the surface of the planet. Ultraviolet rays of the Sun are associated with a number of health-related and environmental issues. Exposure to ultraviolet rays poses an increased risk of developing several types of skin cancers, including malignant melanoma, basal and squamous cell carcinoma. Direct exposure to UV radiations can result in photokeratitis (snow blindness), and cataracts. Effects of UV rays include impairment of the immune system. Increased exposure to UV rays weakens the response of the immune system. Constant exposure to UV radiation can cause photo allergy, which results in the outbreak of rash in fair-skinned people. Ozone chemicals can cause difficulty in breathing, chest pain, throat irritation, and hamper lung functioning.

The discovery of the ozone depletion problem came as a great surprise. Action must be taken now to ensure that the ozone layer is not destroyed. Because CFCs are so widespread and used in such a great variety of products, limiting their use is hard. Also, since many products already contain components that use CFCs, it would be difficult to eliminate those CFCs already in existence. The CFC problem may be hard to solve because there are already great quantities of CFCs in the environment. CFCs would remain in the stratosphere for another 100 years even if none were ever produced again. Despite the difficulties, international action has been taken to limit CFCs. In the Montreal Protocol, 30 nations worldwide agreed to reduce usage of CFCs and encouraged other countries to do so as well.

3.2.6   Health Effects of Several Major Air Pollutants

Air pollutants are composed of a number of components. Some pollutants are very common and may affect human health and/or environment, and are usually regulated by governments on the basis of criteria. Such a group of pollutants are called criteria air pollutants (Table 3.3). In addition, there are some other pollutants related to air quality and human health.

3.2.6.1   Particulate Matter (PM)

Particulate matter (PM), also known as aerosol particles, is a mixture of solid particles and liquid droplets that are suspended in and move with the air. Some PM are large enough to be seen with the naked eyes, such as dust, soot, or smoke; however, other small PM can only be detected by an electron microscope. Some PM occur naturally, such as volcanoes, dust storms, forest fires, and sea spray. The manmade sources of PM include vehicle exhaust, waste incineration, and various industrial activities, etc. The composition of PM depends on their source. The major components of PM are sulfate, nitrates, sodium chloride, ammonia, black carbon, mineral dust and water. It consists of a complex mixture of solid and liquid particles of organic and inorganic substances suspended in the air. Primary PM may transform into secondary particles in the atmosphere as a result of complex reactions of chemicals such as sulfur and nitrogen oxides into sulfuric acid (liquid) and nitric acid (gaseous).

Table 3.3   Overview of Common Criteria for Air Pollutants

Pollutant	Symbol	Example of Source	Health Effects	Environmental Effects
Sulfur Dioxide	SO_2	Burning of fossil fuels; erupting volcanoes	Eye irritation; breathing problems; lung damage; aggravates asthma and chronic bronchitis	Contributes to acid rain, which can corrode building materials and paints, and damage forests and lakes

cottinued

Pollutant	Symbol	Example of Source	Health Effects	Environmental Effects
Ozone	O_3	Formed by chemical reaction of pollutants (NOx and VOCs)	Cardiac system damage; eye irritation; respiratory tract irritation	Reduces vegetation growth; damages materials such as rubber, masonry and paint; reduces visibility
Particulate Matter	PM_{10} $PM_{2.5}$	Combustion processes, such as wood and diesel burning; non-combustion activities, such as earthworks	Lung damage; eye irritation; aggravates asthma; carcinogenic	Causes haze; reduces visibility; discolor buildings and statues
Nitrogen Oxides	NO_x	Vehicles; industrial boilers; industrial processes; power plants; Burning of fossil fuels	Aggravates respiratory diseases, particularly asthma; lung damage	Contributes to acid rain; forms ozone and other pollutants (smog)
Lead	Pb	Burning of leaded fuels; metal refineries	Affects nervous system, kidney function, immune system, reproductive and developmental systems and the cardiovascular system.	Persists and accumulates in environment, decreased growth and reproductive rates in plants and animals, and neurological effects in vertebrates
Carbon Monoxide	CO	Incomplete burning of fuel; dry cleaners	Reduces the oxygen carrying capacity of blood and damages heart and brain.	Contributes to smog; reduces visibility

PM refers generically to a mixture of particles that can vary in size. The size of particles is directly linked to their potential for causing health problems. PM_{10} (with aerodynamic diameter generally equal or less than 10 micrometers) can be inhaled and cause serious health problems, and therefore also are known as inhalable particles. Of these, $PM_{2.5}$ or fine particles (with aerodynamic diameters generally 2.5 micrometers or smaller) have the capability to bypass the body's normal defenses and can be inhaled deeply into the lungs where they are deposited, and some may even get into bloodstream.

Numerous scientific evidences have linked PM exposure to a variety of health problems, including: premature death in people with heart or lung disease, nonfatal heart attacks, irregular heartbeat, aggravated asthma, decreased lung function, increased respiratory symptoms (e. g. irritation of the airways, coughing or difficulty breathing). Researches also show that PM is carcinogenic, and is associated with elevated risk of adverse pregnancy outcomes, such as low birth weight.

PM pollution is a worldwide problem. Based on the modelled data for the year 2014, 92% of the world population are exposed to $PM_{2.5}$ air pollution concentrations that are above the annual mean WHO Air Quality Guidelines (AQG) levels of 10 $\mu g/m^3$, and in 2012, ambient air pollution from PM was responsible for about 3 million deaths and 85 million disability adjusted life years (DALYs). Children, older adults, and people with heart or lung diseases, are the most likely to be affected by PM exposure.

3. 2. 6. 2   Sulfur Dioxide (SO₂)

Sulfur dioxide (SO_2) is a toxic gas with a burnt match smell. The largest source of SO_2 in the atmosphere is the burning of fossil fuels, such as coal, by power plants and other industrial facilities. Smaller sources of SO_2 emissions include: industrial processes such as extracting metal from ore, ships and heavy equipment that burn fuel with a high sulfur content. It is also released naturally by volcanic activity.

Sulfur dioxide is a major air pollutant and has significant impacts upon human health. SO_2 is a water-soluble irritant gas. As such, it is absorbed predominantly in the upper airways and, as an irritant, can stimulate the respiratory tract and increases the risk of tract infections. It causes coughing, mucus secretion and aggravates conditions such as asthma and chronic bronchitis. Short-term exposures to SO_2 can harm the human respiratory system and make breathing difficult. Children, the elderly, and those who suffer from asthma are particularly sensitive to the effects of SO_2. High concentrations of SO_2 in the air generally also lead to the formation of other sulfur oxides (SO_x). SO_x can react with other compounds in the atmosphere to form sulfuric acid small particles that may penetrate deeply into sensitive parts of the lungs and cause additional health problems.

At high concentrations, gaseous SO_x can harm trees and plants by damaging foliage and decreasing growth. SO_2 and other sulfur oxides can play an important role in the production of acid rain which can harm sensitive ecosystems.

3. 2. 6. 3   Nitrogen oxides (NO_x)

Nitrogen oxides (NO_x) may refer to gases made up of a single molecule of nitrogen combine with varying numbers of molecules of oxygen, or a mixture of such compounds. Nitrogen oxides in the atmosphere usually describes a mixture of nitric oxide (NO) and nitrogen dioxide (NO_2), which are gases produced from natural sources, motor vehicles, and other fuel burning processes. NO_2 is used as the indicator for the larger group of nitrogen oxides. Nitrogen oxides can react with volatile organic compounds (VOC) to form photochemical smog. They are also major components of acid rain.

Compared with nitric oxide, the toxicity of nitrogen dioxide is much higher, so the health impact assessment of nitrogen oxides mainly comes from the research results of nitrogen dioxide. Breathing air with a high concentration of NO_2 can irritate airways in the human respiratory system. Such exposures over short periods can aggravate respiratory diseases, particularly asthma, leading to respiratory symptoms (such as coughing, wheezing or difficulty breathing). NO_2 creates ozone which can cause eye irritation and exacerbates respiratory conditions. Long-term exposure to elevated concentrations of NO_2 may contribute to the development of asthma and potentially increase susceptibility to respiratory infections. NO_2 may also affect the senses, for example, by reducing a person's smell ability. People with asthma, as well as children and the elderly are generally at greater risk for the health effects of NO_2.

3.2.6.4　Carbon Oxides (CO_x)

Carbon Oxides is a chemical compound consisting only of carbon and oxygen. The simplest and most common carbon oxides are carbon monoxide (CO) and carbon dioxide (CO_2).

CO_2 is a trace gas in Earth's atmosphere. The concentration of CO_2 has risen due to human activities. Most CO_2 from human activities is released from burning coal and other fossil fuels. CO_2 content in fresh air varies between 0.036% (360 ppm) and 0.041% (410 ppm). CO_2 is an asphyxiating gas. In concentrations up to 1% (10,000 ppm), it will make some people feel drowsy and give the lungs a stuffy feeling. Concentrations of 7% to 10% (70,000 to 100,000 ppm) may cause suffocation, even in the presence of sufficient oxygen, symptoms such as dizziness, headache, visual and auditory dysfunction, and unconsciousness within a few minutes to an hour. CO_2 is the primary greenhouse gas, responsible for about three-quarters of emissions.

CO is a gas formed when substances containing carbon (such as petrol, gas, coal and wood) are burned with an insufficient supply of air. CO can bind to hemoglobin to form carboxyhemoglobin, and reduce the oxygen-carrying capacity of blood. CO has 210 times more affinity for binding with hemoglobin than oxygen does. Exposure to high levels of CO can result in death or serious health consequences, such as visual disturbances and impairment of mental and physical functioning. Inhaled carbon monoxide may also aggravate coronary heart disease, as well as circulatory, lung, and respiratory diseases.

3.2.6.5　Ozone (O_3)

Ozone is formed naturally through the interaction of solar ultraviolet (UV) radiation with molecular oxygen (O_2) in the upper atmosphere (the stratosphere). This "ozone layer" reduces the amount of harmful UV radiation reaching the Earth's surface. Although some ozone can move from the stratosphereinto the troposphere, most of the tropospheric ozone (ground level ozone) is the result of reactions of man-made VOCs and NOx. Tropospheric or ground-level ozone contributes to "smog" or haze.

Ozone affects human health in either good or bad ways depending on where it is in the atmosphere. Stratospheric ozone reduces human exposure to harmful UV radiation that causes skin cancer and cataracts. At ground level, elevated ozone concentrations can affect the cardiac system and lead to respiratory difficulties such as reduced lung function, local irritation of eyes and respiratory tract, and reduction of the ability to fight off colds and related respiratory infections.

3.2.6.6　Metals

In the air, metals occur naturally in small quantities, and can exist as vapor or particles. Mining, metal casting and other industrial processes contribute to metal emissions to the air. Some metals, such as lead (Pb), can cause adverse health effects.

Major sources of lead in the air are ore and metals processing and piston-engine aircraft operating on leaded aviation fuel. Other sources are waste incinerators, utilities, and lead-acid battery manufacturers. The highest air concentrations of lead are usually found near lead smelters. As a result of efforts to remove lead from motor vehicle gasoline, levels of lead in the air has reduced significantly in urban areas.

Young children are most susceptible to the effects of lead, particularly affecting the development of the brain and nervous system, and can suffer profound and permanent adverse health effects, such as behavior and learning problems, lower intelligence quotient (IQ) and hyperactivity, slowed growth, hearing problems, and anemia. Lead also causes long-term harm in adults, including increased blood pressure and incidence of hypertension, decreased kidney function, and reproductive problems. Exposure of pregnant women to high levels of lead can cause miscarriage, stillbirth, premature birth, low birth weight, and damage to the baby's brain, kidney's, and nervous system.

3.2.6.7 Polycyclic Aromatic Hydrocarbons (PAHs)

PAHs are organic compounds containing only carbon and hydrogen, composed of multiple aromatic rings. PAHs are ubiquitous in the environment and can be formed from either natural or manmade combustion sources. The dominant sources of PAHs in the environment are from human activity: wood-burning and the incomplete burning of organic material, of which dung or crop residues contribute more than half of annual global PAHs emissions. PAHs are typically found as complex mixtures. Lower-temperature combustion, such as wood-burning or tobacco smoking, usually generate low molecular weight PAHs. On the contrary, high-temperature industrial processes tends to generate PAHs with higher molecular weights.

Human health effects from environmental exposure to low levels of PAHs are unknown. Exposure to high concentrations PAHs may irritate the eyes, skin and respiratory tract and at high levels may cause headaches, nausea, vomiting, and abdominal pain. Cancer is a primary human health risk of exposure to PAHs, including skin, lung, bladder, liver, and stomach cancers. Adult exposure to PAHs has been linked to cardiovascular diseases. In utero exposure to PAHs has been linked with poor fetal growth, reduced immune function, and poorer neurological development, including lower IQ.

Benzo[a]pyrene (BaP) is the best studied and one of the most toxic of all PAHs. People are usually exposed to mixtures of PAHs and there is little information on human exposure to any single, pure PAH. BaP is often used as an indicator for this group of pollutants. BaP is associated with lung cancer, with the risk increasing in the presence of other substances, such as in the case of tobacco smoke. Other carcinogenic PAHs includes benz[a]anthracene, benzo[b]fluoranthene, benzo[k]fluoranthene, chrysene, dibenz[a,h] anthrancene, indeno[1,2,3-cd]pyrene.

3. 2. 6. 8　Dioxins

The chemical name for dioxin is: 2, 3, 7, 8-tetrachlorodibenzo-p-dioxin (2, 3, 7, 8-TCDD). Dioxins refers to a group of toxic chemical compounds that share certain chemical structures and biological characteristics, for example polychlorinated dibenzo-p-dioxins (PCDDs) and polychlorinated dibenzofurans (PCDFs). Certain dioxin-like polychlorinated biphenyls (PCBs) with similar toxic properties are also included under the term "dioxins". More than 400 types of dioxin-related compounds have been identified, about 30 of them are considered to have significant toxicity.

Dioxins can result from natural processes, such as forest fires and volcanic eruptions. Dioxins are also unwanted by-products of a wide range of manufacturing processes including smelting, chlorine bleaching of paper pulp and the manufacturing of some herbicides and pesticides. In terms of dioxins release into the environment, they are mainly formed as a result of combustion processes such as waste incineration or from burning fuels (like wood, coal or oil), due to incomplete burning. Cigarette smoke also contains small amounts of dioxins.

Dioxins are persistent environmental pollutants (POPs), and can accumulate in the food chain, mainly in the fatty tissue of animals. Because of the omnipresence of dioxins, all people have background exposure and a certain level of dioxins in the body, leading to the so-called body burden. Current normal background exposure is not expected to affect human health on average. Short-term exposure to high levels of dioxins may result in skin lesions, such as chloracne and patchy darkening of the skin, and damaged liver function. Long-term exposure is linked to impairment of the immune system, the endocrine system, the developing nervous system, and reproductive functions, and also cause cancer. The most studied and most toxic of all dioxins is TCDD. Based on animal and human epidemiology data, TCDD was classified by the WHO's International Agency for Research on Cancer (IARC) as a "known human carcinogen". However, TCDD does not damage genetic material and there is a level of exposure below which cancer risk would be negligible. The developing fetus is most sensitive to dioxin exposure. Newborn may also be more vulnerable to certain effects.

3. 2. 7　Indoor Air Pollution

3. 2. 7. 1　Indoor Air Quality (IAQ)

Indoor Air Quality (IAQ) refers to the air quality within and around buildings and structures, especially as it relates to the health and comfort of building occupants, including the quality of the air in a home, school, office, or other building environment. Indoor air pollution has been described by the US EPA to be four to five times worse than outdoor air and even greater. On average, most people spend about 90% of their time indoors. The very young and older adults with cardiovascular or respiratory disease tend to spend even more time indoors.

Outdoor air pollutants can enter buildings through doors, windows, and ventilation systems. Some pollutants, such as radon in the ground, come indoors through building foundations. However, most pollutants affecting indoor air quality come from sources inside buildings (Figure 3.7). Combustion sources, including tobacco, heating and cooking appliances, and fireplaces, can release harmful byproducts such as carbon monoxide and particulate matter directly into the indoor environment. Widespread use of household chemicals will introduce a lot of different chemicals directly into the indoor air. Building materials and furnishings are also potential sources, for example, asbestos fibers released from building insulation, radon in natural stone, and chemical off-gassing from pressed wood products. Inadequate ventilation, high temperature and humidity levels can increase indoor pollutant levels.

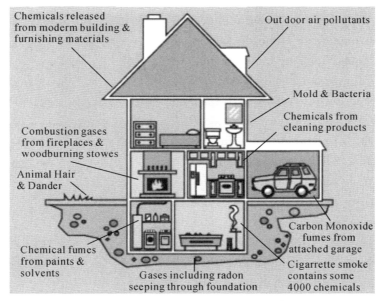

Figure 3.7　Indoor Air Pollution Sources
Source: US Environmental Protection Agency, 2010.

Health effects of indoor air pollutants may occur soon after exposure or years later. Immediate effects may show up after a single exposure or repeated exposures, and are usually short-term and treatable. Certain immediate effects are similar to those in colds or other diseases, and it is difficult to determine they are a result of exposure to indoor air pollution. Under such circumstance, it is important to observe the time and place symptoms occur. If the symptoms fade or go away once a person away from home, indoor air sources may be possible causes. And if the pollutant can be identified, sometimes the simplest treatment is just eliminating the person's exposure to the source of the pollution. Long-term health effects may show up either years after exposure or after long time repeated periods of exposure, which include respiratory diseases, heart disease, and cancer, can be severely debilitating or fatal.

3. 2. 7. 2　Indoor Use of Solid Fuel

Worldwide, more than three billion people burn solid fuels, including biomass (wood, charcoal, dung and crop residues) and coal, to meet their most basic energy needs (cooking, boiling water and keeping warm) in their homes, especially in developing countries. The inefficient burning of solid fuels on an open fire or traditional stove (figure 3. 8) can create pollutants, primarily PM and CO, but also NOx, benzene, butadiene, PAHs and many other toxic chemicals. In some areas, coal may also contain sulfur, arsenic and fluorine, thus these additional contaminants may also be present in the air. Burning solid fuels produces extremely high levels of indoor air pollution. For example, typical 24-hour levels of PM_{10} in biomass-using homes in range from 300 to 3,000 $\mu g/m^3$, and peaks during cooking may reach10,000 $\mu g/m^3$.

Certain health effects have been linked with exposure to indoor air pollution caused by burning solid fuels. Inhaling indoor smoke doubles the risk of pneumonia and other acute infections of the lower respiratory tract among children under five years of age, triples the risk of chronic obstructive pulmonary disease (COPD), such as chronic bronchitis or emphysema, among women. Burning of coal also doubles the risk of lung cancer, particularly among women. A 2009 report by WHO estimates that the indoor air pollution from typical household cooking fires causes nearly 2 million premature deaths annually-mostly of young children and their mothers. And according to the report, indoor smoke from solid fuel causes about 21% of lower respiratory infection deaths worldwide, 35% of chronic obstructive pulmonary deaths and about 3% of lung cancer deaths. Of these deaths, about 64% occur in low-income

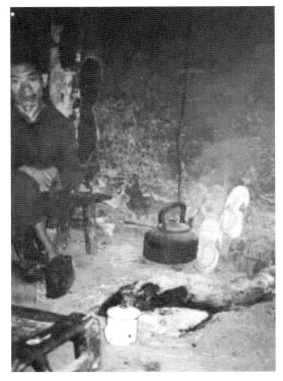

Figure 3. 8　Indoor Air Pollution Hazards in Home: Open Fires

countries, especially in South-East Asia and Africa. A further 28% of global deaths caused by indoor smoke from solid fuels occur in China. Moreover, some researchers have linked exposure to indoor smoke to asthma; cataracts; tuberculosis; adverse pregnancy outcomes, in particular low birth weight; ischemic heart disease; interstitial lung disease, and nasopharyngeal and laryngeal cancers.

The problem of indoor air pollution has been around since the Stone Age, yet only in recent years has the international community realized its health hazards. Some efforts are beginning to improve use of affordable, reliable, clean, efficient and safe home cooking stoves, in order to protect millions from unhealthy indoor air.

3. 2. 7. 3 Secondhand Smoke (SHS)

Secondhand smoke (SHS), contains more than 7,000 substances, is a mixture of the smoke given off by the burning of tobacco products, such as cigarettes, cigars or pipes and the smoke exhaled by smokers. It is also used interchangeably with environmental tobacco smoke (ETS). In contrast with the intended "active" smoking, exposure to secondhand smoke is called involuntary or passive smoking. In restaurants, waiting rooms, international airliners, and other encloses areas where there are cigarette smokers, nonsmokers may have to be exposed to secondhand smoke.

Secondhand smoke causes the same health effects as direct smoking, including disease, disability, and death. The IARC concluded in 2004 that "Involuntary smoking (exposure to secondhand or environmental tobacco smoke) is carcinogenic to humans." SHS can increased risk of some cancer, such as lung, breast, cervical, and bladder cancer. The link between SHS and several health outcomes, such as heart disease (e. g. atherosclerosis and stroke), lung problems (e. g. asthma and COPD), cognitive impairment and dementia (e. g. cognitive impairment and dementia in adults 50 and over, general cognitive and intellectual deficits in children) have long been established. Females exposed to SHS while pregnant may have higher risks of delivering a child with congenital abnormalities, smaller head circumferences, and low birth weight.

SHS is one of the most serious and most widespread exposures in the indoor environment. Globally, more than one third of all population are regularly exposed to the SHS in practically every region of the world. The World Health Organization states that secondhand smoke causes about 600,000 deaths per year, and about 1% of the global burden of disease. In 2017, secondhand smoke was considered to cause of about 900,000 deaths a year, which is about 1/8 of all deaths caused by smoking.

The health risks of SHS have been a matter of scientific consensus. These risks are a major motivation for smoke-free laws in workplaces and indoor public places. Many countries have begun to introduce smoking bans in public areas, including restaurants, bars and night clubs, as well as some open public spaces. These efforts will help to protect the public's health by reducing exposure to SHS.

3. 2. 7. 4 Household chemicals

Household chemicals refer to chemical products used in daily life and living environment of families, including cosmetics, detergents, chemical disinfectants, adhesives, coatings, household pesticides, and other macromolecule products, rubber products, textiles, etc.

Household chemicals can release a variety of air pollutants when they are used and stored. The major air pollutants are formaldehyde, volatile organic compounds, aerosols, ammonia, chlorine, lead and mercury, that can cause harm if inhaled, swallowed, or absorbed through the skin.

Formaldehyde is a colorless, flammable gas at room temperature and has a pungent odor. In the residential environment, formaldehyde exposure comes from a number of different routes. It can be released into the air (off-gas) from composite wood products, building materials and insulation, and may also be found in household products (e. g. glues, permanent press fabrics, paints and coatings, lacquers and finishes, paper products, some medicines, cosmetics, dishwashing liquids, fabric softeners, and pesticides). Exposure to formaldehyde may cause adverse health effects. At concentrations above 0. 1 ppm in air, formaldehyde can irritate the eyes and mucous membranes. Inhalation of formaldehyde at this concentration can cause headaches, a burning sensation in the throat, difficulty in breathing, and may trigger or aggravate asthma symptoms. The IARC in 1995 classified formaldehyde as a probable human carcinogen associated with nasal sinus cancer and nasopharyngeal cancer

Volatile organic compounds (VOCs) are organic chemicals that have a high vapor pressure at ordinary room temperature. VOCs are numerous, varied, and ubiquitous. Concentrations of many VOCs are higher indoors (up to 10 times higher) than outdoors. VOCs are emitted by a wide array of products, including household products (e. g. paints and paint strippers, wood preservatives, aerosol sprays, cleansers and disinfectants, moth repellents and air fresheners, stored fuels and automotive products, dry-cleaned clothing, and pesticides), building materials and furnishings, office equipment (e. g. copiers and printers, correction fluids and carbonless copy paper), graphics and craft materials (e. g. glues and adhesives, permanent markers and photographic solutions). Health effects of VOCs include eye, nose, and throat irritation; allergic skin reaction; headaches; loss of coordination; nausea; and damage to the liver, kidney, and central nervous system. Some VOCs are suspected or known to cause cancer in humans.

3. 2. 7. 5　Sick Building Syndrome and Building-Related Illness

Sick Building Syndrome (SBS) describes a medical condition where people in a building suffer from symptoms of illness or feel unwell for no apparent reason, but no specific illness or cause can be identified. It is also called "building-related symptoms". Sick Building Syndrome may occur in offices, apartment houses, nurseries and schools.

The WHO has classified the reported symptoms into broad categories, including: mucous membrane irritation (eye, nose, and throat irritation), neuro-toxic effects (headaches, fatigue, and irritability), asthma and asthma-like symptoms (chest tightness and wheezing), skin dryness and irritation, gastrointestinal complaints and more. Several of these symptoms are experienced simultaneously and tend to increase in severity with the time people spend in the building, and improve over time or even disappear when people are away from the building. In some cases, particularly in sensitive individuals, there can be long-term health effects. Because these illnesses may happen in the building or other places, it was initially difficult to be attributed to the building.

SBS occurs, frequently but not always, in the building with flaws in the heating, ventilation, and air conditioning systems. The suspected causes include chemical contaminants from indoor or outdoor sources (combustion products, household chemicals), biological materials, traffic noise, and lighting; they are exacerbated by the effect of poor ventilation.

In contrast to SBS, the term "building related illness" (BRI) refers to symptoms of diagnosable illness that are identified and can be attributed directly to airborne building contaminants (Table 3.4). This group of illnesses consists of well-documented conditions with defined diagnostic criteria and generally recognizable causes. These illnesses typically call for a conventional treatment regimen, since simply exiting the building where the illness was contracted does not readily reverse the symptoms. BRI include infectious diseases (e. g. legionellosis, humidifier fever), chemical poisoning (e. g. lead from paint), allergies (e. g. hypersensitivity pneumonitis, asthma, allergic rhinitis and sinusitis), contact dermatitis, and other diseases (e. g. cancer from radon, asbestos-related diseases, and hearing loss from noise).

Table 3. 4   Sick Building Syndrome (SBS) and Building-Related Illness (BRI)

Health effect	SBS	BRI
Symptoms	Acute discomfort, such as headache; eye, nose, or throat irritation; dry cough; dry or itchy skin; dizziness and nausea; difficulty in concentrating; fatigue; and sensitivity to odors, etc.	Cough; chest tightness; fever, chills; and muscle aches, etc.
Causes	Unknown	Clearly identifiable
Outcome	Relief soon after leaving the building	Prolonged recovery after leaving the building

3. 2. 8   Guideline Values for Air Pollutants and Air Quality Index

WHO and many countries have set recommended limits or standards for health-harmful concentrations of key air pollutants both outdoors and inside buildings and homes. This section only presents guideline values for ambient air pollutants and Air Quality Index.

3. 2. 8. 1   Ambient Air Quality Standards

The WHO Air Quality Guidelines (AQG) offer guidance on threshold limits for key air pollutants in reducing the health impacts of them. First AQG was published in 1987 and revised in 1997. The 2005 update represents the most current assessment of air pollution health effects, based on an expert evaluation of the scientific evidence. The guidelines offer recommended exposure levels for particulate matter (PM_{10} and $PM_{2.5}$), ozone, nitrogen dioxide and sulfur dioxide. In addition, AQG also provide interim targets for concentrations of PM_{10} and $PM_{2.5}$ aimed at promoting a gradual shift from high to lower concentrations. It is estimated that reducing annual average PM_{10} concentrations from levels of 70 $\mu g/m^3$, common in many developing cities, to guideline level of 20 $\mu g/m^3$, could reduce air pollution-related deaths by around 15%.

The WHO AQGs are intended for worldwide use. While, air quality standards, as an important component of national risk management and environmental policies, are set by each country to protect the public health of their citizens. National standards may vary according to the approach adopted for balancing health risks, technological feasibility, economic considerations and various other political and social factors, which depend on the level of development and national capability in air quality management. Therefore, national standards may differ from country to country and may be above or below the respective WHO guideline value (Table 3. 5).

Table 3. 5　Guideline Values or Standards for Principal Air Pollutants

Pollutant	WHO	U. S. A (Primary)	Europe	China (grade Ⅱ)
CO		$40mg/m^3$ [1 hr^a] $10mg/m^3$ [8 hr^b]	$10mg/m^3$ [8 hr]	$10mg/m^3$ [1 hr] $4mg/m^3$ [24 hr^c]
O_3	$100\mu g/m^3$ [8 hr]	0. 12ppm [1 hr] 0. 075ppm [8 hr]	$120\mu g/m^3$ [8 hr]	$200\mu g/m^3$ [1 hr] $160\mu g/m^3$ [8 hr]
$PM_{2.5}$	$25\mu g/m^3$ [24 hr] $10\mu g/m^3$ [1 yr^d]	$35\mu g/m^3$ [24 hr] $12\mu g/m^3$ [1 yr]	$25\mu g/m^3$ [1 yr]	$75\mu g/m^3$ [24 hr] $35\mu g/m^3$ [1 yr]
PM_{10}	$50\mu g/m^3$ [24 hr] $20\mu g/m^3$ [1 yr]	$150\mu g/m^3$ [24 hr]	$50\mu g/m^3$ [24 hr] $40\mu g/m^3$ [1 yr]	$150\mu g/m^3$ [24 hr] $70\mu g/m^3$ [1 yr]
NO_2	$200\mu g/m^3$ [1 hr] $40\mu g/m^3$ [1 yr]	100ppb[1 hr] 53ppb[1 yr]	$200\mu g/m^3$ [1 hr] $40\mu g/m^3$ [1 yr]	$200\mu g/m^3$ [1 hr] $80\mu g/m^3$ [24 hr] $40\mu g/m^3$ [1 yr]
SO_2	$500\mu g/m^3$ [10 min] $20\mu g/m^3$ [24 hr]	75ppb[1hr]	$350\mu g/m^3$ [1 hr] $125\mu g/m^3$ [24 hr]	$500\mu g/m^3$ [1 hr] $150\mu g/m^3$ [24 hr] $60\mu g/m^3$ [1 yr]
Lead		1. 5$\mu g/m^3$ [rolling 3 mo^e]	0. 5$\mu g/m^3$ [1yr]	0. 5$\mu g/m^3$ [1yr]

^{a}1hour average; ^{b}8 hour average; ^{c}24 hour average; ^{d}Annual average; ^{e}Rolling 3 month average

3. 2. 8. 2　Air Quality Index (AQI)

Air quality index (AQI) is an index for reporting daily air quality. It is used by government agencies to communicate to the public how clean or polluted the air currently is and also forecast the air quality. It is difficult for the public to understand pollutant concentrations data because of the complexity related to these data. AQI converts measured pollutant concentrations into index values, thus make it easier to interpret air quality data. The index value is the pollutant concentration expressed as a proportion of national air quality standards. AQI values are typically grouped into ranges, and each range is assigned a descriptor, a color code, and a standardized public health advisory. Different countries have their own air quality indices, corresponding to different national air quality standards. Some countries use the term Air Quality Index (AQI), for example, China, India, the United States, etc. Other countries or areas may have different name, such as Air Quality Health Index (AQHI, Canada and Hong Kong), Air Pollution Index (API, Malaysia), and Pollutant Standards Index (PSI, Singapore). Usually, as the index value increases, an increasingly large percentage of the population is likely to experience increasingly severe adverse health effects.

The US National Air Pollution Control Administration is the first to develop an air quality index. The AQI currently used in the United States is established by the Environmental Protection Agency (EPA), based on the five "criteria" pollutants regulated under the EPA National Ambient Air Quality Standards (NAAQS): ground-level ozone, particulate matter, carbon monoxide, sulfur dioxide, and nitrogen dioxide. The AQI is a piecewise linear function of the pollutant concentration, and is divided into six categories indicating increasing levels of health concern (Table 3. 6).

Table 3. 6　AQI of the United States

AQI Values	Levels of Health Concern	Colors	Meaning
0—50	Good	Green	Air quality is considered satisfactory, and air pollution poses little or no risk
51—100	Moderate	Yellow	Air quality is acceptable; however, for some pollutants there may be a moderate health concern for a very small number of people who are unusually sensitive to air pollution
101—150	Unhealthy for Sensitive Groups	Orange	Members of sensitive groups may experience health effects. The general public is not likely to be affected
151—200	Unhealthy	Red	Everyone may begin to experience health effects; members of sensitive groups may experience more serious health effects
201—300	Very Unhealthy	Purple	Health alert: everyone may experience more serious health effects
301—500	Hazardous	Maroon	Health warnings of emergency conditions. The entire population is more likely to be affected

In China, Ministry of Ecology and Environment is responsible for monitoring the level of air pollution. The AQI is computed based on the level of six atmospheric pollutant: SO_2, NO_2, PM_{10}, $PM_{2.5}$, CO and O_3. An individual score (Individual Air Quality Index, IAQI) can be computed for each pollutant and the final AQI is the highest of these six scores. The final AQI value can be calculated either per hour or per 24 hours. It is also divided into six categories (Table 3. 7).

Table 3. 7　AQI and Health Implications of China

AQI Value	Air Pollution Level	Air Pollution Category	Colors	Health Implications
0—50	I	Excellent	Green	No health implications
51—100	II	Good	Yellow	Some pollutants may slightly affect very few hypersensitive individuals
101—150	III	Lightly Polluted	Orange	Sensitive individuals will be slightly affected to a larger extent, and healthy people may experience slight irritations and
151—200	IV	Moderately Polluted	Red	Sensitive individuals will experience more serious conditions. The hearts and respiratory systems of healthy people may be affected
201—300	V	Heavily Polluted	Purple	People with respiratory or heart diseases will be significantly affected and will experience reduced endurance in activities. Healthy people will commonly show symptoms
>300	VI	Severely Polluted	Maroon	Healthy people will experience reduced endurance in activities and show noticeably strong symptoms. Other illnesses may be triggered in healthy people

3. 2. 9　Air Pollution Control

Within certain regions, when the air contains certain substances in concentrations high enough and for durations long enough to cause harm or undesirable effects, including effects on human health, property, and atmospheric visibility, it is considered to be polluted. Since the Industrial Revolution in 19th century, increasing use of fossil fuels has intensified the severity and frequency of air pollution episodes. However, it was not until the mid-20th century that meaningful and sustained efforts were made to regulate or limit the emission of air pollutants from stationary and mobile sources and to control air quality on both regional and local scales. The best way to protect air quality is to reduce the emission of pollutants through regulation and new technology.

3. 2. 9. 1　Laws, Rules, and Regulation

Air pollution is a global problem. To protect the human environment against air pollution and to gradually reduce and prevent air pollution, great efforts have been made by international organizations. In terms of universality, one of the most successful example is the Vienna Convention for the Protection of the Ozone Layer (1985), which provided frameworks necessary for international reductions in the production of chlorofluorocarbons, and to create regulatory measures in the form of the Montreal Protocol (1987). The

Convention on Long-Range Transboundary Air Pollution (1979) was ratified and has been extended by eight protocols, such as Helsinki Protocol on the Reduction of Sulphur Emissions (1985), Nitrogen Oxide Protocol (1988), Volatile Organic Compounds Protocol (1991), Protocol on Heavy Metals (1998), and Aarhus Protocol on Persistent Organic Pollutants (1998). Another example is The Kyoto Protocol, which extends the 1992 United Nations Framework Convention on Climate Change (UNFCCC) that restrict the greenhouse gas emissions of state parties. While not binding agreements, these treaties act as framework for the international efforts to control air pollution.

Various countries have also set their own laws, rules, and regulations to improve air quality. In United States, the 1955 Air Pollution Control Act was the first federal legislation that pertained to air pollution. While, the 1963 Clean Air Act, amended in 1965, 1966, 1967, 1969, 1970, 1977 and 1990, is a federal law designed to control air pollution on a national level, and is considered one of the most comprehensive air quality laws in the world. The Clean Air Act gave the US EPA and other agencies the power to set rules, regulations, standards, and pollution limits, with the goal of reducing the proportion of people exposed to air that does not meet the standards. To prevent and control atmospheric pollution, protect and improve ecological environment, safeguard human health, and promote the sustainable development of economy and society in China, Law of the People's Republic of China on the Prevention and Control of Atmospheric Pollution has been in force since 1988, and revised in 1995, 2000, 2015, 2018.

3.2.9.2   General Control Strategy

Many examples of successful policies have reduced air pollution. For example:

(1) Urban planning: reasonably arranging industrial layout, adjusting industrial structure and improving urban greening system; improving the energy efficiency of buildings and thus energy efficient;

(2) Industry: cleaner fuels; appropriate air-cleaning technologies that reduce industrial emissions; energy recycling and reuse, including capture of methane gas emitted from waste sites as an alternative to incineration (for use as biogas);

(3) Transport: prioritizing rapid urban transit; shifting to cleaner heavy duty diesel vehicles and low-emissions vehicles and fuels;

(4) Power generation: using low-emissions fuels and renewable combustion-free power sources such as solar, wind, or hydropower;

(5) Waste management: strategies for waste reduction, waste separation, recycling and reuse or waste reprocessing; combustion technologies with strict emission controls.

3.2.9.3   Sustainable Living

Sustainable living refers to a lifestyle that attempts to reduce an individual's or society's use of natural resources to reduce environmental impact. Its practitioners can alter their lifestyle in many ways. For example:

(1) Shelter: sustainably designed houses (e. g. oriented to the sun so that it creates the best possible microclimate); using non-toxic and renewable, recycled, reclaimed, or low-impact building materials; rooftop solar power generation;

(2) Food: choosing local, seasonal and organic foods; reducing meat consumption; urban agriculture from community gardens to private home gardens;

(3) Transportation: walking, cycling or using public transportation; new energy vehicle;

(4) Waste: reduce, reuse and recycle.

3.3　Water Environment and Health

Water is essential for life. The existence of life, from the largest mammals to the smallest microbes, depends on water. It involves in all physiological and biochemical activities in the human body, such as regulation of body temperature, metabolism of nutrients and waste excretion. About 60% of the human body is water, and we cannot survive for more than a few days without it. The daily water requirement of adults is about 2.5—3 liters. Numerous health risks can be linked to a deficit in water intake including risks for different types of cancers, childhood and adolescent obesity, and the overall health of the elderly. Water is not only a physiological requirement for human beings, but also closely related to daily life. Water also plays an important role in maintaining personal hygiene and improving living environment. In addition, water is also a dominant factor for socioeconomic development and human civilization.

Water is one of the most abundant natural resources. Nearly 70% of the total area on the earth is covered by water, but less than 3% is fresh water, and only a tiny fraction of this is surface water easily available for human use (Figure 3.9). The rising industrialization around the globe, along with the growing population, is increasing the demand of water. An area is experiencing water stress when annual water supplies drop below 1,700 m³ per person. When water supply drops below 1,000 m³ per person per year, people face scarcity; below 500 m³, they face absolute

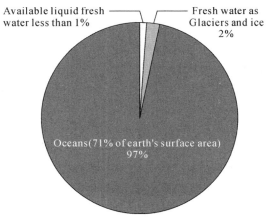

Figure 3.9　Water Distribution on the Earth

scarcity. Whether a water supply is adequate or not depends on the balance that exists among water availability, population, and the ways in which people use water. In many parts of the world, population pressure places a severe strain on water resources. According to the United Nations "Water of Life" water scarcity web page report, there are around 700 million people in 43 countries currently suffer from water scarcity and 1.8 billion people will live in countries or regions with absolute water scarcity by 2025. With the existing climate change scenario, almost half the world's population will be living in areas of high water stress by 2030, including between 75 million and 250 million people in Africa.

3.3.1   Types of Water Resources and Its Hygienic Features

Water resources refer to the amount of water available to human survival and development, mainly refer to the amount of fresh water that can be updated annually. In the nature, there are three types of water resources available, namely, precipitation, surface water and ground water.

3.3.1.1   Precipitation

Water evaporates from oceans, rivers and lakes and rises into the atmosphere where it condenses to form clouds. Precipitation then falls to the earth in the form of rain or snow where it flows into oceans, rivers and lakes. This hydrological process repeats again. The hygienic features of precipitation are as follows: pure water; low mineral salt content; in landing process, water quality varies with the level of air pollution.

3.3.1.2   Surface Water

Surface water is formed by the collection of rainfall runoff when precipitation landed on the ground. It includes all water naturally open to the atmosphere (seas, rivers, lakes, reservoirs, ponds, streams, impoundments, estuaries, etc.). The amount of water varies greatly with seasons, precipitation and other factors. Annual change is divided into wet and dry seasons. Surface water quality is mainly affected by geological environment and human activities. Surface water is usually characterized by large quantity, low mineral salt content, high turbidity, high bacteria content, high dissolved oxygen, and strong self-purification ability. The slow-flowing water in lakes and reservoirs contributes to the deposit of suspended substances in water, so the turbidity is low and the water is clear. Generally, surface water is abundant, soft and easy to access, therefore it can be used as a drinking water source.

3.3.1.3   Groundwater

Groundwater refers to water hidden beneath the Earth's surface, usually in aquifers. The main source is gathered by precipitation and surface water seeping into the underground through soil, riverbeds and lakes. Permeable layer is composed of loose sand with large gaps, gravel, sandy soil, etc., and it not only seeps water but also stores water. Impermeable layer, which is composed of clay with small particles and rocks, etc., cannot seep water. Permeable layer and impermeable layer interlace and hold each other (Figure 3.10). According to the location and the direction of water flow, groundwater can be classified into shallow groundwater, deep groundwater and spring water.

Groundwater quality is directly affected by surface water quality and geological environment. Groundwater and surface water are not independent of each other and an overlap category is also recognized: groundwater is directly influenced by surface water. Groundwater usually has features such as: small quantity, high mineral salt content, few pollution opportunities, low dissolved oxygen, low bacteria content, and weak self-purification ability.

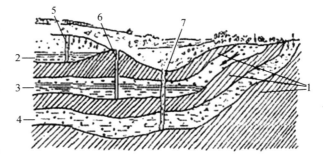

Figure 3. 10　Water-Bearing Formation
1. impermeable layer; 2. shallow ground water;
3. deep ground water; 4. confined water;
5. shallow well; 6. deep well; 7. artesian well

(1) Shallow Groundwater

Shallow groundwater hides beneath the surface and above the first impermeable layer, generally a few meters to dozens of meters away from the surface. The water is greatly influenced by precipitation and is susceptible to pollution. The sensory property of the water in this layer is better and its bacterial content is small, but water hardness is generally higher than surface water, because of soluble minerals in the soil. It relatively has less dissolved oxygen in the water and poor self-purification ability.

(2) Deep Groundwater

The water hiding beneath the first impermeable layer is called deep groundwater. Water in this layer is not easy to be polluted and is a good source of drinking water because of its good quality and stable quantity. But if aquifers of the deep groundwater contain high level of salts and minerals, the water hardness is high.

(3) Spring Water

Spring water is the water flowing out of the surface crack on its own from shallow or deep groundwater. According to the direction of water flow, spring water can be classified into two types, namely, gravity springs and pressure springs. Due to crustal movements, such as natural subsidence, closure in valleys or mountains, aquifer is exposed, the water flows out on its own by gravity. This kind of spring is called gravity spring. Such spring generally comes from shallow groundwater, and it is in small quantity, greatly affected by natural factors. Through collecting and protecting, it can be used as a scattered supply of water source.

Water gushing from layer cracks by itself is called pressure spring or artesian well, which comes from deep underground confined water. With advantages of large quantity, good quality and stability, if it can be collected and protected, it will be a good source of drinking water.

3.3.2　Water Quality-Criteria and Standards

Pure water contains H_2O molecule only. However, natural water inevitably contacts with other substances and impurities, which greatly change the characteristics of water. Water quality can be evaluated with various parameters.

3. 3. 2. 1   Physical Parameters

Water has many physical parameters, such as pH, color, turbidity, taste and odor. These physical parameters are used to judge whether the sensory properties of water quality are good or bad, and to indicate whether the water is contaminated.

(1) Water temperature

Water temperature affects aquatic organisms, water self-purification and the use of water. The temperature of surface water varies with seasons and climatic conditions, with a range of about 0. 1—30℃. Thermal pollution of water leads to low level of dissolved oxygen, which harms the growth and reproduction of aquatic organisms.

(2) pH Value

The pH value of natural water is 7. 2—8. 5. When the pH of water becomes too alkaline, many dissolved material settle out of the water. These materials may clog pipes and affect the taste of the water. On the other hand, water with very low pH can leach metals from pumps, piping, and fixtures. Water that is too acidic has the capability of "eating away" plumbing systems. Metals that can be leached include copper, lead, cadmium and zinc.

(3) Color

Clean water is colorless. When too much humus is in the water, it is tan and clays that make it become yellow. In stagnant water, water color is different because of the multiplication of algae. For example, chlorella makes water become green, diatom makes it brownish green, dinoflagellate makes it dark brown, blue-green algae makes it turquoise, and so on. After water is polluted by industrial wastewater, it will present the specific color of the pollutant.

(4) Odor and Taste

Odor and taste sometimes are difficult to separate completely. Clean water is odorless and tasteless. Lake water has fishy or rotten smell because of the multiplication of algae or excessive organic matters. Water containing hydrogen sulfide may smells of rotten egg. Water may tastes bitter if it contains too much sodium sulfates or magnesium sulfates. Water containing excessive iron or zinc salt may tastes astringent. When it contains proper amount of calcium carbonates and magnesium carbonates, water may has sweet and delicious taste. High oxygenated water tastes slightly sweet. If it is polluted by domestic sewage or industrial wastewater, water will present the odor and tastes of the specific pollutant.

(5) Turbidity

Turbidity mainly depends on the type, size, shape and refractive index of colloidal particles, but has small relation to the concentration of suspended sediment in water. Turbidity of water is an apparent index used to judge whether water was polluted. Turbid surface water is caused by silts, clays, and organic matters in water. Groundwater is generally clear. If water contains divalent iron salt which is in contact with air, ferric hydroxide will be generated. Consequently, water will become brownish yellow.

However, some pollutants are colorless, tasteless, odorless, and dissolved in water. Therefore, water with good physical characteristics is not necessarily safe and healthy water.

3.3.2.2　Chemical Parameters

The chemical characteristic of water quality is very complex, thus many evaluation indexes are adopted to clarify the chemical nature of water quality and the level of pollution.

(1) Total Solid

The total solid refers to the amount of dry residue after the sample water evaporated slowly at a certain temperature, including dissolved and suspended solids in the water. After the sample water is filtered, the filtrate is evaporated, and the residue is dissolved solids which content depends on the amount of mineral salts and dissolved organic matters in the water. Suspended solids are the dry weight of solids which cannot pass through the filter. After burning, all the organic matters of total solids in water have occurred oxygenolysis and volatilized, and the remains are minerals. After burning, the loss can roughly show the content of organic matter in water. The higher the content of total solid is, the more serious the water pollution.

(2) Water Hardness

Water hardness refers to the total content of dissolved minerals which are usually calcium and magnesium. Hardness of water is generally classified into carbonate hardness (calcium, magnesium bicarbonate, and carbonate) and non-carbonate hardness (calcium, magnesium sulfate, chloride, etc.). After boiling, the former generates carbonate sediment, so it is called temporary hardness, while the latter cannot be removed from boiling water, as such it is called permanent hardness.

(3) Nitrogen Compounds

Nitrogen compounds include organic nitrogen, protein nitrogen, ammonia nitrogen, nitrite nitrogen, and nitrate nitrogen. When protein nitrogen and organic nitrogen increases, it indicates that the water is recently polluted by organisms. If ammonia nitrogen increased, it is likely to be newly polluted by human and animal feces. If nitrite nitrogen increases, it indicates that the mineralization of organic matters in water has not been completed and the pollution hazard still exists. If the content of nitrate nitrogen is high while the level of ammonia nitrogen and nitrite nitrogen is not high, it indicates that the water has been polluted by organic matters but self-purified presently. If ammonia nitrogen, nitrite nitrogen and nitrate nitrogen are increased, it shows that the water has been polluted both in the past and present, or water pollution has happened but self-purification is in progress. According to content changes of ammonia nitrogen, nitrite nitrogen and nitrate nitrogen in water, we can make a comprehensive analysis to judge the condition of water pollution.

(4) Dissolved Oxygen

Dissolved oxygen (DO) refers to the dissolved oxygen content in water. DO content of clean surface water is close to saturation, so DO can be regarded as the indirect index to evaluate the organic pollution water and the degree of its self-purification.

(5) Chemical Oxygen Demand

Chemical oxygen demand (COD) refers to the oxygen consumption which is consumed by the organics in the oxidized water with a strong oxidant such as potassium permanganate and potassium dichromate. It is an indirect index that reflects the water body polluted by organics and stands for the total amount of the oxidized organics and reducing inorganics.

(6) Biochemical Oxygen Demand

Biochemical oxygen demand (BOD) refers to the dissolved oxygen consumption when the organics are decomposed by the aerobe in water under the aerobic conditions. Biological oxidation process is associated with the water temperature. In practice, when the water is cultured for 5 days at 20℃, the reducing dissolved oxygen consumption in 1 L water equals to 5-day biochemical oxygen demand. It is an important index to evaluate the water pollution and the effect of water pollution treatment. Generally, the BOD of clean water is less than 1 mg/L.

(7) Chloride

Natural water contains chlorine. In the same area, the content of chloride in the water body is relatively stable. When the content of chloride suddenly increases, it indicates that the water may be contaminated by human and animal excreta, domestic sewage or industrial wastewater.

(8) Sulfate

Natural water contains sulfate and its content is mainly affected by geological conditions. When the content of sulphate is suddenly increased, it indicates that the water may be polluted by domestic sewage, industrial wastewater or ammonium sulphate fertilizer, etc.

(9) Total Organic Carbon

Total organic carbon (TOC) is the amount of carbon bound in all organic compounds in water. It does not identify specific carbon-containing compounds, but represent the presence of unwanted organic compounds in pure water. It is often used as a non-specific indicator of aerobic organic pollution in water.

(10) Other Harmful Chemicals

Harmful substances mainly refers to the heavy metals and the toxic substances in water, such as mercury, cadmium, arsenic, chromium, lead, phenol, cyanide. In recent decades, emerging pollutants such as organochlorine, polychlorinated biphenyls, pesticides, polybrominated diphenyl ethers, pharmaceutical and personal care products in water have been widely concerned.

3.3.2.3 Biological Parameters

There are various living organisms in the natural water and some indicative bacteria can be used to reflect the biological contamination of water bodies.

(1) Bacterial Count

Bacteria count refers to the bacterial colony count of 1 mL water when it is cultured in the ordinary agar medium in 37℃ for 24 hours. It reflects the degree of biological pollution of water body. The more the bacteria count there is, the more serious the water pollution will be. However, the number of bacteria found in the artificial medium can only stand for the bacteria adapted to the laboratory conditions, but not for all the bacteria and pathogenic agents existing in water body. Therefore, the bacteria count can only be taken as the reference index which reflects the water polluted by microorganisms.

(2) Coliform Bacteria

Coliform bacteria refers to a group of aerobic and facultative anaerobic Gram-negative bacillus which can make lactose fermented at 37℃ or 44℃, and produce acid and gas within 24 hours. There are two kinds of coliform in water. One is fecal coliform in human and warm-blooded animal intestine, the other is coliform in natural environment. We can distinguish fecal coliform and natural coliform by increasing the cultural temperature because fecal coliform can survive at 44℃, while this is not the case with natural coliform. Therefore, fecal coliform can be used as the indicative bacteria to reflect the contamination of water by excreta. Meanwhile, it can also be taken as an important indicator to measure whether the drinking water quality is safe in the context of epidemiology.

3.3.3 Water Pollution and Health Hazards

3.3.3.1 Definition of Water Pollution

Pollutants inevitably enter into the water bodies because of the natural or anthropogenic reasons. Water pollution is defined as the presence of physical, chemical and biological pollutants in water body that exceed the self-purification capacity of water and poses a threat to human and ecological environment.

3.3.3.2 Source of Water Pollutants

Water pollutants mainly come from anthropogenic activities. Discharge of domestic and industrial effluent wastes, leakage from water tanks, marine dumping, radioactive waste and atmospheric deposition are the major causes of water pollution. According to the way that the pollutants enter the water, the sources of pollution can be divided into point source pollution (with a fixed outlet) and non-point source pollution (rainwater runoff, etc.).

(1) Industrial Waste Water

Industries produce huge amount of waste which contains toxic chemicals that can cause water pollution. The types and quantities of pollutants in different industrial wastewater vary greatly. Waste water from steel and coking plants contains phenols and cyanides; waste water from chemical industry and pesticide plants contains mercury, chromium, pesticides, etc.; while paper mills produce waste water containing a large amount of organic matter. The toxic chemicals from industrial waste water have the capability to change the color of water, increase the amount of minerals, and pose serious hazard to water ecosystem.

(2) Domestic Sewage

Domestic sewage is the washing waste water, fecal and urinary waste water in daily life. It carries a lot of organic substances and microorganisms, such as intestinal pathogens, viruses, parasite and its eggs, which can cause serious health problems. The sewage water also contains large number of inorganic compounds such as chloride, sulfate, phosphate, ammonium salt, nitrite, nitrate, and so on.

When sewage rich in nitrogen, phosphorus and other nutrients flows into receipt water bodies, it is easy to cause eutrophication. Eutrophication is a phenomenon of rapid reproduction of algae and other plankton, decrease of dissolved oxygen, water quality deterioration, massive death of fish and other organisms. In an outbreak of eutrophication, the colors of the dominant planktonic algae are different, the surface often appears blue, red, brown, ivory, etc. It is usually called "bloom" in rivers and lakes, while known as "red tide" in the gulf.

(3) Agricultural Waste Water

Agricultural wastewater is generated from a variety of farm activities including animal feeding operations and the processing of agricultural products. Additionally, runoff from croplands can contribute sediment, fertilizers, and pesticides into surface water. Agricultural waste water is an important source of eutrophication because it usually contains high level of nitrogen, phosphorus and other plant nutrients.

(4) Other Sources

Water pollutants may also come from other sources, e. g. hospital pollution, improper waste disposal, marine dumping, accidental leakage, and atmospheric deposition.

3.3.3.3 Major Types of Water Pollutants

According to the nature of the pollutants, water pollutants can be divided into three categories:

(1) Biological Pollutants

Biological pollutants mainly refer to a large number of pathogens and other microorganisms. In addition, algae and its toxins from eutrophication caused by pollution of phosphorus and nitrogen also belong to biological pollution.

(2) Chemical Pollutants

Water pollutants include inorganic and organic substances. Inorganic pollutants include heavy metals, arsenic, nitrogen, phosphorus, cyanide and acid, alkali, salt, etc., while organic pollutants consist of benzene, phenol, oil and its products. According to the statistics, 2221 kinds of organic chemicals have been identified from the global water. A total of 324 kinds of organic compounds have been identified in the British river. The

Jiangyin Section of Yangtze River in China contains 150 kinds of organic compounds. More than 500 kinds of organic compounds have been found in the Huangpu River of Shanghai. With the continuous improvement of testing technology level, more kinds of organic pollutants in water body will be found.

(3) Physical Pollutants

The most common physical pollutants are waste heat and radioactive substances (uranium, plutonium, strontium and cesium). Heat pollution is mainly from industrial cooling water, while radioactive pollution results from natural radionuclides and nuclear industry.

3.3.3.4　Health Effects of Water Pollution

There is a significant association between water pollution and health problem. According to the WHO, 80% of diseases are water borne, 3.1% of deaths occur due to the unhygienic and poor quality of water. Health risk associated with polluted water includes various diseases such as cancer, diarrheal disease, neurological disorder and cardiovascular disease.

(1) Biological Pollution and Its Health Effects

Biological pollution usually refers to bacteria, viruses, parasites, algae and its toxin in water. The main adverse health effects of biological pollutants in water are waterborne disease and eutrophication resulted toxicity.

① Waterborne disease: Waterborne diseases are conditions caused by pathogenic microorganisms that are transmitted in water. Diseases can be spread while bathing, washing or drinking water, or by eating food exposed to contaminated water. The most common symptoms of waterborne illness are diarrhea and vomiting, and other symptoms include skin, ear, respiratory, or eye problems. Surface water and shallow water are so vulnerable to contaminate with the pathogens of infectious diseases that it leads to waterborne infectious diseases. According to the WHO, waterborne diseases account for an estimated 3.6% of the total disability-adjusted life years (DALY) global burden of disease, and cause about 1.5 million human deaths annually. The WHO estimates that 58% of that burden, or 842,000 deaths per year, is attributable to lack of safe drinking water supply, sanitation and hygiene. It should be noted that these data are likely to underestimate significantly the actual burden of waterborne diseases.

The pathogens of waterborne infectious diseases can be mainly classified into three categories:

● Bacteria, such as salmonella typhi, paratyphoid salmonella typhi, vibrio cholera, dysentery bacillus shiglla spp., campylobacter spp., leptospira spp., legionella, mycobacterium avium;

● Viruses, such as hepatitis A virus, hepatitis E virus, norovirus, rotavirus, coxsackie virus, polio virus and adenovirus;

● Protozoa, such as giardia, entamoeba histolytica, schistosome, cryptosporidium, cyclospora, naegleria fowleri, acanthamoeba.

They mainly come from human and animal excreta, domestic sewage, the wastewater of hospitals and livestock slaughtering, leather, and the food industry, etc.

The epidemic characteristics of the waterborne infectious disease are as follows:

• After a severe water pollution, the disease can represent epidemic outbreak, and the onset date of the most patients are in the same incubation period. If the water has been polluted for several times, the patients will appear continuously;

• The cases distribution is consistent with the scope of water supply. Most of the patients have drunk or touched the same water;

• Once the pollution is controlled, the purification and disinfection of water are strengthened, the disease can quickly get under control.

The most frequent waterborne disease is diarrheal disease caused by the intestinal infection. Diarrheal cases are about 4 billion and result in 2.2 million deaths globally each year, mostly in developing countries. About 15% of children under five years old died of diarrhea. Of 0.5—1.8 million children die of diarrhea, about 40% to 50% of them died of the rotavirus infection.

The most typical case of waterborne disease documented in the history happened in New Delhi, India. During the period of December 1, 1955 to January 20, 1956, the infectious hepatitis outbroke because of the centralized water supply polluted by domestic sewage. Among the 1.7 million people, 29,300 people suffered from jaundice. Another typical example of waterborne disease is cryptosporidiosis. The drinking water or the source of it polluted by cryptosporidium will lead to the prevalence of cryptosporidiosis in humans and animals. In 1987, the epidemic of the disease occurred in somewhere in Georgia, United States. Among the 64,900 local residents, there were more than 13,000 people infected with this disease and experienced diarrhea as the main clinical symptom. The cryptosporidium capsule has been detected from the patient's excreta and the drinking water. In 1993, the outbreak of cryptosporidiosis affected 403,000 people and spread by tap water in Wisconsin of the United States.

② Eutrophication resulted toxicity: Eutrophication results from the pollution of nitrogen, phosphorus and other nutrients in water. In eutrophication outbreaks, a large number of algae which gather into clouds and float in the water are dissolved by microbes after the death and consume large amounts of dissolved oxygen. Meanwhile, the anaerobic bacteria multiply in a large quantity, dissolve organics, produce harmful gases such as ammonia, methane, hydrogen sulfide, deteriorate the sensory properties of water and reduce the use value of water. Many algae of eutrophication can produce toxins. The toxins not only harm the aquatic animals, but also poison human, livestock and poultry. Research shows that different kinds of algae produce different toxins. For example, microcystis aeruginosa produces polypeptide toxin that can cause deadly poisoning in wild animals and livestock. Pathological examination shows the liver congestion, edema, the necrosis of the centrilobular portion of liver, and the damage of the endothelial cell in liver cell. The electron microscopic examination shows the damage of the subcellular ingredients such as the endoplasmic reticulum of liver cells, the mitochondria, and the expansion of hepatic sinus. In serious cases, cell disintegrate can occur. A recent study shows that the micro capsule coarse cyanobacterial toxin can obviously increase the toxicity of 3-methylcholanthrene and cell malignant transformation started by organic dye. The anabaena in the water bloom can produce alkaloid toxin. For example, the anabaena toxin is a very strong nicotinic neuromuscular depolarizing blocker.

(2) Chemical Pollution and Its Health Effects

Acute or chronic intoxication and various adverse effects to the human may be caused by direct contact or consumption of water contaminated with poisonous chemical pollutants.

① Mercury and methyl mercury: In the nature, mercury exits in the form of metallic mercury, inorganic mercury and organic mercury. Organic mercury consists of methyl mercury, dimethylmercury, phenylmercury, and methoxyethyl mercury. Inorganic mercury may turn into more poisonous organic mercury by the action of microorganism while metallic mercury is almost insoluble in water. The amount of mercury in natural water is usually very little less than $0.1\mu g/L$.

Most liquid mercury comes from water emitted from factories of chemistry, instrument, plastic, metallurgy, battery and chlor-alkali. Gaseous mercury and grainy mercury may drift away with wind and subsequently drop to water on the Earth while the mercury in the earth can evaporate to the air and then drop down with rain.

Part of mercury is soluble to water while the rest may be absorbed in colloidal particles, suspended solids or planktons and falls down into either bottom mud or living bodies. The mercury in bottom mud can become soluble under suitable conditions and also can turn into methyl mercury under the action of anaerobic bacteria, which is more poisonous than inorganic mercury and easier to bioaccumulate through food chain. According to tests, the concentration of methyl mercury in the muscles of some carnivorous fishes, such as catfish, is as 40—50 thousand times as that in the water. Minamata disease found in Minamata, Kumamoto in Japan is a kind of chronic methyl mercury poisoning which was caused by eating fishes or shellfishes contaminated with high level of methyl mercury.

Mercury in water is mainly absorbed through digestive tract. The absorptivity of inorganic mercury is below 15% while that of alkyl mercury is above 90% among which the absorptivity of methyl mercury is above 95%. When inorganic mercury is absorbed in blood, most of it distributes in blood plasma which accumulates in kidney, liver and spleen. However, methyl mercury mainly distributes in red blood cells and flows with the blood to the whole body. It can cross the blood brain barrier and accumulate not only in brain tissues, but also outside the kidney and liver. Most of inorganic mercury excretes through kidney, and a small part of it eliminates through intestinal tract, gland and hair. The main way of eliminating methyl mercury is to intestinal tract through bile, in which 50% of methyl mercury turns into inorganic mercury and then discharges while the non-conversed one is reabsorbed in intestinal tract. Its average half-time period in organism is 74 days while 240 days in brain tissues.

Chronic intoxication manifestations of inorganic mercury are kidney damage, enterorrhagia or ulcer. Methyl mercury mainly damages central nerve system and the clinical manifestations of intoxication are as follows: first, the sense of numb or pricking around the body terminal or the mouth; then sensory disturbance of the hands, dyskinesia, disability, tremor, language barrier, concentration contract of the vision, hearing loss and motion disorder of supply; the serious ones as total paralysis, insaneness, and even death. Besides, methyl mercury leads to fetal malformation because it can cross the placental barrier.

Mercury can combine with sulfur and turn into mercuric sulfide at normal temperature so to reduce its toxicity.

In China, the limit of mercury in drinking water is 0.001 mg/L, and the range of the total mercury in surface water is 0.00005—0.001mg/L while methyl mercury is 0.00005—0.001 mg/L.

② Phenols: Phenols refer to the compounds generated from hydrogen atom of benzene ring in arenes that are replaced by hydroxyl. Phenol is also known as carbolic acid which is a kind of white acicular crystal with unpleasant fragrance. There are more than 2,000 kinds of phenols in the nature which can be divided into volatile phenol and involatile phenol, according to its volatility with vapor. Volatile phenol is more harmful and its compounds usually have special odors and are soluble to water and easy to be oxidized. Phenols which have hygiene significance are phenol, cresol, pentachlorophenol (PCP) and its sodium salt that are widely used for sterilization, snail eradication, anticorrosion, mold prevention and etc.

Phenols in water mainly come from the discharge of phenolic waste water such as industrial enterprises of coking and oil refining in which the phenol content can reach 1500—5000 mg/L. Others come from domestic sewage, for example, the phenol content in excrement and nitrogenous organic compound is about 0.1—1.0 mg/L.

Phenol is a chemical protoplasmic poison with moderate toxicity which can be absorbed through respiratory tract, skin and gastrointestinal tract. It mainly spreads in liver, blood, kidney, and lung. In liver it is oxidized into hydroquinone and hydroxyquinol first, and subsequently combines with glucuronic acid and loses its toxicity. Finally, it ejects with urine. Absorbed phenol can complete supersession in 24 hours and doesn't accumulate in the body but has accumulative poison, because phenol is a protoplasmic poison which can coagulate protein without combination. When cells are damaged and become necrosis, phenol can separate from the cells and permeate to deep tissues which bring necrosis to them.

The main manifestations of acute phenolic intoxication are as follows: profuse sweating, pulmonary edema, dysphagia, damage to liver and hematopoietic organ, melanuria, collapse and even death. Long-time consumption of water containing phenol can cause chronic poisoning with symptoms of hypomnesis, rash, pruritus, dizziness, insomnia and anemia.

Phenol is a kind of tumor promoter which has weak carcinogenesis when reaching a certain concentration. Carcinogenic tests of animals' skin show that 20% of the phenol has weak carcinogenesis and PCP has teratogenicity. Recent researches show that PCP, octylphenol, nonylphenol and biphenol A have the function of endocrine disruption. What's more, animal experiments indicate that PCP can disturb the normal function of thyroid, but the effect on the function of estrogen and testosterone is inconspicuous. However, epidemiological investigations show that it has interference function on women's endocrine system that causes harm to children's growth.

Phenol pollution deteriorates the sensory properties of water and reduces the value of water. When phenol in water reaches a certain concentration, which will threat the survival of aquatic organisms and cause fishes and shellfishes to have the smell of kerosene. Irrigation of farmland with water containing high concentration of phenols will lead to the decay of the crop roots.

In China, volatile phenol cannot exceed 0.002 mg/L in drinking water, 0.01 mg/L in surface water, and 1 mg/L in irrigation water of farmland.

③ Cyanide: Natural water doesn't contain cyanide which usually comes from waste water of various industries such as coking, mineral separation, electroplate, dyeing medicine and plastic.

Long-time drinking water containing hydride whose concentration is about 0.14 mg/L will lead to chronic intoxication. When a large doze of hydride enters into the body, it is hydrolyzed into hydrocyanicacid under the function of gastric acid. Cyanogens will combine with ferric iron of cytochrome oxidase and generate cyanide ferricytochrome oxidase, making ferric iron lose the ability of transmitting electronic. Therefore, respiratory chain will break off, cells will lack oxygen soon and death by suffocation. Because central nerve system is sensitive to hypoxia, and cyanide is not only soluble in lipoids but also has special affinity to nerve system, nerve system symptoms usually appear in chronic and acute intoxications.

When the concentration of hydride in water reaches 0.04—0.1 mg/L, fish will die. Cyanide waste water can reduce agricultural products and even causes death in domestic animals. The limit of cyanide in drinking water in China is 0.05 mg/L.

④ Chrome: The average content of chrome in surface water is 0.05—0.5 μg/L. One source of water pollution is chromate waste water and residues ejected by the production of electroplate, tanning, smelting, refractory material and dyestuff, etc.

Among the compounds of chrome, trivalent chromium is necessary for human being, in which it participates in the metabolism of both glucose and fat. Deficiency of chrome may cause near sightedness and the symptoms of hypertension, coronary heart disease, and diabetes.

With strong irritation and corrosivity, excessive chrome can also cause intoxication.

Chrome is an allergen of skin which leads to allergic dermatitis and eczema lasting for a long period of time. Therefore, it is ranked as forbidden material in cosmetics by China and some European countries.

Hexavalent chromium is the most poisonous one which can lead to symptoms of ulcer and bleeding of gastrointestinal mucosa, nausea, stomachache, even headache, dizziness, polypnea, cyanotic lips, speeded pulse rate, bloody stools, dehydration, oliguria or anuria. Besides, it can also disturb the activity of various enzymes and influence the oxidation process, deoxidation process and hydrolytic process inside the body. The most serious damage is that it can combine with nucleic acid and nucleoprotein to induce cancer. It can penetrate into cells and combine with macromolecules as nucleic acid and nucleoprotein that causes the change of genetic codes and subsequently causes cancer. In addition, chrome can lead to hemoglobin denaturation and thus reduce oxygen carrying capability of red blood cells. Only 5 g of hexavalent chromium is sufficient to kill people.

The limit of hexavalent chromium in drinking water in China is 0. 05 mg/L.

⑤ Arsenic: Arsenic is a semimetallic element naturally present in the environment. It can take the form of inorganic compounds when combined with elements such as oxygen, chlorine, and sulfur; organic compounds when combined with carbon and hydrogen; and highly flammable arsine gas when combined with hydrogen. All these forms are dangerous to human health. Inorganic arsenic is the most significant contaminant in drinking water globally, which affects over 200 million people's drinking water safety, particularly in developing countries such as Bangladesh, Pakistan, India, China and Northern Chile.

The kidney is the main organ for arsenic excretion so that the concentration of urinary arsenic can sensitively reflect the internal exposure level of arsenic in the body. Arsenic can also be excreted through skin, sweat glands, hair and nails. Measurement of inorganic arsenic in the urine is the best way to determine recent exposure, while measuring inorganic arsenic in hair or fingernails may be used to detect high-level exposures that occurred over the past 6—12 months.

The immediate symptoms of acute arsenic poisoning include vomiting, nausea, diarrhea, abdominal pain, central and peripheral nervous system disorders. These are followed by numbness and tingling of the extremities, muscle cramping and death, in extreme cases. Chronic oral exposure to elevated levels of inorganic arsenic has resulted in gastrointestinal effects, anemia, peripheral neuropathy, skin lesions, hyperpigmentation, and liver or kidney damage in humans. Inorganic arsenic exposure of humans, through the inhalation route, has been shown to be strongly associated with lung cancer, while ingestion of inorganic arsenic by humans has been linked to a form of skin cancer and also to bladder, liver, and lung cancer. Long-term chronic exposure to arsenic in drinking water is also linked to diabetes, cardiovascular disease, chronic cough and other diseases. In utero and early childhood exposure has been linked to negative impacts on cognitive development or behavior, and increased deaths in young adults. Emerging data now shows that arsenic exposure also affects the developing fetus and causes adverse pregnancy outcomes including lower birth weight, smaller neonatal size, spontaneous abortion, stillbirth and neonatal deaths in pregnant women.

Skin is one of the major target organs for arsenic and skin lesions are specific signs of chronic arsenic poisoning, with clinical symptoms initiating within a few years of exposure. Arsenic-induced skin lesions usually begin with pigmentation anomalies, including hyperpigmentation, hypopigmentation, raindrop lesions, and café au lait spots. These non-malignant lesions are followed by pre-malignant hyperkeratosis, malignant basal cell carcinoma, Bowen's disease, and squamous cell carcinoma. In rodents, chronic arsenic exposure in drinking water alone will not induce skin cancer, but will enhance carcinogenesis in two-stage models using dimethylbenzanthracene or ultraviolet light as initiators.

Inorganic arsenic is a confirmed human carcinogen of group A. The proposed modes of action in arsenic carcinogenesis include inhibition of DNA repair, co-mutagenicity, altered epigenetics, oxidative stress and aneuploidy. Although many mechanisms have been proposed, no definite model can be given for the mechanisms of chronic arsenic poisoning. The prevailing events of toxicity and carcinogenicity might be quite tissue-specific.

In China, the limit of arsenic is 0.01 mg/L in drinking water, and the range of the total arsenic is 0.05—0.1 mg/L in surface water.

(3) Physical Pollution and Its Health Effect

Physical pollution of water consists of thermal and radioactive pollution. Industrial cooling water is the main source of thermal pollution. Water temperature rises with the emission of waste water. This accelerates the chemical reaction of the water body, reduces the dissolved oxygen, and affects the survival and reproduction of fishes and living beings.

Radioactive pollution in water mainly comes from the emission of radioactive elements in the soil, the decay products, and artificial radioactive substances, such as cooling water from nuclear power plants, radioactive wastes of nuclear tests and wars, nuclear fuels leaking from nuclear ship accidents, and so on.

Consumption of water with radioactive contamination can lead to inner radiation inside the human body. Some radioactive substances absorbed into blood may evenly distribute to the whole body, others may accumulate in a certain organ. For example, ^{131}I accumulates in thyroid while ^{235}U in kidney. All these increase the incidence of some diseases, even cancers. For example, ^{235}U does great harm to liver, marrows, and hematopoietic function while ^{90}Sr may result in bone tumor and leukemia.

In China, the limit of total alpha radioactivity is 0.5 Bq/L and total beta radioactivity is 1 Bq/L in drinking water.

3.3.4 Hygienic Significance of Drinking Water and Water Quality Standards

As previously described, the unsafe drinking water may be great harmful to human health, such as waterborne communicable diseases, chemical toxic diseases, cancer, microelements and endemic diseases. To control the hazards of water pollution, a series of hygienic standards of water quality are formulated in many counties. For example, China has integrated wastewater discharge standard, and hygienic standard for surface water, drinking water, mineral water, and so on. Hygienic standard for drinking water and its hygiene significance are described below.

3. 3. 4. 1   Guidelines for Drinking Water Quality

The primary purpose of the guidelines for drinking water quality is to protect public health. The recommendations in the guidelines for managing the risk include not only hazards that may jeopardize the safety of drinking water, but also the sources that are exposed to these hazards, such as waste, air, food and consumer products. According to the World Health Organization Guidelines for drinking water quality, safe drinking water does not represent any significant health risk over lifetime consumption, including different sensitivities that may occur during different life stages.

3. 3. 4. 2   Hygiene Standards for Drinking Water

(1) The Basic Health Requirements of Drinking Water

① Safety on epidemiology: Drinking water should not contain various pathogens to avoid transmitting waterborne communicable diseases.

② No harmful chemical composition: The chemical properties and radioactive substances contained in the water should not lead to the acute and chronic poisoning and potential hazards during long-term drinking.

③ Good sensory properties: Colorless, tasteless, odorless, transparent, no visible substance to the naked eyes.

④ Sufficient water: Adequate water supply makes it easy for people to get access to water.

(2) The Quality Standards for Drinking Water

To limit the amount of harmful substances in water, to make sure the safety of drinking water, a series of hygienic standards of water quality are formulated in different countries or regions.

① In China, Standards for Drinking Water Quality (GB 5749-2006) was revised and published in 2006 and put in practice on July 1, 2007, which covers a total of 106 enforced index and 28 reference index. The enforced index is made up of 42 items of regular indices and limitations and 64 items of non-regular indices and limitations.

② As one of the earliest countries in the world to set the standard of drinking water quality, the US has revised the standards for more than 10 times since 1914. The EPA (Environmental Protection Agency) has developed a series of primary standards and secondary standards. Designed to protect human health from both naturally occurring and human-made contaminants. The primary standards include maximum contaminant level goals (MCLGs) for selected inorganic contaminants, volatile organic chemicals, and radioactive materials, as well as limits for the presence of coliform organisms. Designed to ensure that drinking water is aesthetically pleasing in terms of temperature, color, taste, and odor. The secondary standards include limits for iron, which can discolor clothes during laundering; sulfates and dissolved solids, which can have the same effect as a laxative; and minerals that can, for example, interfere with the taste of beverages.

③ Drinking water quality standards of the European Union (EU), also called Drinking Water Directive, was established in 1980. The standards covered a total of 61 items including microbiological index, index of poisonous and harmful substances, sensory index and physiochemical index. In 1998, the EU revised its Drinking Water Directive (DWD) (98/83/EC), which concerns the quality of water intended for human consumption and is required for all the EU number states to comply with. Its objective is to protect human health from adverse effects of any contamination of water intended for human consumption by ensuring that it is wholesome and clean. In 2000, the EU passed the Water Framework Directive, an overarching piece of legislation that brings together all existing EU legislations on water resources. Comparisons of regular indices and limitations among China, America and European Union are listed in Table 3.8.

Table 3.8   Regular Indices and Limitations of Water Quality Among China,

America and European Union

Index	Limitations		
	GB5749-2006 (China)	MCL(MCLG) (America)	DWD (European Union)
1. Microbiological index			
Total coliforms (MPN/100mL or CFU/100mL)	Negative	5	
Thermotolerant coliforms (MPN/100mL or CFU/100mL)	Negative		
Escherichia coli(MPN/100mL or CFU/100mL)	Negative		0
Total plate count(CFU/mL)	100		
2. Toxicology index			
Arsenic (As)(mg/L)	0.01	0.01	0.01
Cadmium (Cd) (mg/L)	0.005	0.005	0.005
Chromium-6 (hexavalent [Cr(Ⅵ)])(mg/L)	0.05	0.1	0.05
Lead (Pb)(mg/L)	0.01	0.015	0.01
Mercury (Hg) (mg/L)	0.001	0.002	0.001
Selenium (mg/L)	0.01	0.05	0.01
Cyanide (mg/L)	0.05		0.05

(**to be continued**)

continued

Index	Limitations		
	GB5749-2006 (China)	MCL(MCLG) (America)	DWD (European Union)
Fluoride (mg/L)	1.0	4.0	1.5
Nitrate (calculated as N)(mg/L)	Groundwater source limit is 20	10	50
Trichloromethane(mg/L)	0.06		
Carbon tetrachloride (mg/L)	0.002	0.005	
Bromate (when using ozone, mg/L)	0.01		0.01
Formaldehyde (when using ozone, mg/L)	0.9		
Chlorite (when using chlorine dioxide to disinfect, mg/L)	0.7		
Chlorate (when using chlorine dioxide disinfection, mg/L)	0.7		

3. Sensory properties and general chemical index

Index	GB5749-2006 (China)	MCL(MCLG) (America)	DWD (European Union)
Chroma (Unit of platinum cobalt color)	15	15	User acceptable and no smell
Turbidity / NTU	1	N/A	User acceptable and no smell
Smell and taste	Odorless odor		User acceptable and no smell
Visible substance	Negative		
pH	6.5-8.5	6.5-8.5	6.5-9.5
Aluminum(mg/L)	0.2	0.05-0.2	0.2
Iron(mg/L)	0.3	0.3	0.2
Manganese(mg/L)	0.1	0.05	0.05
Copper(mg/L)	1.0	1.3	2.0
Zinc(mg/L)	1.0	5	
Chloride(mg/L)	250	250	250
Nitrate(mg/L)	250	250	250
Total dissolved solid (mg/L)	1000	500	
Total hardness (with $CaCO_3$, mg/L)	450		
Oxygen consumption (calculated as O_2, mg/L)	3		5
Volatile phenols (calculated as phenol, mg/L)	0.002		

（**to be continued**）

continued

Index	Limitations		
	GB5749-2006 (China)	MCL(MCLG) (America)	DWD (European Union)
Anionic detergent (mg/L)	0.3		
4. Radioactivity index			
Total α radioactivity (Bq/L)	0.5		
Total β radioactivity (Bq/L)	1		

① MPN represents the most likely number; CFU stands for total coliforms. When water samples detected total coliform bacteria, strains and bacterium or heat-resistant coliform bacteria should be further tested. If Water samples did not check out the total coliform bacteria, no test needed on coli bacterium or heat-resistant coliform bacteria.

② If radioactive indicators exceed guideline values, nuclide analysis and evaluation should be undertaken to determine whether to drink.

3.3.4.3　Water Quality Monitoring

Water quality monitoring is the process of measuring various index data, which can reflect the environmental quality of water body. The purpose of water quality monitoring is to determine whether the environmental quality of water is consistent with the corresponding environmental quality standards and to provide basic data for rational use and protection of water resources. Through understanding the distribution, sources, pollution pathways and migration rule of pollutants in water, the development trend of water pollution can be predicted. The possible water pollution degree, its impact on human health, and the evaluation of the practical effects of control measures can be judged by water quality monitoring, which can provide a scientific basis for formulating the pollutants discharge standards.

Water monitoring covers a wide range of uncontaminated and contaminated natural water (river, lake, ocean and groundwater) as well as various industrial drains. Since the latter is not the source of drinking water, it is not included in this section. Main monitoring items can be divided into three categories: first is a comprehensive indicator reflecting water quality natural traits, such as temperature, chromaticity turbidity, pH, conductivity, suspended solids, hardness; second is a general hygiene indicator, such as dissolved oxygen, chemical oxygen demand (COD), biochemical oxygen demand (BOD) and total coliforms (TC); third is toxic substances such as phenol, cyanide, arsenic, lead, chromium, cadmium, mercury and organic pesticides. Water quality monitoring can provide data for environmental management, and a basis for assessing the quality of surface water and groundwater. The rules and regulations of the spots-setting, sampling, monitoring methods, and data processing of surface/wastewater or groundwater monitoring are set in accordance with the ＜ Technical Specifications Requirements for Monitoring of Surface

Water and Waste Water> (HJ/T 91—2002, China) and < Technical Specifications for Environmental Monitoring of Groundwater> (HJ/T 164—2004, China), respectively. This specification applies to groundwater monitoring, but does not apply to underground hot water, mineral water, and brine.

3.3.5   Purification, Disinfection and Special Treatment for Drinking Water

There are two kinds of water supply in China, centralized water supply and decentralized water supply. The former is mainly available in large, medium and small city, while the latter in the village. There are two categories for selected source water, surface water and groundwater. Regardless of the kind of water used as drinking water, it requires purification and disinfection, and sometimes special treatments before it can meet the requirements of sanitary standard for drinking water. Here, we take the centralized water supply as an example to introduce the source selection, protection, cleaning, disinfection and special treatment.

Centralized water supply is the way to water users by water distribution network after water abstraction, water purification, disinfection and meeting the health requirements. Its advantages are to facilitate the selection and protection of water source; easily to take the improvement of water quality, ensure good water quality; use water conveniently; easily supervise and manage the hygiene. However, once polluted, the centralized water supply poses great and wide harm.

3.3.5.1   Selection and Protection of Water Sources

(1) Selection Principles

① Adequate water sources: It is generally required that 95% low flow assurance rate is greater than the total design water consumption.

② Good water quality: Sensory properties indicators and general chemical indicators can reach the requirement of drinking water through the present treatment technology; water toxicology index and radioactive indicators must comply with the standards for drinking water quality requirements; When the water contains hazardous chemical materials, its concentration should not exceed the maximum allowable concentration as stipulated; COD in water should not exceed 4 mg/L; BOD5 should not exceed 3 mg/L; when the water iodine content is lower than 10 μg/L, iodine supplementation measures can be taken according to specific situations; water sources with the appropriate amount of fluoride will be selected in drinking water type fluorosis endemic areas, and when no proper water sources, fluoride removal measures should be taken.

③ Being convenient to protect: Groundwater should be preferred when conditions permit. When surface water is used as the water source, the water intake point should be set in the upstream of towns and industrial mining enterprises in order to prevent water pollution.

④ Being technically and economically reasonable: When selecting water sources, we should base on the analysis and comparison of different water content, water quality, further combine water quality and water abstraction, purification, distribution and other specific conditions, and consider the basic construction minimum investment solution.

(2) Health Protection of Water Sources

① Health protection of surface water: No pollution can be found within 100 meters around water abstraction points. Industrial wastewater and domestic sewage shall not be discharged into the waters from 1,000 meters upstream to 100 meters downstream of the water abstraction points. No waste residue shall be stacked within its coastal protection area, no warehouses or stacks of toxic or harmful chemicals shall be set up, no wharves shall be set up for loading and unloading garbage, faeces and toxic and harmful chemicals, no industrial waste water or domestic sewage shall be used for irrigation and application of pesticides that are difficult to degrade or highly toxic.

② Health protection of groundwater sources: No pollution sources can be found within the radius of 30 meters around the well. It's not allowed to discharge industrial wastes in the form of seepage pits. Water quality of artificial recharge should meet the drinking water quality requirements.

3.3.5.2 Purification and Disinfection of Water

No matter where the water sources of drinking water come from, it contains various impurities to varying degrees. Without purification and disinfection, water quality often fails to meet the requirements of sanitary standards for drinking water. The purpose of purification is to remove suspended matter, colloidal particles and bacteria from the raw water. There are three kinds of purification treatments for drinking water, such as conventional purification, deep purification and special purification. And four stages of water treatment in most plants include coagulation, sedimentation, filtration, and disinfection (Figure 3.11).

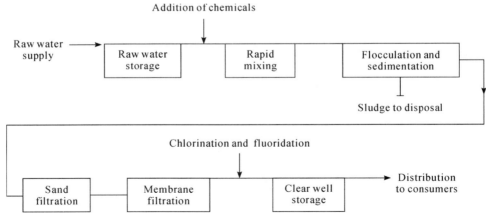

Figure 3.11   Principal Steps in the Water Purification Process

(1) Coagulation Sedimentation

Natural water often contains a variety of suspended particles and colloidal substances. Since the colloidal particles are difficult to precipitate naturally, coagulant is required to coagulative precipitation. Raw water+water treatment chemicals→mixing→reaction→alum water. The commonly used coagulants are metal salt coagulants (such as aluminum salts and iron salts) and polymer coagulants (such as polyaluminum chloride and polyacrylamide).

Precipitation refers to the process in which floccule formed in the coagulation stage depends on the gravity to separate from water, and the process is finished in the sedimentation pool. Water flows into the sedimentation area, then slowly to the exit area, and particles sediment is left at the bottom of the pool.

(2) Filtration

Filtration is the process in which water intercepts and adsorb the suspended impurities and microorganisms in the water through the quartz sand filtering layer. Three functions of filtration: ① Water quality turbidity after filtration reaches the drinking water quality requirements; ② After filtration, most of the pathogens, such as bacteria, viruses and parasitic protozoa and worms are removed from the water. Especially amoebic cysts and Cryptosporidium oocysts, they have the strong resistance to disinfectant, mainly depending on the removal of filtration; ③ After filtration, the residual microorganism loses the protective effect of suspended solids, which provides conditions for disinfection. Filter layer thickness and particle size, filter speed, water quality and filter type are the main factors affect the filtration effect.

(3) Disinfection

Disinfection of drinking water is a very important process to kill pathogen in water, and guarantee the water quality safety of epidemiology. Some groundwater without purification treatment is allowable, but it usually needs disinfection. The purpose of disinfection is to consider the contamination of pathogenic mircroorganism in all aspects of the water supply process, and to prevent the occurrence and spread of infectious diseases by disinfecting the path of transmission of pathogenic microorganisms in drinking water quality. Disinfection methods for drinking water can be divided into two categories: physical disinfection and chemical disinfection. The former adopts several disinfecting methods, such as boiling, ultrasonic, the latter disinfects with chlorine, chlorine dioxide, ozone, peroxide, ultraviolet, and so on.

① Chlorination disinfection Chlorination refers to the way of disinfection which applies liquid chlorine or chlorinated products to drinking water. Chlorine preparations for disinfecting drinking water mainly include liquid chlorine, bleaching powder [$Ca(OCl)Cl$], bleaching powder detergent [$Ca(OCl)_2$] and organochlorine preparations. A kind of chlorine named active chlorine has a strong bactericidal action. If the valence number of chlorine content in chlorinated compounds is greater than—1, such chlorine will be active chlorine. The newly-produced bleaching powder and bleaching powder concentrate respectively contains 25%—30% active chlorine and 60%—70% active chlorine. With the extension of storage time, the active chlorine will fall gradually, and lose its effectiveness when it is below 15%.

- The principle of chlorination.

The following reaction occurs when chlorine is dissolved in water:

$$Cl_2 + H_2O \longrightarrow HOCl + H^+ + Cl^- \qquad HOCl \Longrightarrow H^+ + OCl^-$$

Bleaching powder and bleaching powder detergent are turned into hypochlorous acid in the water:

$$2Ca(OCl)Cl + 2H_2O \longrightarrow Ca(OH)_2 + 2HOCl + CaCl_2$$
$$Ca(OCl)_2 + 2H_2O \longrightarrow Ca(OH)_2 + 2HOCl$$

Both liquid chlorine and chlorine compounds can be turned into hypochlorous acid volume in the water which is small in size and neutral in charge. The hypochlorous acid is a kind of strong oxidizer that can damage the cell membrane, increase its permeability, cause the leakage of materials such as proteins, RNA and DNA in the cell, interfere with a variety of enzyme system (especially the thiol oxidation of glucose phosphate dehydrogenase stops sugar metabolism), and consequently lead to the bacterial death. The chlorine effect on virus is mainly that chlorine acts on the nucleic acid of the virus and causes the lethal damage to virus.

- Factors affecting chlorination effect.

Chlorine dosage and the contact time: The experimental results show that enough disinfectant added to water and sufficient contact time can ensure the effect of chlorination. The contact time is not less than 60 minutes in winter and 30 minutes in summer. Chlorine demand refers to the amount of available chlorine consumed by the oxidation of organic matters and reduced inorganic matters in a liter of water, sterilization as well as some chlorination reaction. Residual chlorine refers to the rest of active chlorine in water after adding chlorine to disinfect for a certain period of time, including free residual chlorine and combinative residual chlorine. Free residual chlorine is HOCl, OCl$^-$; Combinative residual chlorine is monochloroamine (NH$_2$Cl) and dichloramine (NHCl$_2$). The limited value of residual chlorine in the water is related to its properties. Chlorine dosage refers to the amount of active chlorine added when using chlorine to disinfect. It is the sum of the amount of chlorine demand and residual chlorine. Chlorine dosage varies from one water quality to another.

The pH of water: The lower the pH value is, the better the sterilization effect. Hypochlorous acid is a weak electrolyte, forming hypochlorous acid (HOCl) and hypochlorous acid root (OCl$^-$) in water, the amount of which is related to the pH value of water. According to the experiment with colibacillus, hypochlorous acid is 83 times more than hypochlorous acid root in sterilization efficiency. Therefore, the pH value of the water should not be too high when chlorinating.

Water temperature: The higher the water temperature is, the better the sterilization effect is. Every 10℃ increased in the water temperature, the sterilization rate can be improved by 2—3 times.

Water turbidity: Suspended particles can absorb microorganisms and subsequently agglutinate them. The disinfectant is not easy to act on microorganisms, so the disinfection effect is reduced.

The type and amount of microorganisms in water   The resistance to chlorine varies from one microorganism to another. In general, the resistance to chlorine in ascending order is colibacillus, virus, and protozoa cyst.

- Common methods of chlorination.

Ordinary chlorination: With low turbidity and light organic pollution, the proper amount of chlorine is added to the water for at least 30 minutes when there is no phenolic compound in the water. Short time is needed for this method, and the effect is reliable. The residual chlorine in the water is mainly the free residual chlorine (HOCl, OCl⁻). The disadvantage is that such chlorination by-products as tri-halomethanes are produced after disinfection when the source water contains organic compounds or humus.

Chloramine disinfection: Ammonia (ammonium sulfate, ammonium chloride) is first added to the water, and then chlorine. The proper proportion between ammonia and chlorine is 1 : 3 to 1 : 6. The advantages of this approach are as follows: reduction of the tri-halomethanes formation; prevention of chlorophenol odor with the way of adding chlorine after ammonia, stable combinative residual chlorine for long time. The disadvantages are as follows: long contact time, the more costly, complex operation and the poorer sterilization effect.

Break point chlorination: The method has the advantages that the disinfection effect is reliable, the Mn, Fe, phenol and organic matter content can be significantly reduced, the odor and the chromaticity can be reduced. Disadvantages: Chlorine consumption is high, and it will produce more chlorinated by-products; it is necessary to determine the amount of chlorine added in advance, which is more troublesome; sometimes the break point of water is not obvious, the pH of the water will be too low. Therefore, alkali need to be added for adjustment if necessary.

Superchlorination: Large amount of chlorine is added to water to make the amount of residual chlorine achieve 1—5 mg/L within short time when the organic pollution is serious, or when you work in the field, or there is an accident. The dechlorination of water after disinfection can be done by sodium sulfite, sodium hydrogen sulfite or activated carbon.

Chlorine dioxide disinfection: ClO_2 is a kind of orange gas at normal temperature. It dissolves and volatilizes easily in water, but it does not react with water. It is explosive when the concentration of ClO_2 in the air is more than 10% or the water concentration is greater than 30%. In the alkaline solution, there will be disproportionation reaction on ClO_2: $2ClO_2 + 2OH^- \longrightarrow ClO_2^- + ClO_3^- + H_2O$.

Chlorine dioxide is a kind of good disinfectant of drinking water, with better antiseptic effect than liquid chlorine, effectively killing bacteria, viruses, fungi spores.

- The mechanism of killing pathogens.

ClO_2 has better adsorption and permeation to cell walls. It can oxidize enzyme containing sulfenyl in the cell, react with cysteine, tryptophan and free fatty acids, rapidly control the biological protein synthesis and enhance the permeability of the membrane. It also can change the viral capsid structure, killing the virus. The oxidation of ClO_2 is better than that of liquid chlorine. The oxidized organic matters mostly degrade into products that mainly contain the oxygen radicals (carboxylic acids) without chlorinated by-products. The strong oxidization of ClO_2 also appears as such quinoid structure which can oxidize carcinogen B(a)P to substances without carcinogenicity.

- Advantages and disadvantages of ClO_2 disinfection.

Advantages: It can reduce such chlorinated by-products as tri-halomethanes in water. The intensity of oxidation disinfection is unchanged when there is ammonia in water. The effect of killing pathogens in water is not influenced by pH value. The residual chlorine remains stable after disinfection. It can remove different colors and smells from water, not forming chlorophenol odor. It has strong ability to remove ferrum and manganese from water. Disadvantages: ClO_2 is explosive, so it needs site preparation and immediate use. The process is complex and costly. The disproportionated compounds of ClO_2 can cause diseases such as hemolytic anemia and hemoglobin denaturation to animals.

② Ozone disinfection As a kind of strong oxidizer, the solubility of O_3 is 13 times higher than that of oxygen in water. It is an unstable gas which has to be produced at the point of use. As a matter of fact, the adding dosage is no more than 1 mg/L and the contact time required is 10—15 min.

- The mechanism of killing pathogens.

The mechanism of killing pathogens: After contacting with water, ozone can produce hydroxyl radicals, a more powerful oxidant than ozone, which works on bacteria. It can enhance the permeability of cell membrane and leak the cellular contents. It also can affect the viral capsid protein, killing virus.

- Advantages and disadvantages of ozone disinfection.

Advantages: Ozone disinfection has better effect than ClO_2 disinfection and Cl_2 disinfection. With little amount and short contact time, it can purify water color, smell, taste and remove ferrum, manganese, and phenol from water without producing of haloform. It is not affected by the sensory properties of water and can strengthen the flocculation effect before pretreatment, reducing the dosage of coagulant. Disadvantages: It needs large investment and high cost. The ozone in water is unstable, so higher technologies are needed for control and detection. In addition, ozone can corrode the water pipe, so the finished water does not contain O_3 and cannot kill bacteria continuously. As a result, it needs another disinfectant. It also can react with ferrum, manganese and organic matters to form micro floc, which increases the water turbidity. Regular indices and requirements of disinfectant in drinking water are listed in Table 3. 9.

Table 3. 9   Regular Indices and Requirements of Disinfectant in Drinking Water

Name of Disinfectant	Contact Time in Water	The Factory Water Limit	The factory Water Residue	Residue in Direct Provide Water
Chlorine and free chlorine preparation (free chlorine, mg/L)	at least 30 min	4	$\geqslant 0.3$	$\geqslant 0.05$
Monochloramine (total chlorine, mg/L)	at least 120 min	3	$\geqslant 0.5$	$\geqslant 0.05$
ozone(O_3, mg/L)	at least 12 min	0.3		0.02 If using chlorine, total chloride 0.05 or higher
chlorine dioxide (ClO_2, mg/L)	at least 30 min	0.8	$\geqslant 0.1$	$\geqslant 0.02$

③ UV disinfection   Ultraviolet light with a wavelength of 200—295 nm has a bactericidal effect, and the UV at 254 nm has the strongest effect.

• The mechanism of killing pathogens.

When the microorganisms are irradiated, ultraviolet rays can penetrate into the microorganisms and act on nucleic acids, protoplasmic proteins and enzymes, making adjacent thymidine which bonds on the DNA synthesized into two bodies, so that DNA loses the transcription ability and protein synthesis is prevented, resulting in the death of pathogenic microorganisms.

• Advantages and disadvantages of UV disinfection.

Advantages: With short contact time and high sterilization efficiency, UV disinfection has broad-spectrum disinfection effect on pathogenic microorganisms, especially on Cryptosporidium. During the disinfection, it can reduce odor, taste and degradation of trace organic pollutants without producing harmful substances. Moreover, its disinfection effect is less affected by water temperature and pH. Disadvantages: UV disinfection does not have lasting disinfection effect, and it needs to cooperate with chlorine use, the price is higher.

(4) Special Treatment

① Common methods of fluorine removal.

• Activated alumina method.

As a kind of white granular porous adsorbent, activated alumina has larger specific surface area, and is an amphoteric substance with the isoelectric point of about 9. 5. when the water pH is normal, it has great choice to absorb fluorine.

• Bone carbon method.

It's also called calcium phosphate method, which is effective, convenient and economical. The main constituent of bone carbon is hydroxyl calcium phosphate that can react with fluorine as following:

$$Ca_{10}(PO_4)_6(OH)_2 + 2F^- \rightleftharpoons Ca_{10}(PO_4)_6F_2 + 2OH^-$$

- Electrodialysis method.

Under the effect of dc electric field, the soluble ion in the raw water migrates, achieving separation through ion exchange membrane without adding agents.

② Algae removal and odor removal: Algae reproduction in water not only produces odor and toxin, but also is a typical kind of the chloride by-product precursors. In the process of disinfecting tap-water, algae can react with chlorine to generate a variety of harmful by-products such as chloroform, increasing the mutagenic activity of water.

- Physical methods.

Flotation technology is widely used at home and abroad to remove algae with good effect and high removal rate of 70%—80%. Moreover, as a kind of large green algae, hydrodictyaceae can also be used to remove the algae with its stronger reproduction ability than cyanophycoae. Hydrodictyaceae can absorb large amount of phosphorus in water in its growth process, and nitrogen keeps cyanophycoae from multiplying in water, so as to achieve the goal of controlling algae.

- Chemical methods.

Aluminum sulfate and copper sulfate are used as the algaecides to remove most algae. Ferric salt also can be used to remove algae, because it can form heavier alum flowers with water, increasing the coagulation effect and improving the removal rate of algae.

- Biological methods.

Honeycomb tube is vertically placed in the reaction tank to gradually generate biological membranes when the raw water runs through the honeycomb tube, which can absorb the impurities in water and remove pollutants and algae in raw water.

③ Iron removal and manganese removal: The Fe^{2+} in the water can be removed by aeration filtration. The role of aeration is to increase dissolved oxygen in water; and increase CO_2 in order to increase the pH of water and subsequently oxidize Fe^{2+} to Fe^{3+}. The effect of filtration is to remove flocculation formed by Fe^{3+}; Fe^{2+} which has not been oxidized is contacted and adsorbed on the filter material. When the filter material forms an iron filter, the catalytic oxidation of MnO_2 and the ion exchange of iron oxyhydroxide are used to achieve the purpose of iron removal. The manganese removal method is the same as above.

3.3.5.3　Approaches for Water Treatment

For the prevention of water pollution, especially the sanitary status of urban drinking water sources and the health of residents, water sanitary protection should be strengthened. Promoting "cleaner production" technology and turning terminal treatment to source prevention are fundamental measures to prevent water pollution. In addition, dealing properly with the utilization and treatment of industrial wastewater and domestic sewage also plays an important role in protecting and improving the health of water bodies.

(1) Industrial Wastewater Treatment

The treatment of industrial wastewater can be divided into three levels: Primary treatment can remove the floating substance and most suspended state pollutants, the pH of the water can be regulated. Through the treatment, the degree of corrosion of wastewater and subsequent processing load will be reduced. However, if the degree of purification of the primary treatment is not suitable enough for discharge, secondary treatment, which can remove the organic pollutants, must be carried out. After that, the biochemical oxygen demand in wastewater can be generally removed by 80%—90%, which can generally meet the standards for discharge to water bodies, or for wastewater reuse and farmland irrigation. Tertiary treatment is used to further remove the pollutant leftover after the secondary treatment, including organic matter of failure microbial degradation, as well as phosphorus, nitrogen, and soluble inorganic substances. Considering wastewaters from industrial operations contain a wide range of contaminants, treatment methods, either solely or in combination, should include physical, chemical, physical-chemical, and biological treatments.

(2) Sanitary Sewage Treatment

Domestic sewage refers to people's daily washing wastewater and fecal sewage, etc., more than 99% is water, and solid materials are generally less than 1%, the latter is mainly composed of cellulose, oil, protein, and its decomposition products. Its treatment methods commonly include physical treatment (grid, screen mesh, sedimentation tank, etc.) and biological treatment (activated sludge process, biological filter method), the principle and equipment of which are the same as industrial wastewater treatment (Figure 3.12). Domestic sewage usually contains a certain amount of nitrogen, phosphorus, potassium, and other fertilizer ingredients. Under suitable natural conditions, the treated domestic sewage can be used for farmland irrigation to increase soil fertility and water content, increase crop yield, and purify sewage by biological oxidation.

(3) Approaches to Wastewater Treatment

In recent years, additional technologies have been developed and applied in the purification of water not only for the efficiency of treatment but also for environmental protection.

① UV radiation: Being effective against bacteria, viruses, and parasites, UV radiation is now being applied in more than 2,000 wastewater-treatment installations in the US. Since turbidity can severely reduce the effectiveness of UV radiation, it is often used to filter the sewage prior to applying the UV process.

② Membrane bioreactor (MBR): Developed in the late 20th century, MBR is a new technology that combines membrane separation technology and biological technology with the advantages of good effluent quality, simple operation management and small floor space. It can improve active sludge concentration and control hydraulic retention time (HRT) and sludge retention time (SRT) respectively by using membrane separation device to activate

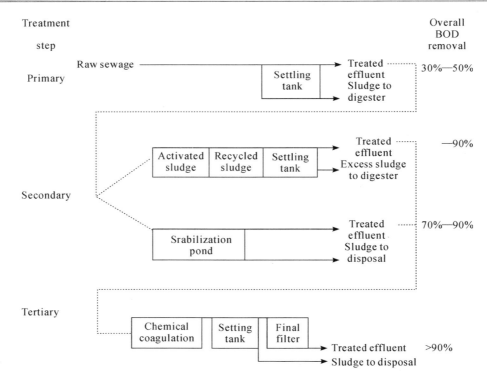

Figure 3. 12   Primary, Secondary, and Tertiary Stages in the Treatment of Municipal Sewage

sludge and macromolecular substance in the biochemical reaction tank. Most of the bacteria, microorganisms, heat source, the carriers of the virus can be trapped in sewage for further disinfection. Some tertiary treatment processes such as advanced oxidation and activated carbon filtration have been shown to be rather effective in micropollutant removal in drinking water, but in many cases these techniques are cost-prohibitive and not sustainable. To some extent, bioaugmentation is a viable alternative for micropollutant removal in drinking water and further studies are warranted to fill knowledge gaps and bring the concept to practical implementation.

③ Magnetic separation technology Cryptosporidium oocysts is an efficient, cost-effective, high separation efficiency, no-secondary pollution, and easy operation, green and economic separation technology. Magnetic separation technology Cryptosporidium oocysts also shows potential in the field of water treatment. Due to these advantages, the magnetic separation technology is receiving more attention in the research and application in water treatment, especially the high gradient magnetic separation (HGMS) and superconducting magnetic separation (SMS). In addition, on the basis of continuous improvement of the new type filler and equipment, research and development of high mass transfer biological packing and equipment will also improve the efficiency of biological membrane method sewage treatment process.

3. 4   Geological Environment and Health

The geological environment, also known as geoenvironment, is part of the lithosphere which directly influences the conditions of the existence and development of the society which man exploits and converts. The basic components of the geoenvrionment are rocks, relief, water and atmosphere, but in this part, soil and water are mainly discussed. The study of geological environment and human health also partly belongs to the science of "Medical Geology".

Rocks and minerals comprise the fundamental building blocks of the planet and contain the majority of naturally occurring chemical elements. Many elements are essential to plant, animal, and human health in small doses. Most of these elements are taken into the human body via food, water, and air. Rocks, through weathering processes, break down to form the soils on which crops and animals are raised. Drinking water travels through rocks and soils as part of the hydrological cycle and much of the dust and some of the gases contained in the atmosphere are of geological origin. Hence, through the food chain and inhalation of atmospheric dusts and gases human health is directly linked to geology.

The periodic table of elements, as an indicator of the roles played by the elements in the biosphere, is the basis for our understanding. The periodic table currently has a total of 118 elements. It is now known that an increasing number of the 92 naturally occurring elements on Earth are essential to humans and other vertebrate species. In addition to the eleven main constituents (C, H, N, O, Na, Mg, P, S, Cl, K, Ca), ten elements present in trace quantities are generally accepted to have necessary functions in the human body. These essential trace elements are Mn, Cr, Fe, Co, Cu, Zn, Se, Mo, F, and I. Meanwhile, they are dangerous via inhalation or ingestion, and their effects usually accumulate over time to cause health problem when they exceed a certain threshold. So, either too much or too little consumption will be harmful to our health. Biogeochemical diseases are closely associated with these trace elements.

In this section, both nonhuman, natural geological environment and the anthropogenic chemical contamination due to the industrialization, urbanization, and waste disposal will be discussed.

3. 4. 1   Biogeochemical Disease

Biogeochemical disease is due to the uneven distribution of chemical elements on earth's crust, so that in some areas the element is too much or too little, leading to certain specific diseases in a particular region. Biogeochemical diseases mainly include the following: iodine deficiency disorders(IDD) endemic fluorosis, endemic arsenism, keshan disease and kaschin beck disease.

Usually, the biogeochemical disease has four characteristics: ① Distinct regional distribution; ② Associated with the environmental element level; ③ A clear dose-response relationship between some chemical elements and geological diseases; ④ Correlation can be explained by modern medical theory. There are several factors affecting the prevalence of biogeochemical diseases: ① Nutritional conditions: In epidemic areas, the intensity of epidemic can be reduced by improving people's living conditions and nutrition. ② Living habits: For example, in Tibet, Inner Mongolia and other regions, residents are used to drinking brick tea. Brick tea has a high content of fluorine, causing brick-tea drinking fluorosis. ③ Combined action of multiple elements: The geological environment with high fluorine and low iodine, high fluorine and low arsenic increases the complexity of the impact on population health. In some mountain areas, both endemic fluorosis and iodine deficiency disorders are prevalent. Studies have shown that in low iodine areas, the presence of high fluorine can cause early onset of fluorosis in the population.

3.4.1.1 Iodine Deficiency Disorders

(1) Iodine Ecology

Iodine is widely but unevenly distributed in the earth. Most iodide is found in the oceans. The concentration of iodide in sea water is approximately 50 $\mu g/L$. Iodide ions in seawater are oxidized to elemental iodine, which volatilizes into the atmosphere and is returned to the soil by rain, completing the cycle. However, iodine cycling in many regions is slow and incomplete, leaving soils and drinking water iodine depleted. Crops grown in these soils will be low in iodine, and humans and animals consuming food grown in these soils become iodine deficient. The dry weight of crops grown in iodine-deficient soils may be as low as 10 $\mu g/kg$, compared with approximately 1 mg/kg in crops from iodine-sufficient soils. The iodine content in water is closely related to the prevalence of IDD. In IDD areas, the iodine content in water is less than 10 $\mu g/L$.

Iodine-deficient soils are common in mountainous areas (e.g., the Alps, Andes, Atlas, and Himalayan ranges) and areas of frequent flooding, especially in South and Southeast Asia (for example, the Ganges River plain of northeastern India). Although many inland areas, including central Asia and Africa, and central and eastern Europe are iodine deficient, iodine deficiency may also affect coastal and island populations.

(2) Iodine and Health

Iodine is an essential trace element for humans because it is part of the chemical structure of thyroid hormones [thyroxine (T_4) and triiodothyronine (T_3)]. The thyroid hormones act at target organs by influencing many different chemical reactions, usually involving manufacture of proteins. Iodine is especially important during pregnancy, infancy and childhood. Nevertheless it is also important during adult life, for normal metabolism and function.

In 1983, the term iodine deficiency disorders (IDDs) was coined to emphasize that iodine deficiency can affect human beings at all stages of the life cycle and have a broad spectrum of adverse effects, including mental and physical impairment, disturbed thyroid function and goiter (Table 3. 10).

Table 3. 10   Health Consequences of Iodine Deficiency

Physiological groups	Health Consequences of Iodine Deficiency
All ages	Goiter; hypothyroidism; increased susceptibility to nuclear radiation
Fetus	Spontaneous abortion; stillbirth; congenital anomalies; perinatal mortality
Neonate	Endemic cretinism including mental deficiency with a mixture of mutism; spastic diplegia; squint; hypothyroidism and short stature Infant mortality
Child and adolescent	Impaired mental function; delayed physical development; iodine-induced hyperthyroidism
Adults	Impaired mental function; iodine-induced hyperthyroidism

(3) Epidemiology

In 2011, iodine intake is inadequate in 32 countries, adequate in 71, more than adequate in 36, and excessive in 11. Over one-half of the children with low intakes are in two regions: 78 million children in South-East Asia and 58 million children in Africa. The smallest proportions with low intakes are in the Americas (13.7%) and the Western Pacific (19.8%), whereas the greatest proportions of children with inadequate iodine intake are in European (43.9%) and the African (39.5%) regions. Inferring from the proportion of school aged children (SAC, between 6 to 12 years old) to the general population, 1.92 billion people globally have inadequate iodine intakes.

① Goiter: The most visible consequence of iodine deficiency is goiter. Goiter means "an enlarged thyroid" (Figure 3. 13a).

The process begins as an adaptation in which the thyroid is more active to make enough thyroid hormone for the body's needs, despite the supply of iodine is limited. If this adaptation is successful and iodine deficiency is not too severe, the person may only have thyroid enlargement but no other apparent damage from the iodine deficiency. Older individuals with goiters may develop nodules (lumps) in their thyroid gland, and sometimes too much thyroid hormone may be produced when they are suddenly exposed to iodine. This result occurs because these nodules are independent of usual controls, and they make thyroid hormone at their own rate which may be overproduced when more iodine is supplied. In addition, the nodular goiters in iodine deficiency are also called "follicular cancer." Goiters can sometimes enlarge enough to produce compression of other neck structures and may need surgical removal.

• Etiology

Iodine deficiency is the main cause of endemic goiter, but other dietary substances (termed goitrogens) that interfere with thyroid metabolism can aggravate the effect (Table 3. 11). Most goitrogens do not have a major clinical effect unless there is coexisting iodine deficiency.

Table 3. 11   Goitrogens and Their Mechanism

Goitrogens	Mechanism
Food	
Cassava, lima beans, linseed, sorghum, sweet potato	Contain cyanogenic glucosides; they are metabolised to thiocyanates that compete with iodine for thyroidal uptake
Cruciferous vegetables such as cabbage, kale, cauliflower, broccoli, turnips, rapeseed	Contain glucosinolates; metabolites compete with iodine for thyroidal uptake
Soy, millet	Flavonoids impair thyroid peroxidase activity
Nutrients	
Selenium deficiency	Accumulated peroxides might damage the thyroid, and deiodinase deficiency impairs thyroid hormone synthesis
Iron deficiency	Reduces haeme-dependent thyroperoxidase activity in the thyroid and might blunt the efficacy of iodine prophylaxis
Vitamin A deficiency	Increases TSH stimulation and goitre through decreased vitamin A-mediated suppression of the pituitary TSH β gene

TSH＝thyroid-stimulating hormone.

Source: ZIMMERMANN M,B, JOOSTE P L, PANDAY C S. Indine-deficiency Disorders[J]. Lancet, 2008, 372(9645): 1251-1262.

• Morphology.

Regarding morphology, goiters may be classified either as the growth pattern or as the size of the growth:

Growth pattern

a. Uninodular (struma uninodosa): can be either inactive or a toxic nodule

b. Multinodular (struma nodosa): can likewise be inactive or toxic, the latter called toxic multinodular goitre

c. Diffuse (struma diffuse): the whole thyroid appearing to be enlarged.

Size

a. Class Ⅰ (palpation struma): in normal posture of the head, it cannot be seen; it is only found by palpation.

b. Class Ⅱ: the struma is palpative and can be easily seen.

c. Class Ⅲ: the struma is very large and is retrosternal; pressure results in compression marks.

② Cretinism: Cretinism is a very severe form of in utero brain damage due to iodine deficiency, marked by permanent mental retardation, and other developmental defects such as deaf-mutism, short stature and muscle spasticity.

• Types of cretinism.

There are two main types of cretinism-neurological cretinism and hypothyroid cretinism.

Neurological cretinism: Worldwide this is the common type in areas of severe iodine deficiency (Figure 3.13b). Neurological cretinism is characterised by mental retardation, deaf mutism, squint, spastic diplegia, and disorders of stance and gait.

Hypothyroid cretinism: Hypothyroid cretinism is less common and characterised by mental retardation, dwarfism, and hypothyroidism with associated physical symptoms. Severe or long-standing hypothyroidism is predominant in this type with the following features: dwarism, myxoedema, dry swollen or thickened skin, sparseness of hair and nails, deep hoarse voice, sexual retardation, retarded maturation of body parts, skeletal retardation, weak abdominal muscles, inactive bowel function and delayed tendon relexes. A typical feature is incomplete maturation of the face: wide-set eyes, saddle-nose deformity with retarded maturation of nasoorbital conigurations, mandibular atrophy and thickened lips (Figure 3.13c).

The different features of the two types are summarized in Table 3.12.

Table 3.12   Comparative Clinical Features in Neurological and Hypothyroid Cretinism

Features	Neurological Cretinism	Hypothyroid Cretinism
Mental retardation	Present, often severe	Present, less severe
Deaf mutism	Usually present	Absent
Cerebral diplegia	Often present	Absent
Squint	Often present	Absent
Stature	Usually normal	Severe growth Retardation usual
General feature	No physical signs	Coarse dry skin Husky voice
Reflexes	Excessively brisk	Delayed relaxation
ECG	Normal	Small voltage QRS Complexes and other abnormalities of hypothyroidism
X-ray limbs	Normal	Epiphyseal dysgenesis
Thyroid hormones	No effect	Improvement

Source: CHEN Z P, HETZEL B S. Cretinism Revisited[J]. Best Pract Res Clin Endocrinol Metlab, 2010, 24(1): 39-50.

• Iodine requirement.

Several methods have been used to estimate the requirement for iodine. Daily uptake and turnover of radioactive iodine can be used to estimate the requirement for iodine, provided that the subjects tested have adequate iodine status and are euthyroid. Table 3.13 shows recommendations for daily iodine intake by age group.

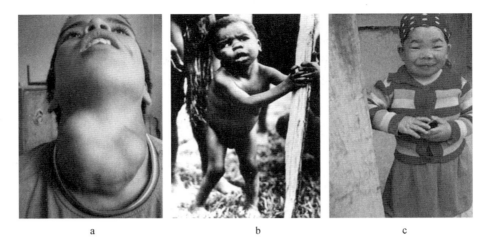

a   b   c

Figure 3. 13   a. Large nodular goiter in a 14-year-old boy photographed in 2004 in an area of severe IDD in northern Morocco, with tracheal and esophageal compression and hoarseness, likely due to damage to the recurrent laryngeal nerves. b. Child with severe neurological cretinism associated with brain damage, squint, deaf mutism and ataxia, as such that he is dependent on the stick he is holding (Papua New Guinea). c. Child with hypothyroid cretinism showing thickened features, dry skin and growth retardation (Xinjiang, China).

Table 3. 13   Recommendations for Iodine Intake by Age or Population Group

	Iodine Intake (μg per day)
US Institute of Medicine recommendations	
Infants 0—12 months *	110—130
Children 1—8 years	90
Children 9—13 years	120
Children ≥14 years+adults	150
Pregnancy	220
Lactation	290
WHO recommendations	
Children 0—5 years	90
Children 6—12 years	120
Children ≥12 years+adults	150
Pregnancy	250
Lactation	250

* Adequate intake.

Source: ZIMMERMANN M.B, JOOSTE P L, PANDAY C S. Indine-deficiency Disorders[J]. Lancet, 2008, 372(9645): 1251-1262.

● Assessment of iodine nutrition.

Four methods are generally recommended for assessment of iodine nutrition: urinary iodine concentration, goiter rate, serum TSH, and serum thyroglobulin. These indicators are complementary, in that urine iodine concentration is a sensitive indicator of recent iodine intake (days) and thyroglobulin shows an intermediate response (weeks to months), whereas changes in the goiter rate show long-term iodine nutrition (months to years).

● Prevention of cretinism.

a. Salt fortification with iodine: In nearly all regions affected by iodine deficiency, the most effective way to control iodine deficiency is through salt iodization. WHO/UNICEF/ICCIDD recommends that iodine is added at a level of 20−40 mg iodine/kg salt, depending on local salt intake. Iodine can be added to salt in the form of KI or potassiumiodate (KIO_3).

b. Other fortification vehicles: Bread can be an effective vehicle for iodine by including baker's salt enriched with iodine. Although iodizing drinking water or irrigation water can also be effective, the higher cost and the complexity of monitoring are the disadvantages. Iodine-containing milk is a major adventitious source in countries such as Switzerland and the United States, due to the use of iodophors in the dairy industry, rather than to the deliberate addition of iodine. In Finland, iodine-fortified animal fodder has increased the iodine content of foods derived from animal sources. In countries affected by IDD, whenever possible, iodine should be routinely added to complementary foods for weaning infants to provide approximately 90 μg of iodine per day.

c. Iodine supplementation: In some regions, iodization of salt may not be practical for control of iodine deficiency, at least in the short term. This may occur in remote areas where communications are poor or where there are numerous small-scale salt producers. In these areas, iodized oil supplements can be used. Iodized oil is prepared by esterification of the unsaturated fatty acids in seed or vegetable oils, and addition of iodine to the double bonds. Iodine can also be given as KI or KIO_3 in drops or tablets. Single oral doses of KI monthly (30 mg) or biweekly (8 mg) can provide adequate iodine for school-age children.

d. Education: Educate the public through various media (television, internet) to create awareness of the importance of iodine for health and consequences of inadequate iodine intake, especially for pregnant women, infants and children.

e. Propaganda: Let the public know which foods are rich in iodine.

● Toxic effects of excess iodine intake.

Iodine excess can also cause thyroid underactivity, because large amounts of iodine block the thyroid's ability to make hormone. Individuals vary widely in their tolerance to iodine. Most people can handle large amounts satisfactorily, but there are exceptions. People with a tendency towards so-called autoimmune thyroid diseases, such as Graves' disease or Hashimoto's thyroiditis, or who have family members with these problems, may be more sensitive to iodine. In fact, high iodine intakes in a population are associated with an increased incidence of these autoimmune thyroid diseases. Also, high levels of iodine in the population may increase the incidence of papillary thyroid cancer, although this is not well established.

3.4.1.2　Endemic Fluorosis

Endemic fluorosis is a form of damage to teeth and bones caused by an excessive intake of fluoride occurring in high level of fluoride regions.

(1) Fluorine

Fluorine is a highly toxic gas that usually occurs in combination with other elements, forming fluorides. At an estimated 0.065% of the Earth's crust, fluorine is roughly as plentiful as carbon, nitrogen, or chlorine. Many minerals contain small amounts of the element, and it is found in both sedimentary and igneous rocks. Typical concentrations of fluoride in soils are around 20—500 mg/kg. Fluoride in water is mostly of geological origin. Waters with high levels of fluoride content are mostly found at the foot of high mountains and in areas where the sea has made geological deposits. Concentrations in natural waters span more than four orders of magnitude, although values typically lie in the 0.1—10 mg/L range.

Well known fluoride belts on land include: one that stretches from Syria through Jordan, Egypt, Libya, Algeria, Sudan and Kenya, and another that stretches from Turkey through Iraq, Iran, Afghanistan, India, northern Thailand and China. There are similar belts in the Americas and Japan.

(2) Fluoride and Health

Fluorine is an essential trace element needed for the healthy development of teeth and bones. Deficiency in fluorine has long been linked to the incidence of dental caries. The detrimental effects of ingestion of excessive doses of fluorine are also well documented. Chronic ingestion of high doses has been linked to the development of dental fluorosis, and in extreme cases can lead to skeletal fluorosis.

(3) Prevalence and Endemic Area Type

The latest information shows that fluorosis is endemic in at least 25 countries around the world. The total number of people affected is unclear, but a conservative estimate will reach tens of millions. In 1993, 15 of India's 32 states were identified as endemic for fluorosis. In Mexico, 5 million people (about 6% of the population) are affected by fluoride in groundwater. Fluorosis is prevalent in some parts of central and western China, not only because of drinking fluoride in groundwater but also by breathing airborne fluoride released from the combustion of fluoride-containing coal. In addition, brick tea-type fluorosis was also discovered in China in 2000. The fluoride content in brick tea is very high, generally more than 100 mg/kg.

(4) Clinical Manifestations

Dental fluorosis is a developmental disturbance of dental enamel caused by excessive exposure to high concentrations of fluoride during tooth development. The H. T. Dean's

Index (Table 3.14) is used as a measurement of dental fluorosis (Figure 3.14). It was created in 1934 by H. T. Dean.

Table 3.14 H. T. Dean's Fluorosis Index

Classification	Description of Enamel
Normal	Smooth, glossy, pale creamy-white translucent surface
Questionable	A few white flecks or white spots
Very Mild	Small opaque, paper white areas covering less than 25% of the tooth surface
Mild	Opaque white areas covering less than 50% of the tooth surface
Moderate	All tooth surfaces affected; marked wear on biting surfaces; brown stain may be present
Severe	All tooth surfaces affected; discrete or confluent pitting; brown stain present

Source: DEAN H T. The Investigation of Physiological Effects by the Epidemiological Method (Report No. 44) [R]. Washington, DC: American Association for the Advancement of Science, 1942.

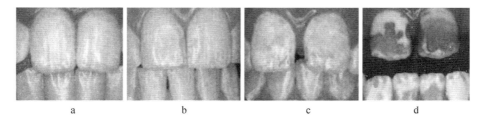

a   b   c   d

Figure 3.14 Dental Fluorosis

a. Mild with slight accentuation of the perikymata; b. Moderate, showing a white opaque appearance; c. Moderate, white opaque enamel with some discoloration and pitting; d. Severe.
Source: DENBESTEN P, LI W. Chronic Fluoride Toxicity: Dental Fluorosis[J]. Monogr Ord Sci, 2011, 22:81-96.

Skeletal fluorosis is a bone disease caused by excessive consumption of fluoride. In advanced cases, skeletal fluorosis causes pain and damage to bones and joints (Figure 3.15, Figure 3.16).

Skeletal fluorosis has a number of stages (Table 3.15).

Table 3.15 Stages of Skeletal Fluorosis

Osteosclerotic Phase	Symptoms and Signs
Normal Bone	Normal
Preclinical Phase	Asymptomatic; slight radiographically-detectable increases in bone mass
Clinical Phase I	Sporadic pain; stiffness of joints; osteosclerosis of pelvis and vertebral spine
Clinical Phase II	Chronic joint pain; arthritic symptoms; slight calcification of ligaments' increased osteosclerosis and cancellous bones; with/without osteoporosis of long bones
Clinical Phase III	Limitation of joint movement; calcification of ligaments of neck vertebral column; crippling deformities of the spine and major joints; muscle wasting; neurological defects/compression of spinal cord

Source: http://en.wikipedia.org/wiki/Skeletal_fluorosis.

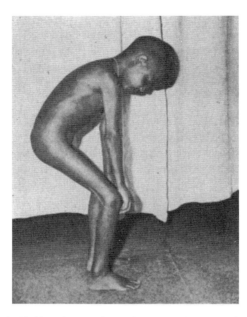

Figure 3. 15　A Child with Crippling Fluorosis, Showing Clinical Invalisism with
Marked Deformities of the Sine and Joints.

Source: TEOTIA M,TEOTIA S P, KUNWAR K B. Endemic Skeletal Fluorosis[J].
Arch Dis Child, 1971, 46(249): 686-691.

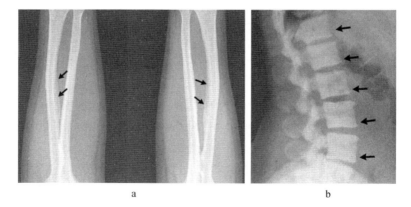

a　　　　　　　　　　　　　　　　　　　b

Figure 3. 16　Skeletal Fluorosis Interosseous Membrane Calcifications (Panel A, arrows), and
Radiography of the Spine Revealed a Tuggerjersey Appearance (Striated Pattern of Increased Density in the
Upper and Lower Zones of the Vertebrae) (Panel B, arrows).

Source: KAKUMANU N, RAO S D. Images in Clinical Medicine: Skeletal Fluorosis due to
Excessive Tea Drinking[J]. N Engl J Med. , 2013, 368(12):1140.

(5) Recommendations of Water Fluoride

Drinking water is particularly sensitive because large variations in fluoride concentration
exist in water supplies in different areas. Table 3. 16 shows guideline values for fluoride in
drinking water.

Table 3.16　Guideline Values for Fuoride in Drinking Water in Diverse Institutions/Nations

Institution/nation	Limit/guideline	Value (mg/L)	Comment
WHO	Guideline value(GV)	1.5	2004 guidelines
U.S. EPA	Primary standard	4	Enforceable
U.S. EPA	Secondary standard	2	Guideline to protect against dental fluorosis; not enforceable
EC	Maximum permissible value	1.5	1998 regulations
Canada	National standard	1.5	No comment
India	National standard	1	Lowered from 1.5 mg/L in 1998
China	National standard	1	No comment
Tanzania	National standard	8	Interim standard

(6) Prevention

① Removal of excessive fluoride from drinking-water is difficult and costly. The preferred option is to find a supply of safe drinking-water with safe fluoride levels. Where access to safe water is already limited, de-fluoridation may be the only solution. Methods include: use of bone charcoal, contact precipitation, use of Nalgonda or activated alumina (Nalgonda is called after the town in South India, near Hyderabad, where the aluminium sulfate-based defluoridation was first set up at a water works level).

② In coal-born fluorosis regions, improved stoves or avoid using high-fluoride coal is recommended.

③ A low-fluoride brick tea is suggested for tea drinkers, alternatively they should adapt to preparing tea using tender leaves that contain lower fluoride levels.

3.4.1.3　Endemic Arseniasis

Arsenicosis is a chronic health condition arising from prolonged ingestion (not less than 6 months) of arsenic above a safe dose, usually manifested by characteristic skin lesions in high levels of arsenic areas.

(1) Arsenic and Arsenicosis Prevalence

Arsenic (As) is a naturally occurring element widely distributed in the Earth's crust. In the environment, arsenic is combined with oxygen, chlorine, and sulfur to form inorganic arsenic compounds. Arsenic occurs naturally in soil and minerals and may enter the air, water, and land from wind-blown dust and may get into water from runoff and leaching. As has two primary oxidation states: As^{3+} and As^{5+}. The average abundance in the earth's crust is $1-2$ mg/kg. Excepting localized sources of anthropogenic contamination, the highest aqueous arsenic concentrations tend to be found in groundwater because of natural water-rock interaction processes and the high solid/solution ratios found in aquifers. Groundwater therefore poses the greatest overall threat to health.

Over 137 million people in more than 70 countries are probably affected by arsenic poisoning from drinking water. Exposure to groundwater with high levels of As has been reported in Argentina, Chile, China, Ghana, Hungary, India, Mexico, Thailand, the United Kingdom, and the United States. In China, over 2 million people live in areas of high geological As concentrations (drinking water and combustion of coal with high concentrations of As), and more than 17,000 arsenicosis patients in 21 counties of five provinces or Autonomous Regions have been identified.

(2) Arsenic and Health

① Effects of short-term exposure: The substance may cause effects on the gastrointestinal tract, resulting in severe gastroenteritis, loss of fluid, and electrolytes, cardiac disorders, shock and convulsions. Exposure far above the OEL may result in death. The effects may be delayed. Medical observation is indicated.

② Effects of long-term or repeated exposure: The substance may have effects on the skin, mucous membranes, peripheral nervous system, liver and bone marrow, resulting in pigmentation disorders (Figure 3.17), hyperkeratosis, perforation of nasal septum, neuropathy, anaemia, and liver impairment. This substance is carcinogenic to humans. Animal tests show that this substance possibly causes toxicity to human reproduction or development.

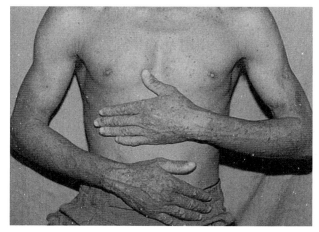

Figure 3.17 Rain-Drop Pigmentation on the Trunk, along with Arsenical Hyperkeratosis Affecting the Dorsa of Hands, Fingers, and Forearm

Source: DAS N K, SENGUPTA S R. Arsenicosis: Diagnosis and Treatment[J]. Indian J Dermatol Venereol Leprol, 2008, 74(6): 571-581.

(3) Diagnosis.

WHO has not yet included the systemic manifestations as diagnostic hallmarks. Residence of the affected person in an endemic zone is an important diagnostic criterion. Consumption of drinking water or contaminated food with an arsenic concentration more than the prevailing national standard for at least 6 months is essential for establishment of elevated exposure to arsenic.

The clinical and laboratory criteria are both essential for the diagnosis of arsenicosis, but principally it can be diagnosed on the basis of its cutaneous manifestations. Melanosis and keratosis are suggested to be the most important marker for detection of arsenicosis at an early stage. Presence of Bowen's disease or squamous/basal cell carcinoma also serves as diagnostic clue for arsenicosis.

Tests are available to diagnose poisoning by measuring arsenic in blood, urine, hair, and fingernails. The urine test is the most reliable test for arsenic exposure within the last few days. Urine test needs to be done within 24—48 hours for an accurate analysis of an acute exposure. Tests on hair and fingernails can measure exposure to high levels of arsenic over the past 6—12 months. These tests can determine if one has been exposed to above-average levels of arsenic.

(4) Treatment

Till date, no effective cure is known. Symptomatic and supportive treatments are mainly used in the clinical practice.

(5) Prevention

① Cessation of exposure to high-level As in drinking water or coal combustion: Finding safe water sources having arsenic level below the 'maximum permissible limit' remains the prime objective. Safe water sources include deep wells, treatment of surface water, and rainwater harvesting. Improved stoves can be used in coal burning areas.

② Removing arsenic from the contaminated water: Many new methodologies are being developed for removing the arsenic content in the water, but they have not yet passed the test of time.

③ Administration of nutritional supplement: People should be encouraged to take food of high calorific value from either animal or plant source. Consumption of polyphenols and extracts of green and black tea have antioxidant effects.

(6) Recommendations

The WHO guideline value for arsenic in drinking water is 0.01 mg/L. Countries which are the worst affected, like India, Bangladesh and China are still following the previous guideline of 0.05 mg/L.

3.4.2 Soil Pollution and Health

Sanitary state of the soil is intimately related to human health. Soil pollution is caused by the presence of xenobiotic chemicals or other alterations in the natural soil environment. It is typically caused by industrial activities, agricultural chemicals, or improper disposals of waste. The most prominent chemical groups of organic contaminants are fuel hydrocarbons, polynuclear aromatic hydrocarbons (PAHs), polychlorinated biphenyls (PCBs), chlorinated aromatic compounds, detergents, and pesticides. Inorganic pollutants include nitrates, phosphates, and heavy metals such as cadmium, chromium, lead, and thallium. There are also some radioactive substances in the soil. If they fail to be completely destroyed by the process of soil self-purification or by sanitary measures adopted in disposing them, they will in turn pollute food and water, and hence will affect human health.

Soil pollution can lead to water pollution if toxic chemicals leach into groundwater, or if contaminated runoff reaches streams, lakes, or oceans. Soil also naturally contributes to air pollution by releasing volatile compounds into the atmosphere. Nitrogen escapes through ammonia volatilization and denitrification. The decomposition of organic materials in soil can release sulfur dioxide and other sulfur compounds, causing acid rain. Heavy metals and other potentially toxic elements are the most serious soil pollutants in sewage. Sewage sludge contains heavy metals and, if applied repeatedly or in large amounts, the treated soil may accumulate heavy metals and consequently become unable to even support plant life. Heavy metal pollution is covert, persistent and irreversible. In addition, chemicals that are not water soluble contaminate plants that grow on polluted soils, and they also tend to accumulate increasingly toward the top of the food chain.

3. 4. 2. 1　Cadmium Poisoning

Cadmium (Cd) is a soft, ductile, silver-white or bluish-white natural element in the Earth's crust. It is usually found as a mineral combined with other elements such as oxygen, chlorine, or sulfur. All soils and rocks, including coal and mineral fertilizers, contain some cadmium. Cadmium is an extremely toxic metal. The IARC classified cadmium as a human carcinogen. In the natural environment, cadmium concentration is generally low. Some typical levels of the natural occurrence of cadmium are as follows: atmosphere 0. 1 to 5. 0 ng/m^3, Earth's crust 0. 1 to 0. 5 mg/g, marine sediments 1 mg/g, and sea water 0. 1 mg/L.

Cadmium is used in pigments, coatings, stabilizers, specialty alloys and electronic compounds, but mostly (about 85%) in rechargeable nickel-cadmium batteries. Environmental exposure levels to cadmium, that are substantially above the background, occur in areas with current or historical industrial contamination, for instance, in regions of Belgium, Sweden, UK, Japan, and China.

Exposure to cadmium occurs through consumption of contaminated food or water, or by inhalation of polluted air. Occupational exposures are found in industries such as electroplating, welding, smelting and refining, pigment production, and battery manufacturing. Other respiratory exposures to cadmium can occur through inhalation of cigarette smoke or indoor dust contaminated with cadmium.

Environmental exposure to cadmium had been particularly problematic in Japan where many people have consumed rice that was grown in cadmium contaminated irrigation water. This phenomenon is known as itai-itai disease (Figure 3. 18). Itai-itai disease was the name given to the mass cadmium poisoning of Toyama Prefecture, Japan, starting around 1912. The term "itai-itai disease" was coined by locals for the severe pain. People with the condition felt severe pain in the spine and joints.

(1) Health Effects

Effects of short-term exposure: The fume is irritating to the respiratory tract.

Inhalation of fume may cause lung edema and metal fume fever. The effects may be delayed. Medical observation is indicated.

Effects of long-term or repeated exposure: One of the main effects of cadmium poisoning is weak and brittle bones. Spinal and leg pain is common, and a waddling gait often develops due to bone deformities caused by the cadmium. The pain eventually becomes debilitating, with fractures becoming more common as the bone weakens. Other complications include coughing, anemia, and kidney failure, leading to death. Cadmium is carcinogenic to humans.

(2) Diagnosis

According to the exact cadmium contact history, typical clinical manifestations, the reference of cadmium in blood/urine or other biological materials, determination of cadmium in, diagnosis of cadmium poisoning can be given.

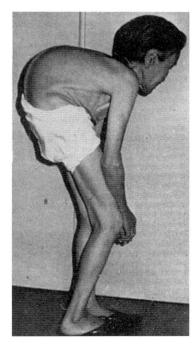

Figure 3.18   Itai-itai Disease with Severe Bone Deformity

Increased concentrations of urinary β2-Microglobulin can be an early indicator of renal dysfunction in persons chronically exposed to low but excessive levels of environmental cadmium. Blood or urine cadmium concentrations provide a better index of excessive exposure in acute poisoning. Cadmium concentrations in healthy persons without excessive cadmium exposure are generally less than 1 $\mu g/L$ in either blood or urine. Persons who have sustained renal damage due to chronic cadmium exposure often have blood or urine cadmium levels in a range of 25—50 $\mu g/L$ or 25—75 $\mu g/g$ creatinine, respectively.

(3) Treatment

There is no effective treatment for cadmium toxicity. Symptomatic and supportive treatments are mainly used in clinical salvage.

3.4.2.2   Thallium Poisoning

Elemental thallium (Tl) is a blue-white metal found in small amounts in the Earth's crust. It can combine with other substances such as bromine, chlorine, fluorine, and iodine. When it's combined, it appears colorless-to-white or yellow. In the past, thallium was obtained as a by-product of smelting other metals; however, it has not been specifically mined or refined in the United States since 1984. It is still used in relatively small amounts in pharmaceutical and electronics manufacturing, the latter being the current major industrial consumer of thallium.

Thallium enters the environment primarily from coal-burning and smelting, in which it is a trace contaminant of the raw materials. It stays in the air, water, and soil for a long time and is not broken down. Some thallium compounds are removed from the atmosphere in rain and snow.

Eating food contaminated with thallium may be a major source of exposure for most people. Other sources include: breathing workplace air in industries that use thallium; smoking cigarettes; living near hazardous waste sites containing thallium; touching or, for children, eating soil contaminated with thallium; breathing low levels in air and water. Endemic Tl poisoning occurred in southwestern China due to Tl contamination in local drinking water and vegetables surrounding the Tl-rich sulfide mineralized areas.

(1) Health Effect

Effects of short-term exposure: Thallium may cause effects on the gastrointestinal tract, nervous system, kidneys and cardiovascular system. It may also cause hair loss and atrophy of nails. Exposure may result in death when ingested. The effects may be delayed. Medical observation is indicated.

Effects of long-term or repeated exposure: Most harmful effects of Thallium were cause by chronic exposure of this element. The main effects include: ①peripheral nerve damage; ②visual impairment or even blindness; ③hair loss; ④teratogenicity and mutagenicity.

(2) Diagnosis

According to the exact thallium contact history, typical clinical manifestations, the reference of thallium in urine or other biological materials, determination of thallium in, and exclusion of other causes of peripheral neuropathy, diagnosis of thallium poisoning are generally not difficult.

(3) Treatment

Thallium poisoning is not reversible. No specific therapeutic has been found, symptomatic and supportive treatments are mainly used in clinical salvage. Prussian blue (six cyanide iron potassium ferrate) is commonly used in clinical treatment.

3.4.2.3 Soil Pollution Control

Numerous attempts are being made to decontaminate polluted soils, including an array of both in situ (on-site, in the soil) and off-site (removal of contaminated soil for treatment) techniques. None of these is ideal for remediating contaminated soils, and often, more than one of the techniques may be necessary to optimize the cleanup effort.

The most common decontamination method for polluted soils is to remove the soil and deposit it in landfills or to incinerate it. These methods, however, often exchange one problem for another: landfilling merely confines the polluted soil while doing little to decontaminate it, and incineration removes toxic organic chemicals from the soil, but subsequently releases them into the air, in the process causing air pollution.

For the removal and recovery of heavy metals, various soil washing techniques have been developed including physical methods, such as attrition scrubbing and wet-screening, and chemical methods consisting of treatments with organic and inorganic acids, bases, salts and chelating agents. For example, chemicals used to extract radionuclides and toxic metals include hydrochloric, nitric, phosphoric and citric acids, sodium carbonate and sodium hydroxide and the chelating agents EDTA and DTPA. The problem with these methods, however, is again that they generate secondary waste products that may require additional hazardous waste treatments.

In contrast to the previously described methods, in situ methods are used directly at the contamination site. In this case, soil does not need to be excavated, and therefore the chance of causing further environmental harm is minimized. In situ biodegradation involves the enhancement of naturally occurring microorganisms by artificially stimulating their numbers and activity. The microorganisms then assist in degrading the soil contaminants. A number of environmental, chemical, and management factors affect the biodegradation of soil pollutants, including moisture content, pH, temperature, the existing microbial community, and the availability of nutrients. Biodegradation is facilitated by aerobic soil conditions and soil pH in the neutral range (between pH 5.5 to 8.0), with an optimum reading occurring at approximately pH 7, and a temperature in the range of 20℃ to 30℃. These physical parameters can be influenced, thereby promoting the microorganisms' ability to degrade chemical contaminants. Of all the decontamination methods, bioremediation appears to be the least damaging and most environmentally acceptable technique.

（Sun Xiance, Wang Xiaoke, Wang Jintao, Wu Jiguo, Zhao Ran, Wu Dongmei）

Exercises

Chapter 4　Occupational Environment and Health

4.1　Introduction

Occupational health is concerned with health in its relation to work and the working environment, both physically and mentally. The International Labor Organization (ILO)/ WHO Committee on occupational health (at its first session in 1950 and revised at its twelfth session in 1995) decided upon broad definition: "Occupational health should aim at the promotion and maintenance of the highest degree of physical, mental and social well-being of workers in all occupations." Occupational health may be defined as the maintenance of the individual worker's state of well-being and freedom from occupationally-related disease or injury. Occupational health has gradually developed from a mono-disciplinary, risk-oriented activity to a multi-disciplinary and comprehensive approach that considers an individual's physical, mental and social well-being, general health and personal development. Occupational hygiene is the practice whereby this is achieved.

As a multidisciplinary activity, occupational health aims at: ① protection and promotion of the health of workers through preventing and controlling occupational diseases and injuries; ② development and promotion of healthy and safe work, work environments and work organizations; ③ enhancement of physical, mental and social well-being of workers; ④ support and promotion of their working capacity, as well as professional and social development at work; ⑤ enabling workers to conduct socially and economically productive lives and to contribute positively to sustainable development.

4.1.1　Interaction of Work and Health

The social and economic importance of work receives considerable attention, because a primary function of work in any society is to produce and distribute goods and services. Far less attention is paid to the importance of work to the individual, yet it is clear from recent research that work plays a crucial and perhaps unparalleled psychological role in the formation of self-esteem and a sense of order. Work is a powerful force in shaping a person's sense of identity. It can lend vitality to existence and establish the cyclical patterns of day, week, month and year. It is believed that work, for which there is no economic gain, such as child care, care for the aged and voluntary work, also has its rewards and contributes to personal gratification.

There is a continuous two-way interaction between a person and the physical and psychological working environment: the work environment may influence the person's health either positively or negatively and productivity is, in turn, influenced by the worker's state of physical and mental well-being. Work, when it is well-adjusted and productive, can be an important factor in health promotion, e. g. partially disabled workers may be rehabilitated by undertaking tasks suited to their physical and mental limitations and, in this way, may substantially increase their working capacity. However, the potential positive influence of work on health has not yet been fully exploited; knowledge of work physiology and ergonomics needs to be further developed and applied to benefit worker's health. When work is associated with health hazards, it may cause occupational diseases, and become one of the multiple causes of other diseases or may aggravate existing ill-health of non-occupational origin. In developing countries, where work is becoming increasingly mechanized, a number of work processes have been developed that treat workers as production tools, putting their health and lives at risk. The occupational health lessons learned during the Industrial Revolution should be borne in mind in planning for improved occupational health in developing countries.

4. 1. 2　Classification of Occupational Hazards

Occupational Hazards is source or situation with a potential for harm in terms of injury or ill health, damage to property, damage to the workplace environment. People at work face a variety of hazards owing to chemicals, physical factors, biological agents, adverse ergonomic conditions, and varied psychosocial factors. Exposure to occupational hazards may have adverse effects on human health. A worker may be exposed to multi-types of hazards, depending on occupation types.

4. 1. 2. 1　Chemical Hazards

Chemicals represent the greatest number of hazards to workplace health. The category of chemicals includes many naturally-occurring substances, such as minerals and cotton, as well as both simple and complex manufactured chemical products. Chemical exposure can be the result of direct use or from by-products. Exposure to chemical hazards may occur through inhalation of airborne contaminants or skin contact. These chemicals are classified according to their physical state, chemical composition or physiological action.

(1) Gases and Vapours

① Asphyxiants: Asphyxiants can cause asphyxia either by replacing oxygen or by other mechanisms. They are classified into: simple asphyxiants and chemical asphyxiants. Simple asphyxiants replace oxygen in the air, e. g. nitrogen, hydrogen and carbon dioxide.

② Irritant gases: They can cause irritation or inflammation of the mucous membranes with which they come into contact. This property depends on their degree of solubility in water.

③ Organometallic compounds.

Arsine (AsH_3): produced during chemical treatment of metals if arsenic is present as an impurity due to nascent hydrogen. It is colourless and has a garlic odour. Exposure results in haemolysis, anaemia, jaundice and anuria in severe cases.

Nickel carbonyl [$Ni(C)O_4$]: a volatile liquid produced during the extraction of nickel, inhalation causes severe pulmonary irritation.

④ Anaesthetic vapours: Many of these have some other systemic effects as well and tend to accumulate in low, closed, poorly ventilated places.

(2) Metals

In industry, metal poisoning usually takes the chronic form and results from the absorption of small amounts over long periods of time. Acute poisoning may result from accidental (or suicidal) intake of large doses of some of the more toxic compounds (like arsenicals).

Metals and their compounds gain access into the body by inhalation, ingestion and, in a few cases, through the skin. A large number of metallic compounds are used in industries with the following being some of the more important.

(3) Organic Solvents

Organic solvents are organic liquids in which substances can be dissolved without changing their chemical composition. They are used in the extraction of oils and fats in the food industries, chemical industry, paint, varnishes, enamel, in degreasing process, dry cleaning, printing and dying in the textile and rayon industries. Organic solvents are volatile: many are inflammable and are considered as fire hazards. Solvents are absorbed mainly through the lungs, *via* the gastrointestinal tract if administered orally, and many of them can be absorbed *via* intact skin.

If the work atmosphere is dusty, dust will inevitably be inhaled. Dust particles below five microns in diameter are called respirable since they have the chance to penetrate to the alveoli. In a dusty environment, a significant amount of dust can be retained in the lungs.

Pneumoconiosis is disabling pulmonary fibrosis that results from the inhalation of various types of inorganic dust, such as silica, asbestos, coal, talc and china clay, e. g. silicosis and asbestosis.

(4) Pesticides

Pesticides are a group of chemicals used to destroy various kinds of pests including insects, rodents, weeds, snails, fungi, etc. The degree of toxicity of different pesticides varies greatly from deadly poisons to slightly harmful pesticides. Exposure to pesticides occurs in industries where the pesticides are manufactured and formulated, and during their application in agriculture. Pesticides are also used at home.

They are classified into several groups, according to their chemical composition. The most frequently used nowadays are organophosphates, carbamates and thiocarbamates, pyrethroids and organochlorine pesticides. Other groups include lead arsenate, organic mercury, thallium compounds, coumarin, bromomethane, cresols, phenols, nicotine, zinc phosphide, etc. Pesticides are absorbed *via* the lungs, gastrointestinal tract and sometimes through the intact skin and eyes (organophosphates).

4. 1. 2. 2   Physical Hazards

All workplaces result in exposure to physical agents which could be harmful, including heat, noise, vibration, repetitive movements, light and other radiation. Increasing mechanisation may decrease heat stress, but increases in industrialisation and greater use of high technology can be accompanied by new hazards.

(1) Noise

Noise is unwanted sound. Workers are exposed to noise in textile and glass industries, ship building, aeroplane manufacturing, engineering industries, manufacture of boilers and pressure vessels, and power plants. Noise is absorbed though the ear; some very low frequency (infrasound) and ultra-sonic sounds are absorbed directly by the body. The effects of noise include two types: One is auditory effect (temporary or permanent hearing loss) and the other is non-auditory effects (nervousness, fatigue, interference with communication by speech, decreased efficiency and annoyance). The degree of injury from exposure to noise depends on a number of factors such as intensity and frequency range, duration of exposure, and individual susceptibility.

(2) Vibration

Workers exposed to whole vibrations include tractor drivers, transport workers, workers involved in drilling for petroleum and those in the textile industry. Whole body vibrations cause various ailments related to congestion of pelvic and abdominal organs.

Segmental vibrations affect workers using pneumatic vibrating tools such as drills and hammers in mining, road construction, shoe manufacture and sawing. Vibration usually affects the hands and arms. Vascular changes in the upper limbs lead to "dead hands" and "white fingers". Exposure to vibration can injure joints of hands, elbow and shoulder joints.

(3) Light

The workers may be exposed to poor or excess illumination. The acute effects of poor illumination include eye strain, eye pain, headache, tearing and eye fatigue. The chronic effects on health include "miners' nystagmus". Exposure to excessive brightness or "glare" is strongly associated with discomfort, annoyance and visual fatigue. Intense direct glare may also result in blurring of vision and lead to accidents. There should be sufficient and suitable lighting, natural or artificial, wherever persons are working.

(4) Heat and Cold

Heat is a common health hazard in industries. The direct effects of heat exposure are heat stroke (sun stroke), burns and heat cramps. Indirect effects of heat are decreased efficiency, increased fatigue and increased chances of accidents. Many industries have local "hot spots"—ovens and furnaces, which radiate strong heat. Radiant heat is the main problem in foundry, glass and steel industries, while heat stagnation is the principal problem in jute and cotton textile. Physical work under such conditions is very stressful and impairs the health and efficiency of the workers. For gainful work involving sustained and repeated effort, a reasonable temperature must be maintained in the work room. Important hazards associated with cold work are chilblains, erythrocyanosis, immersion foot, and frostbite as a result of cutaneous vasoconstriction. General hypothermia is not unusual.

(5) Electromagnetic Non-ionizing Radiation

Ultraviolet radiation in industries like welding can hurt the eyes and can cause conjunctivitis known as "welder's flash". Symptoms of welder's flash are redness of eyes and pain, but disappear in a few days without any permanent damage to the eyes.

Infrared radiation exposure occurs in front of furnaces, in steel mills, in the glass industries, in blacksmiths and in chain manufacture. Exposure of the eyes can cause cataracts or corneal affection. Skin burns can also occur. Complete protection of the eyes can be achieved by wearing special goggles.

(6) Ionizing Radiation

Sources of radiation include radioactive isotopes and X-ray machines. Ionizing radiation is used in medicine, industry, agriculture, research, and atomic warfare. Radiations are either electromagnetic waves, like X-rays and gamma rays, or minute particles, such as alpha, beta and neutrons. Both types cause ionization or excitation of atoms which leads to tissue damage. The effect of ionizing irradiation depends on the dose, type of radiation, whether exposure was continuous or interrupted or it was total body or localized, as well as the type of tissue irradiated. The power of penetration of different types of radiation varies from very high, such as X-ray and gamma ray radiation, to very low, such as alpha radiation. The radiation hazards comprise genetic changes, malformation, cancer, leukaemia, depilation, ulceration, sterility and in extreme cases death. The International Commission of Radiological Protection has set the maximum permissible level of whole body occupational exposure at 5 Rem per year.

4.1.2.3 Biology Hazards

Some workers are subject to health hazards relating to work with biological materials or from working in environments where micro-organisms may abound. These hazards may arise from animal or plant materials, or sometimes the handling or treatment of sick persons. A few biological hazards (e.g. Legionella) exist more widely and affect members of the general working community. Human diseases caused by work associated exposure to microbial agents, e.g. bacteria, viruses, rickettsia, fungi and parasites (helminthes, protozoa), are called occupational infections. An infection is described as occupational when some aspect of the work involves contact with biologically active organisms. Exposure occurs among health care workers in fever outpatient department and laboratories; among veterinarians and agricultural workers in animal husbandry and dairy farms, and pet shops; and among sewerage workers, wool sorters and workers in the leather industry.

4.1.2.4 Ergonomic Hazards

The science of ergonomics studies and evaluates a full range of tasks including, but not limited to, lifting, holding, pushing, walking and reaching. Many ergonomic problems result from technological changes, such as increased assembly line speeds, adding specialized tasks, and increased repetition. Some problems arise from poorly designed job tasks. Any of these conditions can cause ergonomic hazards, such as excessive vibration, noise, eye strain, repetitive motion, heavy lifting problems, poorly designed tools or work areas.

4. 1. 2. 5　Psychosocial Hazards

The psychosocial hazards arise from the workers' failure to adapt to an alien psychosocial environment. Frustration, lack of job satisfaction, insecurity, poor human relationships, emotional tension are the psychosocial factors which may undermine both physical and mental health of the workers. The health effects can be classified in two main categories: psychological and behavioral changes, and psychosomatic illness. The former include hostility, aggressiveness, anxiety, depression, tardiness, alcoholism, drug abuse, sickness absenteeism, and the latter include fatigue, headache; pain in the shoulders, neck and back; propensity to peptic ulcer, hypertension, heart disease and rapid aging.

The physical factors (heat, noise, poor lighting) play a major role in adding to or precipitating mental disorders among workers. The increasing stress on automation, electronic operations and nuclear energy may introduce newer psychosocial health problems in industry. Psychosocial hazards are therefore assumed to be more harmful than physical or chemical hazards.

4. 1. 3　Occupational Adverse Effects

Exposure to occupational hazards may adversely threaten human health. Adverse effects range from asymptomatic physiological and biochemical changes to symptoms of illness, diagnosed diseases, and even death. For some risk factors there is a very clear connection between the exposure and the disease. For example, the primary route of exposure to airborne particulates, gases and vapors is by inhalation, whereby these agents gain access to the respiratory system and are either deposited (in the case of particulates) or enter the circulatory system (gases and vapours). An exposure may cause multiple adverse health outcomes. For instance, exposure to asbestos can result in malignant conditions of the lung, pleura, or peritoneum, and nonmalignant conditions of the lung (asbestosis).

4. 1. 3. 1　Occupational Disease

(1) Definition of Occupational Diseases

There are several definitions for the term "occupational disease". Occupational diseases are adverse health conditions in human being, the occurrence or severity of which is related to exposure to factors on the job or in the work environment. However, for the purpose of the Protocol of 2002 to the Occupational Safety and Health Convention of International Labor Organization (ILO), the term "occupational disease" covers any disease contracted as a result of an exposure to risk factors arising from work activity. The ILO Employment

Injury Benefits Recommendation defines occupational diseases more precisely in the following terms: "Each member should, under prescribed conditions, regard diseases known to arise out of the exposure to substances and dangerous conditions in processes, trades or occupations as occupational diseases." The various definitions, however, have two main mandatory elements in common. The causal relationship between exposure in a specific working environment or work activity and a specific disease; and, the fact that the disease occurs among the group of exposed persons with a higher frequency rate than in the rest of the population, or in other worker populations.

The causal relationship is established on the basis of clinical and/or pathological data, occupational background and job analysis, identification and evaluation of occupational risk factors and of the role of other risk factors. As a general rule, the symptoms are not sufficiently characteristic to allow an occupational disease to be diagnosed without the knowledge of the physical, chemical, biological and/or other risk factors encountered in the exercise of an occupation. The recognition of an occupational disease is a specific example of clinical decision-making or applied clinical epidemiology. Diagnosis of an occupational disease is not a "pure clinical medical science" but rather a judgment based on a critical review of all the available evidence. This should include the strength of association, consistency, specificity, time sequence or biological gradient (the greater the level and duration of the exposure, the greater the severity of the diseases or their incidence).

Reportable occupational diseases is referred to as occupational diseases mentioned in national lists as part of national laws or administrative provisions liable for compensation and subject to prevention measures. Reported occupational diseases are reportable diseases already passed through the legally required reporting process.

(2) Definition of Prescribed Occupational Disease

Certain occupational diseases are prescribed as occupational by law and are thus presumed to be occupational in origin. A prescribed occupational disease is one that has developed because of the type of work you do. It also includes any condition resulting from the disease. In China, if one is suffering from a prescribed occupational disease, he or she may qualify for payment under the Occupational Diseases Prevention and Control Act, P. R. China.

According to the Occupational Diseases Prevention and Control Act, P. R. China, which has been put into effect since May 1st 2002, the List of the Prescribed Occupational Diseases is renewed as follows (No. 132 in 10 categories): Pneumoconiosis, Ionizing Radiation-induced Occupational Illness, Occupational Poisonings, Physical Agents-induced Occupational Diseases, Biological Agents-induced Occupational Diseases, Occupational Dermatoses, Occupational Eye Diseases, Occupational Ear, Nose and Throat Diseases, Occupational Cancers, Other Occupational Diseases.

(3) Characteristics of Occupational Diseases

Five common characteristics for occupational diseases can be summarized: ①

Occupational factors contribute the main cause of the disease, after controlling or eliminating the corresponding occupational harmful factors, the incidence can be reduced or eliminated. ② Most of the causes are detectable, and a dose-response relationship exists between exposure and incidence. ③ Workers exposed to the same occupational factors have often a certain incidence, rarely only individual patients. ④ Most occupational diseases have no effective treatment at present, the later they are found, the worse the curative effect will be. ⑤ Early detection and timely treatment are all beneficial for the recovery and prognosis of the diseases. However, from the etiological point of view, occupational diseases are completely preventable.

4.1.3.2　Work-related Diseases

Work-related diseases are defined as all illnesses that can be caused, worsened or jointly caused by working conditions. A case of work-related illness does not necessarily refer to recognition by an authority whereas occupational diseases have a specific or a strong relation to the occupation, generally with only one causal agent while work-related diseases have a complex etiology. Among their multiple causal agents, factors arising from the work and/or working environment play a role in the development of such diseases. A more precise distinction between occupational diseases and work-related diseases can be made by evaluating their attributable fractions. It is suggested that the attributable fraction of occupational diseases is more than 50% from the work and/or working environment and less than 50% for work-related diseases.

This category has certain characteristics which were identified and stated by a WHO Expert Committee as follows: "Multifactorial diseases", which may frequently be work-related, also occur among the general population, and working conditions and exposures need not be risk factors in each case of any one disease. However, when such diseases affect the worker, they may be work-related in a number of ways: they may be partially caused by adverse working conditions; they may be aggravated, accelerated or exacerbated by workplace exposures; and they may impair working capacity. It is important to remember that personal characteristics, other environmental and sociocultural factors usually play a role as risk factors for these diseases.

Multifactorial "work-related" diseases are often more common than occupational diseases and therefore deserve adequate attention by the health service infrastructure, which incorporates the occupational health services. The work-related diseases which deserve particular attention include behavioral and psychosomatic disorders, hypertension, coronary heart disease, peptic ulcers, chronic nonspecific respiratory disease, and locomotor disorders.

4.1.4　Diagnostic Principles of Occupational Diseases

People face numerous hazards at workplaces, which may result in injuries, hearing loss, cancer, and respiratory, cardiovascular, musculoskeletal, skin, reproductive, neurological and mental disorders. Classifications of occupational diseases have been developed mainly for two purposes: ① notification for labor safety and health surveillance and ② compensation. The majority of the classification systems have the following hierarchy: ③ Diseases classified by occupational hazards, including chemical hazards, physical hazards, biological hazards, etc. ; ④ Diseases classified by target organs, including occupational respiratory diseases, occupational skin diseases, occupational musculoskeletal diseases, occupational cancer, etc.

The classifications contain both categories defined by the causative agent and categories defined by the medical diagnosis. Cases of a given disease may therefore fall into several categories. The absence of general diagnostic criteria and classification reduce the compatibility and comparability of national statistics on occupational diseases. Even for classical occupational diseases like asbestosis, there is heterogeneity in the national statistics and clinical practice in what kind of conditions are coded under the general heading of asbestosis.

Occupational diseases span a broad range of human illnesses, many of which clinically and pathologically are not different from those of non-occupational origins. They are contracted as a result of exposure to risk factors resulting, at least partially, from work activities. The diagnosis of occupational diseases can rarely be established on clinical grounds alone. It is essential to reveal the link between occupation and disease because of the employers' responsibility to prevent occupational diseases and the compensation of ill workers. However, the list of reportable occupational diseases, as well as the related compensation systems, differs from country to country, making comparisons considerably more difficult.

In occupational disease diagnosis, a comprehensive analysis of the following factors shall be conducted: ① the occupational history of a patient; ② a history of exposures to occupational disease hazards and information on occupational disease hazard factors in the work site; and ③ clinical manifestations, results of assistant examination, etc. Where there is no evidence for denying a necessary connection between occupational disease hazard factors and a patient's clinical manifestations, the patient shall be diagnosed with an occupational disease.

4.1.5 Treatment Principles of Occupational Diseases

Clinical occupational health practice encompasses a wide range of services provided by professionals working in multidisciplinary teams. The primary goals are to reduce hazard exposure and to prevent disease and injury. Provision of services to meet these goals include assessment and monitoring of the workplace and the general environment for health and safety hazards, interventions designed to mitigate or eliminate hazardous exposures, case management for injured and ill individuals, and other measures to promote health and prevent disease and injury.

For employees who suffer or may suffer any acute occupational disease hazards, an employer shall organize rescue, treatment, and conduct of health examination and medical observation in a timely manner. Employers shall transfer employees who are found to have suffered health injuries related to their jobs from such jobs and settle such employees appropriately. Employers shall transfer occupational disease patients who are no longer suitable for their original jobs from their jobs and settle them appropriately.

Occupational diseases patients enjoy the occupational disease benefits prescribed by the state. Employers shall, according to the relevant provisions of the state, arrange the diagnosis, rehabilitation, and regular examination of occupational diseases patients. Employers shall provide appropriate job allowances to employees conducting operations with exposure to occupational hazards. The expenses for the diagnosis and rehabilitation of occupational disease patients and the social security of occupational disease patients who are disabled or have lost work ability shall be governed by the state provisions on work related injury insurance.

Medical and health institutions, when discovering patients suspected of occupational diseases, shall inform the employees themselves and notify the employers in a timely manner. Employers and medical and health institutions shall report in a timely manner discovered occupational disease patients or patients suspected of occupational diseases to the local health administrative department and work safety administrative department. If an occupational disease is confirmed, an employer shall also report to the local labor and social security administrative department. The departments receiving such reports shall make dispositions according to law.

4.1.6　Prevention of Occupational Diseases

4.1.6.1　Three Levels of Prevention

(1) Primary Prevention

Primary prevention is accomplished by reducing the risk of disease. In the occupational setting, this is most commonly done by reducing the magnitude of exposure to hazardous substances. As the dose is reduced so is the risk of adverse health consequences. Such reductions are typically managed by industrial hygiene personnel and are best accomplished by changes in production process or associated infrastructure, e. g. the substitution of a hazardous substance with a safer one, or enclosure or special ventilation of equipment or processes that liberate airborne hazards. These are known as engineering controls.

Other methods of exposure reduction include use of personal protective equipment and rotation of workers through areas in which hazards are present to reduce the exposure dose to each worker (However, this method does increase the number of workers exposed to the hazard).

(2) Secondary Prevention

This is accomplished by identifying health problems before they become clinically apparent (i. e. before workers report feeling ill) and intervention to limit the adverse effects of the problem. This is also known as occupational disease surveillance. The underlying assumption is that such early identification will result in a more favorable outcome.

An example of secondary prevention is the measurement of blood lead levels in workers exposed to lead. An elevated blood lead level indicates a failure of primary prevention but can allow for corrective action before clinically apparent lead poisoning occurs. Corrective action would be to improve the primary prevention activities listed above.

(3) Tertiary Prevention

This is accomplished by minimizing the adverse clinical effects on health of a disease or exposure. Typically this is thought of as clinical occupational medicine. An example of tertiary prevention is the treatment of lead poisoning (headache, muscle and joint pain, abdominal pain, anaemia, and kidney dysfunction) by administration of chelating medication. The goal is to limit symptoms or discomfort, minimize injury to the body and maximize functional capacity.

4. 1. 6. 2　Anticipation, Recognition, Evaluation and Control of Occupational Health Hazards

There are four fundamental principles in occupational hygiene-anticipation, recognition, evaluation, and control of occupational health hazards.

(1) Anticipation

Anticipation of problems is considered a vital skill, but while this usually requires considerable experience, assistance is now provided by material safety data sheets (MSDSs) and abundant advice available in the literature, and various electronic databases.

(2) Recognition

Recognition means knowing the hazards, the processes or identifying them through adverse health effects. Inspection is the first step in the process leading to evaluation and control. It entails the identification of materials and processes that have the potential to cause harm to workers. Inspection of the workplace is the best source of obtaining directly relevant data about health hazards. There is no substitute for observation of work practices, use of chemical and physical agents, and the apparent effectiveness of control measures. The primary health care (PHC) worker should be able to recognize major and obvious health hazards and distinguish those that require formal evaluation by the industrial hygienist.

(3) Evaluation

Evaluation means measuring exposures, comparing against standards, and evaluating health risk. Evaluation of health hazards within a plant includes measurement of exposures (and potential exposures), comparison of those exposures to existing standards and recommendation of controls if needed.

(4) Control

Control means providing contaminant or hazard control. The level of protection is based on knowledge of the toxicology or adverse effects produced by known quantitative exposures to the hazard.

Occupational/industrial hygienists recognize that engineering, work practice and administrative controls are the primary means of reducing employee exposure to occupational hazards.

Control of the hazards to health is the most important aspect of the process. Control involves finding ways of reducing the risk factors and providing safe conditions. Control may be directed towards control of hazardous substances or control of hazardous environments.

① Legal requirements: There are occupational health and safety (OH&S) Acts and Regulations in most of the countries over the world. Most of these contain requirements for a general duty of care, plus some directives to manage specific chemicals or agents, such as asbestos, silica, lead, carcinogens. In these Acts and Regulations there is a framework under which the obligations of various parties, including both employers and workers, are well-established. There are obligations of employer towards ensuring the health and safety of their workers by controlling hazards at source. There are also obligations for workers to cooperate with the employer in their own health and safety, plus obligations applying to all traditional safety matters (guarding, electrical, fall prevention, etc.) as well as to the more difficult matter of occupational health and occupational hygiene.

It is not defensible under law to let hazards persist simply because control will be too costly. It is equally indefensible to leave an identified hazard in an uncontrolled state simply because workers seem prepared to tolerate it. In almost all workplaces there is still room for improvement in the control of hazards.

② Control of chemical hazards: It is the basic obligation of manufacturers, importers and suppliers for providing information to workplaces at which their products are used. Employers also have obligations to provide relevant information on hazardous substances in their workplaces, to assess and control risks, to train staff, to undertake health surveillance and keep records where necessary. There are many published guidelines about the management of hazardous substances that contain useful information on the hierarchy of control, but the optimal control strategy for any workplace will depend on the situation in each workplace. Some additional regulations on asbestos, lead and carcinogens detail specific actions to be taken.

③ Elimination/Substitution: Elimination of a hazard in the workplace, by removing a process or a substance completely, is the definitive way of reducing risk. In practical terms, however, the drastic step of eliminating a process central to a workplace may result in the closing down of an industry (e. g. airships which used hydrogen, or domestic fireworks manufacturing). Elimination is often rejected in favor of more practicable control alternatives. Substitution offers multiple ways of controlling health hazards in the workplace. It can involve substitution of materials and/or processes.

④ Administrative controls: Exposure controls by eliminating the material or hazard, or by applying engineering control methods, which alone are absolutely insufficient. So it becomes necessary to change the system of work to achieve the desired level of exposure control. Changes to work methods or systems have been considered administrative controls. It would be simplistic to think that a single control strategy (except complete elimination) would result in satisfactory control of exposure. Sometimes higher-level control mechanisms just do not work, or they cannot be made to work well enough to completely eliminate the hazard. For example, consider the following workplace situations: Working inside a deep freezer; Working inside a hot oven; Working underwater at a depth of 100 m.

In the freezer and the oven, it is rarely practicable to introduce a microenvironment to compensate for the existing thermal environment. Efforts to keep divers at great depths for long times have to be very elaborate.

The use of administrative controls in regulating workplace hazards is an alternative strategy that concentrates on the work processes and systems, and worker behaviors, rather than the workplace hardware. While preference has to be given to engineering solutions, invariably special attention must be given to worker education, behavior or work practices because conventional methods are neither feasible nor adequate to control the hazard. Administrative controls should not be confused with the usual management concepts such as responsibility, audit and review.

A full appreciation of the hazards of a particular workplace is often only achieved if a complete risk assessment is undertaken with involvement of all parties concerned. Most legislative jurisdictions require formal chemical risk assessments. The respective regulations relating to workplace hazardous substances call for the hazards to be identified, mainly based on the hazardous substances. Risk phrases used in material safety data sheets; for exposure routes to be developed while applying the hierarchy of controls, and for all affected staff to be trained in all aspects of the hazard and its controls. These formal risk assessments are an integral aspect of the application of an administrative control in the workplace.

Work procedures such as teamwork can be an effective administrative control process for some dangerous tasks. For example, work in confined spaces is controlled by performing risk assessments and using work permits. The hazards of restricted visibility areas can be reduced by working in pairs or groups. Housekeeping and labeling are two administrative control processes that operate to limit inadvertent (especially skin) exposure to work-place hazards.

The importance of maintaining high standards of housekeeping cannot be overstated. Dirty and untidy workplaces not only increase the likelihood of secondary exposures (e. g. dust raised by draughts and wind, or inadvertent skin contact on dirty surfaces and equipment) but may also send a message to personnel that poor work habits are acceptable. In other words, worker involvement, participation, training and education are critical to the success of administrative control programs.

⑤ Personal protective equipment: At the start of this section, the hierarchy of controls was discussed. At the bottom of the hierarchy is personal protective equipment (PPE). PPE represents the absolute last resort; beyond the PPE is the unprotected worker and inevitable exposure if the PPE is not correctly selected, maintained and used. Even though PPE is on the bottom of the hierarchy it is still widely used and accepted as a back-up and supplement for other controls. There will also be situations where higher level controls cannot be used and PPE will be the only practicable solution.

4.2   Occupational Poisoning

4.2.1   Metals

4.2.1.1   Lead

(1) Physical and Chemical Properties

Lead is a naturally occurring element with symbol Pb which is derived from the Latin word *plumbum*. Its melting point and boiling point are 327℃ and 1740℃, respectively. Lead exists in elemental, inorganic, and organic forms. Lead is soft, malleable, resistant to corrosion, and is characteristics of poor conductivities to heat and electricity. Lead is easily soluble in nitric acid and concentrated sulfuric acid but not water. Most lead compounds are powder and insoluble or weakly insoluble in water. However, lead acetate and lead nitrate are soluble in water. Metallic lead has a bluish-white color after being freshly cut, but it soon tarnishes to a dull grayish color when exposed to air.

(2) Exposure Opportunities

Production and consumption of lead and lead compounds is increasing worldwide. Potentially high levels of lead exposure may occur in the following processes.

Primary production of lead is from lead ores, in which Lead coexists with zinc, silver and copper and co-extracted during its production. The main lead minerals are galena (PbS), cerussite ($PbCO_3$), and anglesite ($PbSO_4$).

Secondary lead production is automobile batteries and secondary application of lead compounds. About half of the total annual production is from recycling. Battery recycling facilities in less developed countries are a serious source of occupational lead exposure.

① Manufacture of storage batteries: The largest use for lead is in storage batteries in cars and other vehicles. More than half of the US lead production is used for automobiles, mostly as electrodes in the lead acid battery.

② Production and application of lead compounds as pigments: Various lead compounds are widely used as pigments in a variety of industries including painting, dyes, printing ink, rubber, plastic, ceramic glazes, stationery, caulk, etc. Lead chromate ($PbCrO_4$), also known as chrome yellow, has a vivid yellow color. Trilead tetraoxide (Pb_3O_4 or $2PbO \cdot PbO_2$), also called red lead, has a bright red or orange color. Given its anticorrosive property, trilead tetraoxide is extensively used to make a reddish brown paint that prevents rust on outdoor steel structures. Lead carbonate hydroxide [$2PbCO_3 \cdot Pb(OH)_2$], is also known as white lead.

③ Production, grinding, molding, spray-painting, flame welding and cutting, blasting, scrapping, or sanding operations of lead containing alloys and coatings: Lead is easily molded and shaped, and lead also can be combined with other metals to form alloys. Lead and lead alloys are commonly found in pipes and weights. Lead paint for anticorrosion purposes may contain up to 70% to 80% lead, flame cutting in metal coated with such paint causes a considerable risk.

④ Manufacture of lead glass: Lead monoxide (PbO) is used extensively in making glass, and the percentage of PbO could be from 12% to 28%.

(3) Absorption, Distribution, Metabolism and Excretion

① Absorption: Exposure to lead and its chemicals can occur through inhalation, ingestion and dermal contact.

Lead may be inhaled as an aerosol, and the respiratory tract provides the most effective route of absorption. The pattern of deposition of inhaled lead in the respiratory tract depends on the particle size.

Absorption of inorganic lead compounds via the gastrointestinal tract of adults is usually about 5% to 10%, and this percentage is higher during fasting or in people with deficiencies of calcium, zinc, or iron, but lower when excess calcium, phosphate, and phytate are present. Lead is readily absorbed in children and pregnant women, because their bodies have a greater demand for calcium and iron, and lead substitutes for calcium. Meanwhile, the immature gastrointestinal tract is relatively permeable to lead, and balance studies in small children have suggested that oral intake may result in absorption rates of 30% to 50%.

Absorption of inorganic lead compounds via skin is to a minor degree. However, the transdermal absorption may be substantial for alkyl lead.

② Distribution: Lead is absorbed into the bloodstream rapidly. Once absorbed, approximate 99% of lead binds to erythrocytes, and the remaining 1% is soluble in blood plasma in the form of lead hydrogen phosphate ($PbHPO_4$) and lead glycerophosphate. Then the absorbed lead is distributed to soft tissues (liver, kidneys, lungs, brain, spleen, muscles, and heart) and bone, where it equilibrates with blood lead. At high blood lead concentrations, the fraction of lead in plasma increases. Among the soft tissues, the liver and the kidney attain the highest concentrations. The distribution within the nervous system is uneven, with high levels in the hippocampus, amygdala, and choroids plexus. Lead is also distributed to the gonads, other parts of the male reproductive system, and ovary. Lead can enter the fetus through the placental barrier, and the developing fetus and fetal nervous system are, therefore, exposed to lead through their mothers. Lead concentrations in cord blood and fetal tissues correlate with maternal blood lead concentration.

After several weeks, most lead moves into bones and teeth, where lead is deposited as insoluble lead phosphate [$Pb_3(PO_4)_2$]. Over 95% of the total body burden of lead of an adult person is located in bones and teeth, while only about 73% for children. The half-life of lead differs from each of the compartments, ranging from 25 to 40 days in erythrocytes, generally about 2 months in soft tissues other than brain, and more than 1 year in brain. Bone lead can be divided into two parts. One is relatively stable state with a half-life of about 20 to 30 years, and the other has metabolic activity with a half-life of about 19 days, which can maintain a dynamic equilibrium between bone and blood or soft tissue.

There is a continuous turnover of the skeleton, which causes a release of lead from the skeleton, making a potential endogenous lead exposure. During periods of stress, fever, infection, alcoholism, hyperthyroidism, prolonged immobilization, pregnancy, and lactation, bone demineralization, or progressive osteoporosis, the skeleton turnover of lead is increased and the lead in the skeleton may mobilize into the bloodstream. The turnover rate of lead in the skeleton is higher in children than in adults.

③ Metabolism: Evidence indicates that certain inorganic lead compounds in water can be methylated via biological (by lake sediment microorganisms) or abiotic process. However, there are no indications of methylation of lead in human body.

④ Excretion: Lead ingested is excreted mainly through the urine (65% to 75%) and feces (25% to 30%), and only a small amount of lead (1%) is stored in bones. There is a correlation between lead levels in whole blood and urine, which has been used widely for biomonitoring. Low concentrations of lead have been detected in saliva, sweat, milk and menstruation.

⑤ Mechanism of toxicity: Lead can affect many biochemical processes by dysfunction of many enzymes through mimicking other biologically important metals, such as calcium, iron and zinc. One of the most important mechanisms of lead toxicity is its effect on various enzymes containing sulfhydryl groups in the heme biosynthetic pathway. Among which, the most sensitive enzyme is delta aminolevulinic acid dehydratase (ALAD), which converts two molecules of delta aminolevulinic acid (ALA) to form the monopyrrole porphobilinogen. ALAD is a zinc dependent enzyme, requiring zinc ions to maintain its enzymatic activity. Lead inhibits ALAD activity by displacing zinc since lead has approximately 20 times higher affinity for ALAD than zinc, resulting in altered thiol bonding and protein structure. The inhibition of the conversion of ALA to porphobilinogen causes accumulation of ALA, which increase in plasma and is excreted into urine. The less sensitive enzyme to lead is ferrochelatase, which incorporates ferrous ion into protoporphyrin IX, which can be inhibited by repressing the oxidation of coproporphyrinogen III through hindering coproporphyrinogen oxidase the oxidation of coproporphyrinogen. When this reaction is inhibited, free erythrocyte protoporphyrin (FEP) is elevated, and zinc substitutes for iron and binds to FEP producing zinc protoporphyrin (ZPP), therefore, FEP and ZPP elevate and can be used as effect biomarkers for lead in clinics. The inhibitions of lead to ALAD, coproporphyrinogen oxidase and ferrochelatase cause ineffective heme synthesis and subsequent hypochromatic anemia.

Lead may also inhibit the activity of alkaline phosphatase and adenosine triphosphatase (ATPase), which results in cellular, mitochondrial and nuclear swelling, abdominal cramp (smooth muscle spasm of intestinal wall or arteriole), and renal tubular dysfunction or damage.

Lead also can affect membrane structure and fluidity via directly attaching to biological membranes. It is of major clinical importance when these occur on blood cells and the nervous system. Once the cell membranes of the erythrocytes are affected, cellular fragility is increased, and thereby hemolysis followed by hemolytic anemia is produced.

Lead may inhibit calcium dependent events by interfering with calcium dependent processes. For example, lead is able to inhibit the release of several neurotransmitters and receptor coupled ionophores in glutamatergic neurons and to activate protein kinase C, calmodulin, and calcium-dependent ion channels.

Lead is able to pass through the endothelial cells at the blood brain barrier because it can substitute for calcium ions and be uptaken by calcium-ATPase pumps. In brain, lead is a potent inhibitor of the N-methyl-D-aspartate (NMDA) receptor and γ-aminobutyric acid (GABA) receptors which are known to play an important role in brain development and cognition. Meanwhile, at lower levels, lead acts as a calcium analog, interfering with ion channels during nerve conduction. Furthermore, buildup of heme precursor ALA may be directly or indirectly harmful to neurons.

(4) Clinical Findings

① Acute lead poisoning: Occupational acute lead poisoning is rare and often caused by eating large amounts of lead compounds by mistake. It is mainly characterized by gastrointestinal system symptoms (such as metallic taste, nausea, vomiting, paroxysmal abdominal pain, constipation or diarrhea), headache, elevated blood pressure, kidney dysfunction (such as oliguria and liver), and spasms, convulsions, coma and circulatory failure in severe cases.

Acute tetraethyl lead poisoning is often caused by inhalation of high concentration of tetraethyl lead or ethyl gasoline in a short time. It is mainly manifested as insomnia, dreams, loss of appetite, nausea and other neurological symptoms, which may be significantly reduced after 72h medical observation.

② Chronic lead poisoning: Chronic lead poisoning is common, which results in multiple systems as listed in the following.

● Nervous system.

Both the central and the peripheral nervous systems are affected. Early symptoms of central nervous system are commonly nonspecific and include headache, dizziness, malaise, fatigue, loss of short-term memory, and sleep disturbances. Later neuropsychiatric effects such as irritability, hostility, depression, difficulty in concentrating, delayed reaction times, and cognitive impairment can occur. In severe cases, lead encephalopathy may occur with or without cerebral edema, headaches with vomiting, lethargy alternating with lucidity, bizarre and aggressive behavior, coordination disorder, ataxia, altered sensorium, seizures, tremor, and coma. Children are more susceptible to the central nervous effects.

Lead has been shown to permanently reduce the cognitive capacity of children at extremely low levels of exposure, and there is no apparent threshold for this effect.

Peripheral neuropathy is classic manifestation of lead toxicity, and both motor and sensory peripheral neuropathies may occur. At lower exposures, symptoms and signs of sensory peripheral neuropathy may include sensory effects in term of tingling or numbness in the extremities, muscle pain, affected sensory and pain perceptions thresholds in fingers, and decreased vibration thresholds in hands and toes. Motor symptoms include mild distal weakness (decreased pinch and grip strength) of the upper limb. The neuropathy is reversible, if adequately handled. At severe exposure, the main clinical disorder is peripheral motor neuropathy with paralysis, manifested as classical symptoms of wrist drop and foot drop. In particular, the dominant hand is affected.

- Digestive system.

In chronic exposure conditions and bad oral hygiene, the accumulation of lead sulfide can cause a formation of a bluish gray seam of the gingival edge, the so-called lead seam, and it is also known as Burton line.

Symptoms from the gastrointestinal tract are often not characteristic. Early symptoms and signs include nausea, loss of appetite, anorexia, dysphagia, constipation, and occasionally diarrhea. In severe cases, contractions of the smooth muscle lining of intestinal walls lead to very intensive, excruciating, and colic like abdominal pain. The abdominal cramps are intermittent, often with pain free intervals, most often localized in the hypogastrium, sometimes in the epigastrium, sometimes radiating to the urinary bladder, scrotum, and kidney. It is known as lead colic.

- Hematopoietic systems.

Anemia is a typical symptom in classic lead poisoning. Anemia occurs from impairment of heme synthesis and shortened life span of circulating erythrocytes. Lead-related anemia is characteristically normocytic and hypochromic. Blood film examination may reveal basophilic stippling of peripheral erythrocytes (dots in red blood cells visible through a microscope).

- Other systems.

Lower lead exposure can cause hypertension and nephropathy, which is usually reversible and characterized by dysfunction of proximal tubule. Higher lead exposure, the nephropathy is irreversible as proximal tubule cells is changed in both function and morphology, including renal tubules atrophy, interstitial nephropathy, interstitial fibrosis and chronic renal failure. Lead is classified as a 2B carcinogen by IARC, which is confirmed in lab rat but is equivocal in human's studies. Lead has direct toxic effects on spermatogenesis, resulting in a decreased sperm count, an increase in the number of abnormal sperms, and a reduction in sperm motility. In pregnant women, elevated blood lead level may lead to miscarriage, prematurity, neonatal deaths, low birth weight, and problems with development during childhood.

(5) Diagnosis and Treatment

The diagnosis of lead poisoning depends on a history of lead exposure, the information on lead in the work site; symptoms and signs compatible with lead toxicity, laboratory tests supporting the diagnosis, and exclusion of other, more reasonable explanations (differential diagnoses).

The principle of treatment:

① Acute tetraethyl lead poisoning.

● On-site treatment: Once acute lead poisoning found, patients should leave the workplace immediately, remove contaminated clothes, shoes and hats, and wash contaminated skin, nails, hair with water or soapy water. At same times, pay attention to heat preservation.

● For those who are exposed to a large amount of tetraethyl lead in a short period of time, medical monitoring is required for 72 hours, and necessary examination and treatment are given, although there is no obvious clinical manifestation or only mild symptoms at that time.

● For patients with obvious psychotic symptoms, rescue according to the principle of acute toxic encephalopathy in GBZ 76—2002, treat according to psychopathy timely, and strengthen nursing to prevent accidents.

② Chronic lead poisoning.

● Expelling lead therapy.

Chelating agents including calcium edetate ($CaNa_2EDTA$) and 2,3-dimercaptosuccinic acid (DMSA) are treated according to the specific circumstances of poisoning.

● Symptomatic therapy.

It is advised the patient to rest properly and strengthen nutrition, and give different drugs depending on the patient's condition, such as those with neurosis treated with sedative, abdominal cramps injected with calcium gluconate or atropine.

(6) Prognosis and Prevention

In most cases, lead poisoning is preventable by avoiding exposure to lead. Of course, the exposure source should be identified immediately and removed. The mainstays of treatment are removal from the source of lead and, for people who have significantly high blood lead levels or who have symptoms of poisoning.

4.2.1.2　Mercury

(1) Physical and Chemical Properties

Mercury is a chemical element with symbol Hg which is derived from its former name hydrargyrum, a Latinized form of the Greek compound word hydrargyros meaning water silver. The atomic number of mercury is 80, its melting point and boiling is $-38.8℃$ and $356.6℃$, respectively.

Mercury exists in elemental, inorganic, and organic forms. Inorganic mercury compounds occur as monovalent mercurous mercury and divalent mercuric mercury. Organic mercury compounds exist at mercuric state. Metallic mercury is the only metal that is liquid at room temperature, in color of silvery white, but rather volatile, and thus exists as liquid metal or as vapor. As compared to other metals, it is a poor conductor of heat, and a fair conductor of electricity. It may evaporate at room temperature forming mercury vapor. Thus, increased amounts will evaporate if mercury is scattered on the floor as small droplets. In the presence of oxygen, metallic mercury is rapidly oxidized to ionic form. Mercuric salts, like halides, sulfates, and nitrates, are water soluble. Mercurous mercury is rather unstable in organisms and undergoes disproportionation to metallic mercury and mercuric mercury. Therefore, among inorganic mercury compounds, elemental mercury and the divalent mercury salt are of interest. Organic mercury compounds are historically important but are of little industrial value.

(2) Exposure Opportunities

Exposure to mercury vapor is the most common form of occupational exposure to mercury. Such exposure occurs in a variety of industries as detailed in the following.

Mercury is produced primarily from mercury ores, which are found either as a native metal or in cinnabar (mercuric sulfide, HgS), corderoite and other minerals, with cinnabar being the most common ore throughout the world. The cinnabar is the main component of the mercury rich ores which may contain up to 70% mercury. HgS in cinnabar can react with O_2 to produce Hg vapor and SO_2. Workers may be exposed to mercury dusts during the process of mining and crushing, and mercury vapor during extracting and smelting.

In chemical industry, approximate 50% of the mined mercury is used for chlorine caustic soda manufacture. Commonly mercury is also used to synthetize mercury compounds, such as mercuric chloride, mercury nitrate, and mercury arsenate and mercury cyanide.

Mercury thermometers and barometers are still widely used for certain scientific applications because of the greater accuracy and working range.

There is mercury exposure during industrial applications in electric lamps, switches, gauges and controls, battery production, and nuclear weapons production.

Mercury dissolves many other metals such as gold and silver to form amalgams, which has been used for centuries in a number of practices such as gold and silver mining, dentistry, cosmetics, and medicine. Dental amalgam is a dental filling material that is used to fill cavities caused by tooth decay. Dental amalgam is a mixture of metals, consisting of liquid mercury and a powdered alloy composed of silver, tin, and copper.

Manufacture of mercury containing medicine and reagents, which are found in topical antiseptics, stimulant laxatives, diaper-rash ointment, eye drops, and nasal sprays. Except for some preparations of influenza vaccine, organomercury compound thiomersal as a preservative has been phased out.

(3) Absorption, Distribution, Metabolism and Excretion

① Absorption: Inhalation of mercury vapor is the main route of occupational exposure to mercury salt or organic mercury. In human, the absorption rate of mercury vapor from respiratory route is approximately up to 80%. Absorption of mercury vapor from skin is minor, with an absorption rate of less than 1%. Liquid metallic mercury is poorly absorbed from the gastrointestinal tract.

Mercuric mercury salts from aerosols may be absorbed through the lungs. Its absorption rate by gastrointestinal tract is usually from 2% to 10% and depended on its solubility. Excessive intake, the corrosive action of mercuric mercury may alter the permeability of the gastrointestinal tract, enhancing absorption. Mercuric mercury may penetrate the skin.

② Distribution: The major part of mercury in blood is found in the erythrocytes during ongoing exposure. Due to its lipophilic and highly diffusible properties, mercury vapor can be released from the cells, pass biological membranes including the blood brain barrier, resulting in considerable deposition in the central nervous system. After entering the brain, mercury is oxidized and will not transfer back across the blood brain barrier, thus continued exposure to mercury vapor results in the accumulation of mercury in the nervous system.

Mercury vapor also penetrates the placental barrier, causing an accumulation of mercury in the fetus when the mother is exposed to mercury vapor. The mercury vapor dissolved in the blood and tissues is rapidly oxidized to mercuric mercury then acts in the same way as mercuric mercury.

The distribution of mercuric mercury varies widely with dose and time lapse after absorption. Mercuric mercury is distributed between plasma and erythrocytes immediately after absorbed. Mercuric mercury has a special affinity for ectodermal and endodermal epithelial cells and glands, thus it can be distributed to almost all tissues in the body, including the epithelial lining of the intestinal tract, the squamous epithelium of the skin and hair, glandular tissues like the salivary glands, thyroid, liver, pancreas, and the sweat glands, as well as subcutaneous organs like the testicles and the prostate. Little mercuric mercury crosses the blood brain barrier or placenta as contrasted with mercury vapor.

In all conditions, the kidney is the primary target organ that takes up and accumulates mercuric ions from the blood. The uptake and accumulation of mercuric species in the proximal renal tubule occur very rapidly after exposure. The next largest mercury pool is liver with high level in the periportal areas.

③ Metabolism: The lifetime of mercury vapor in the body is very limited. The mercury vapor dissolved in the blood and tissues is rapidly oxidized to divalent mercury. In tissues, a small portion of mercuric mercury can be reduced to mercury vapor.

④ Excretion: After exposure to mercury vapor, a small fraction of it can be exhaled, and most are excreted as form of mercuric mercury, which is excreted mainly through the kidney, fecal route, and sweat glands and little by lacrimal glands, mammary glands, and salivary glands. The retention time of accumulated mercury varies widely among different organs. Biological half time varies from a few days to months. The organs with the longest retention time are the brain (about several years), kidneys, and testicles. However, about 80% of mercury accumulated in the body is excreted with biological half time of approximately 60 days.

⑤ Mechanism of toxicity: The toxicity of mercury, in general, depends on the release of the mercuric ion. Mercuric ions have particular affinity for sulfur, sulfhydryl, and selenohydryl groups in proteins and non-proteins. The mercuric ions binding to these groups of various proteins in membranes and enzymes can modify the tertiary and quaternary structure of proteins and alter binding conditions in prosthetic groups in enzymes, thereby interfering with enzyme, receptor, ion channel, and intracellular signal link functions.

Alternatively, mercury-thiol-complexes can mimic endogenous molecules thereby interfere with the functions of endogenous molecules. Meanwhile, mercuric ions have a particular propensity to bind to the sulfhydryl groups on glutathione (GSH), cysteine (Cys), homocysteine (Hcy), N-acetylcysteine (NAC), metallothionein (MT), and albumin.

(4) Clinical Findings

Occupational mercury poisoning is mostly chronic and acute is rare, which often occurs in accidents caused by inhalation of high concentration of mercury vapor in short time.

① Acute mercury poisoning: Inhalation of mercury vapor may cause airway irritation, corrosive bronchitis, interstitial pneumonitis, pulmonary edema, respiratory insufficiency, even respiratory distress in severe cases.

Acute exposure to mercury vapor also results in central nervous system effects, such as headache, tremor, increased excitability, performance deficits in tests of cognitive function, psychotic reactions characterized by delirium, and hallucinations can be displayed as well.

The critical organs for mercuric mercury ingestion are the kidneys and the intestinal tract. The corrosive effect of concentrated mercuric mercury solution on the mucous membranes of the gastrointestinal tract causes extensive precipitation of proteins. Gastric pain and vomiting may ensue. When mercuric mercury passes the lower regions, general abdominal pain and bloody diarrhea with necrosis of the intestinal mucosa will occur. This may lead to circulatory collapse and death.

After the gastrointestinal damage, the critical organ will be the kidney. Within 24 hours, renal failure caused by necrosis of the proximal tubular epithelium may develop, anuria and uremia occur.

Without continuous or heavy exposure, neurologic damage is insignificant since mercuric mercury does not cross blood brain barrier easily.

② Chronic mercury poisoning: Long term exposure to low levels of mercury vapor mainly causes damage both the peripheral and central nervous system.

Early signs are nonspecific neuroid symptoms and autonomic dysfunction symptoms, such as including dizziness, headache, forgetfulness, insomnia, weakness, fatigue, palpitations, and hyperhidrosis. Lately, the major manifestations appear, including excitability, tremor, and stomatitis.

Excitability is characterized by severe behavioral and personality changes, irritability, increased excitability, excessive shyness, insomnia, and depression. In severe cases, delirium and hallucination may occur.

Parallel to the development of excitability, mercurial tremor develops, this appears as fine trembling of the muscles interrupted by coarse shaking movements, and initially involves the fingers and later spreads to eyelids, lips and tongue. In progressive cases, it may develop into a generalized tremor involving the entire body, with violent spasms of the extremities. Furthermore, the tremor is usually perpendicular to the direction of movement and specified as intention tremor, which appears when moving and is aggravated during the movement and disappears after the movement completed. The more a person wants to control it, the more obvious for tremor.

Another characteristic feature of mercury toxicity is excessive stomatitis, such as salivation and gingivitis. Severe exposure to inorganic mercury causes an inflammation of gingiva and oral mucosa, which become tender, reddish, swollen, and bleed easily. With development, the gums are pulled away from the teeth, leaving deep pockets where the bacteria can grow and damage the bone that supports the teeth. The gums also shrink back from the teeth, and the teeth may need to be pulled out, or may become loose and fall out.

Other features can be demonstrated, such as metallic taste in the mouth, loss of appetite, signs of disturbance of gastrointestinal functions, local irritation, and allergic contact dermatitis.

Signs of impaired cognitive skills also can be demonstrated, such as difficulties in concentration, decreased performance on memory tests, and verbal concept formation. In cumulative mercury exposure, peripheral nerve conduction velocity and motor coordination were reduced. Unfortunately, neurological symptoms can remain for decades after exposure has been ceased.

For chronic exposure, kidney is the critical organ. Both glomeruli and tubules can be damaged. In glomeruli, autoimmune reaction is induced, and the basal membrane is damaged. In tubules, mercury accumulation causes necrosis and damage of the proximal tubules, as indicated by an increased excretion of small proteins in the urine.

(5) Diagnosis and Treatment

① Diagnosis: Diagnosis of elemental or inorganic mercury poisoning involves determining the occupational history of exposure, the clinical manifestations and laboratory test, the occupational hygiene survey. Comprehensive analysis can be carried out after excluding similar diseases caused by other causes.

② Treatment: In cases of poisoning, identifying and removing the source of the mercury is crucial. Decontamination requires removal of clothes, washing skin with soap and water, and flushing the eyes with saline solution as needed. Immediate expelling mercury therapy is needed using chelation agents [sodium dimercaptosulfonate (Na-DMPS) or sodium dimercaptosuccinate (Na-DMS)] and symptomatic treatment according to internal medicine.

(6) Prognosis and Prevention

Mercury poisoning can be prevented by minimizing exposure to mercury and mercury compounds. Heating of mercury and mercury compounds that may decompose when heated should be always carried out with adequate ventilation. Containers of mercury should be securely sealed to avoid spills and evaporation. In cases of spills involving mercury, specific cleaning procedures should be used. Protocols call for physically merging smaller droplets on hard surfaces, combining them into a single larger pool for easier removal with an eyedropper, or for gently pushing the spill into a disposable container. Thereafter, fine sulfur, zinc, or activated carbon powder that readily forms an amalgam with mercury at ordinary temperatures can be used to sprinkle over the area before being collected and properly disposed of.

4.2.1.3 Cadmium

(1) Physical and Chemical Properties

Cadmium is a chemical element with symbol Cd, which is a silvery-white metal. It can be slowly oxidized by moist air to form CdO and is readily soluble in dilute HNO_3 but insoluble in HCl and H_2SO_4.

(2) Exposure Opportunities

Production and consumption of cadmium and cadmium compounds is increasing worldwide. Primary production of cadmium is from cadmium ores. The main cadmium minerals are cadmium oxide (CdO), cadmium sulfide (CbS), cadmium chloride (CbCl$_2$), and cadmium sulfate (CbSO$_4$). Potentially high levels of cadmium and its compounds exposure may occur from the smelting and refining of ore, and from its use of cadmium-containing pigments, electroplating, nickel-cadmium batteries, plastic stabilizer, semiconductor component, amalgams, alloys, ceramic glazes, and the manufacture of high speed bearings, solder jewellery, etc. Currently, nearly 86% of the world's Cadmium is used in the manufacture of nickel-Cadmium batteries, 9% for pigments, 4% for coatings, and 1% for alloys, solar panels and stabilizers.

(3) Absorption, Distribution, Metabolism and Excretion

① Absorption: Inhalation of dust or fumes containing cadmium is the main route of occupational exposure to cadmium. In human, the absorption rate of cadmium smoke or dust from respiratory route is approximately up to 50%. However, cadmium salts are poorly adsorbed via the skin (1%) or gastrointestinal tract (3% to 7%). Sometimes, cadmium smoke or dust can also enter the body *via* the gastrointestinal tract when worker eats in the workshop.

② Distribution: The major part of Cadmium in blood is found in the erythrocytes. It mainly accumulates in kidney and liver. About one third of the total Cadmium entering the body distributes in the kidney, while the content of Cadmium in renal cortex accounts for about one third of the total kidney.

③ Metabolism: Cadmium has strong accumulation, and its biological half-life of cadmium in the body is as long as 30 years.

④ Excretion: After exposure to Cadmium dust or fumes, cadmium is mainly excreted by the kidney, the fecal route, hair and nail.

⑤ Mechanism of toxicity: The mechanism of Cadmium poisoning is still unclear. Current available research evidence showing the possible toxicity mechanism as follows.

• Reduce the activity of antioxidase: Many antioxidant enzymes contain thiol group (-SH). Cadmium can compete with these divalent metal ions for inclusion into metalloenzymes, thereby inactivating their activity of SH-based enzymes and reducing the ability to scavenge oxygen free radicals.

• Mitochondrial stress: Cadmium can directly bind to thiol-containing proteins and lead to the membrane permeability vary and mitochondrial dysfunction. In addition, cadmium can interfere with the electron transfer by inhibiting the activity of the electron transport chain enzyme complex MitoQ10, and cause electron leakage and ROS release.

• Disorder of calcium ion metabolism. Cadmium can interfere with calcium ion metabolism, calcium channel, intracellular calcium level, and calmodulin function. In addition, the toxic effect of cadmium on tissues is to bind calmodulin (CaM) by competing with cadmium to interfere with CaM and its regulated physiological and biochemical process.

• Induce cell apoptosis: Cadmium can induce apoptosis by increasing intracellular calcium levels, which in turn activates Ca^{2+}/CaM-mediated apoptosis. Cadmium also can induce apoptosis by causing DNA fragmentation, which in turn activates the death receptor Fas and Caspase-8. Furthermore, Cadmium can also cause apoptosis by inducing autophagy dysfunction and high levels of oxygen free radicals through retarding cellular respiration process or promoting the release of cellular inflammatory factors.

• Others: Cadmium also stimulates catecholamine synthase activity to increase dopamine levels and inhibits Na^+-K^+-ATPase, zinc-containing enzymes, amino acid decarboxylase, histase, amylase, peroxidase, etc. , especially leucyl amino peptide.

(4) Clinical Findings

Acute Cadmium poisoning often occurs in accidents at workplaces and is rare in most countries today. Preventing chronic Cadmium poisoning is of great importance in the field of occupational health.

① Acute Cadmium poisoning.

Cadmium fume fever (caused by inhalation of fumes generated during smelting, welding, plating, soldering, brazing, and nickel-cadmium battery or pigment manufacturing), characterized by fever, headache, cough, wheezing, chills, myalgias, pleuritic chest pain, and sore throat, shortness of breath, typically develops 4 to 12 hours after an acute inhalational exposure and resolves within 1 to 2 days. In severe, pneumonitis or acute lung injury may develop 24 hours or longer after exposure and may progress to respiratory failure, such as bronchitis, emphysema and pulmonary edema. Serious acute cadmium exposure may result in death.

Acute ingestion of large amounts of foods or water contaminated with cadmium-containing fumes and dusts usually causes nausea, vomiting, salivation, diarrhea (sometimes are hemorrhagic), and abdominal pain, which can continue to develop into hypotension, renal failure, and death. Swallowing overdoses of cadmium or its compounds can result in caustic injury to the gastrointestinal tract. However, direct hepatotoxicity and cardiotoxicity are rare.

② Chronic Cadmium poisoning.

Chronic toxicity of cadmium, both at work and in the general environment, mainly includes serious detrimental effects on the kidney, in particular tubular function, bone softening, and hepatic injury.

Kidney is the key target organ for the general and occupational populations exposed to cadmium compounds. After cadmium enters the body, it combines with metallothionein to form a cadmium-metallothionein complex, which is transported to the kidneys through the blood and absorbed by the renal tubules. In the renal tubular cells, the complex is degradated by lysosomes and free cadmium is released and deposits, which then lead to kidney dysfunction, manifested by kidney atrophy, thickening of the glomerular capsule, and glomerular proteinuria, decrease of renal tubular reabsorption function, which in turn leads to nephrolithiasis and osteomalacia.

The bone is another target organ of cadmium or its compounds, which exert a direct effect on bone metabolism, affect bone resorption and formation, and cause osteomalacia and/or osteoporosis. The first clinical manifestations are lumbago, backache, knee pain, and later throughout the body. The pain is unbearable and aggravated during activity. Patients often have pathological fractures, shortened bodies, and severe deformities of the bones. In severe cases, some minor activities or cough can cause fractures. Therefore the "pain" caused by chronic cadmium poisoning was called Itai-itai disease.

In addition, long-term inhalation of cadmium fumes and dusts may also affect the respiratory system. The clinical manifestations are decreased lung function, edema and emphysema. In severe cases, it can lead to lung cancer and prostate cancer. In 1993, cadmium has been classified as Class I carcinogen (a human carcinogen) by the IARC. In American, cadmium is listed as the seventh health hazard by American Toxicology and Disease Registry (ATSDR), and it is also listed as one of the key monitoring indicators for the implementation of total emission control in China.

(5) Diagnosis and Treatment

The diagnosis and treatment of occupational cadmium poisoning follows the national standards GBZ 17—2015.

(6) Prognosis and Prevention

There is no specific antidote for cadmium poisoning, so prevention is the first choice. In order to prevent cadmium poisoning, the workplace where smelting, welding, plating, soldering and other places using cadmium and its compounds, should have good ventilation and hermetic devices. In addition to the above necessary air exhausting equipment, worker should use personal gas mask in the process of welding and plating. Eating, drinking or smoking at the workshop should be avoided.

4.2.1.4 Manganese

(1) Physical and Chemical Properties

Manganese is a chemical element with symbol Mn, which is a silvery-white metal, firm and brittle. In natural mineral, compounds of MnO, $MnCl_2$ and MnO_2 are common, and the stable oxidations of manganese are permanganate such as $KMnO_4$, and manganate such as K_2MnO_4. The compounds of Manganese are readily soluble in water and dilute acid.

(2) Exposure Opportunities

Manganese is widely distributed in nature, and almost all kinds of ore and silicate rocks contain manganese. There are many kinds of manganese ore, in which the most important and economical are pyrolusite (MnO_2), psilomelane ($mMnO \cdot MnO_2 \cdot nH_2O$), manganite ($MnOOH$), manganese in brown ($Mn_2O_3$), hausmannite ($Mn_3O_4$), and rhodochrosite ($MnCO_3$). The content of manganese can reach $50\%-70\%$ in the above manganese minerals. Potentially high levels of manganese and its compounds exposure may occur during the process of mining, smelting, refining, transportation and manufacturing of manganese compounds or alloys. Currently, nearly 90% to 95% of the world's manganese is used in the steel industry, and the remaining 10% to 5% of manganese is used in other industrial fields, such as the chemical industry (manufacturing various manganese-containing salts), light industry (for batteries, matches, paints, soaps) and building materials industry (glass and ceramics).

(3) Absorption, Distribution, Metabolism and Excretion

① Absorption: Manganese is mainly ingested by inhalation of dust or fumes. The main transport of inhaled manganese can be transmitted to brain directly through the olfactory pathway and depositing in the olfactory bulb, olfactory tract, striatum and globus pallidus, or by systemic circulation crossing blood-brain barrier and entering the striatum and globus pallidus. However, manganese is poorly adsorbed via the gastrointestinal tract (1% to 5%). Manganese is rarely absorbed by skin except for a few organic manganese compounds, such as tricarbonyl cyclopentadienyl manganese (MCT), tricarbonyl methyl cyclopentadienyl manganese (MMT), which is a gasoline additive instead of tetraethyl lead, and manganese carbamate, which is used as agricultural pesticide.

② Distribution: Manganese absorbed into the blood can bind to β1-globulin in plasma to form β1-globulin transporter, which is called transmanganese. Manganese mainly deposits in brain, muscles and kidneys. A small part of Manganese enters the red blood cells to form manganese porphyrin or bind to hemoglobin, which is rapidly transferred to mitochondria-rich cells and accumulates in liver, pancreas, kidney, heart and brain in the state of insoluble trivalent Manganese.

③ Metabolism: After Manganese enters the body, the chemical valence state is mostly $+2$ and $+4$. Plasma ceruloplasmin can oxidize Mn^{2+} (binding to macroglobulin) to Mn^{3+} (binding to transferrin), and cause the retention of Manganese in the body, because the serum clearance rate of Mn^{2+}-macroglobulin is much faster than that of transferrin-Mn^{3+}.

④ Excretion: Most of the Manganese is mainly excreted by the feces up to 90%, and a small amount is excreted with the urine. Manganese in the lenticular nucleus and cerebellum of brain has a long storage time.

⑤ Mechanism of toxicity: According to studies, the possible mechanisms of manganese poisoning are the following.

• Oxidative stress and mitochondrial damage: Manganese has a special affinity for mitochondria, and leads to dysfunction of oxidative phosphorylation, energy production, and oxidative stress. Manganese can also exert its neurotoxicity by reducing the level of dopamine and 5-serotonin and increasing the accumulation of acetylcholine. At the same time, Manganese can also interact with mitochondrial permeablity transition pore (mPTP) and result in mitochondrial oxidative damage.

• Affecting immune function: Excessive manganese exposure can inhibit protein synthesis by suppressing RNA-dependent DNA polymerase and lymphocyte proliferation or the activity of NK cells by competing with Ca^{2+} and Mg^{2+}.

• Causing an inflammatory response: Manganese can lead to inflammatory response by facilitating the release of inflammatory factors (IL-6, IL-1β, IFN-γ and TNF-α), activating of microglia in the nervous system, promoting the expression of nitric oxide synthase and NO in astrocytes.

• Affecting trace element homeostasis: Manganese can compete with other metal ions and affect their metabolism. For example, excessive manganese can bind to divalent metal ion transporter-1 (DMT-1), transferrin and its receptor to inhibit the transmembrane transport of iron and reduce the absorption of manganese by the lungs. Manganese can also bind to the calcium channel in the heart to block Ca^{2+} influx and affect the heart function. In addition, manganese can compete with Ca^{2+} in the mitochondria to inhibit its efflux and lead to changes in mitochondrial membrane permeability, ultrastructural and mitochondrial swelling.

• Others: Manganese can damage the male reproductive system. At the same time, dysfunction of autophagy and arginine homeostasis imbalance may be implicated in the pathophysiology of neurological disorders.

(4) Clinical Findings

Occupational chronic manganese poisoning is a disease with nervous system damage mainly caused by long-term exposure to manganese dust, and the most obvious clinical manifestation is extracorporeal damage accompanied by mental and emotional disorders. Acute manganese poisoning is rare. According to clinical manifestations, chronic manganese poisoning is divided into observation object, mild poisoning, moderate poisoning and severe poisoning.

Chronic Manganese poisoning is mainly characterized by neuroid symptoms (dizziness, fatigue, forgetfulness) and autonomic dysfunction (loss of appetite, runny, sweating, palpitations, heavy feeling). Then symptoms of extramedullary nerve damage (muscle tone increasing, obvious tremor of the fingers, hyperreflexia, and neuroemotional changes) will be discovered. In severe patients, extra-pyramidal neurological disorders are prominent, which often manifest as Parkinson's disease-like symptoms and signs of toxic psychosis, such as feelings of indifference, involuntary crying, obsessive attitudes and impulsive behaviors.

(5) Diagnosis and Treatment

The diagnosis and treatment of occupational manganese poisoning follow the national standards GBZ 3—2006.

(6) Prognosis and Prevention

In the workplace, Manganese exists mainly in the form of fume or dusts, so it is important to prevent manganese from entering the body through the respiratory tract. First, the workplace where blasting, smelting, refining, welding and cutting or sanding operations of manganese or its compounds, should have good ventilation and hermetic devices. In addition to the above necessary air exhausting equipment, worker should be worn with a personal gas mask when working, and changes clothes and bathe frequently. At the same time, workers should conduct a pre-job occupational health examination to find occupational contraindications timely and regular on-the-job and off-the-job examination to detect early health damage. Furthermore, it is necessary for workers to accept occupational health education before starting work.

4.2.1.5　Other Metals of Workplace Concern

(1) Aluminum

Aluminum is a kind of silver white light metal and widely used. Inhalation of dust or fumes containing aluminum is the main route of occupational exposure. Similar to manganese, there are two ways in which aluminum can be ingested by inhalation entering CNS. First, the particulates of aluminum and its compounds can be absorbed by systemic circulation. Second, the inhaled fume containing aluminum can be transferred into brain tissue directly via the olfactory neurothe. In addition, a small part of aluminum is ingested by oral absorption. The adverse effects of aluminum exposure include multiple tissues and organs damage. At the early stage of aluminum exposure, the first symptom is anemia. Second, long-term inhalation of aluminum fumes can result in aluminum pneumoconiosis. Third, extensive occupational aluminum exposure can lead to adverse neurological symptoms or signs such as Alzheimer's disease. In addition, aluminum can also cause osteomalacia, inhibit the activities of acetylcholine and multiple enzymes of the reproductive system, and contract of smooth muscles of the digestive tract. The treatment, prognosis and prevention of aluminum pneumoconiosis are similar to pneumoconiosis in Chapter 4. 3. 6.

(2) Arsenic, Zinc and Copper

Zinc and copper except arsenic are essential trace elements of the body. In industrial environment, they often exist in the form of fumes and dust, and cause metal smoke heat, which is a systemic disease characterized by a typical sudden rise in temperature and an increase in the number of white blood cells caused by inhalation of new metal oxide smoke. The diagnostic criteria and treatment principles for metal smoke heat caused by zinc, copper, arsenic, silver, iron, cadmium, lead, arsenic and other minerals is according to national standard GBZ48−2002. Similar to lead, the diagnostic principles of occupational cadmium and manganese poisoning include five parts: the history of occupational metal oxide smoke exposure, the typical clinical symptoms (sudden rise in body temperature and increase of white blood cells number), the working environment detection, comprehensive analysis, and elimination of similar diseases. Generally, no special medication is needed. In severe cases, symptomatic treatment is given according to the condition.

4. 2. 2　Organic Solvents

Organic solvents are defined as carbon-based substances capable of dissolving or dispersing one or more other substances. Many classes of chemicals are used as organic solvents, including aliphatic hydrocarbons, aromatic hydrocarbons, amines, esters, ethers, ketones, and nitrated or chlorinated hydrocarbons.

(1) Classification

Most organic solvents can be classified into chemical groups based on the configuration of the hydrogen and carbon atoms and the presence of different functional groups. Chemical groups that are commonly used are straight or branched chains of carbon and hydrogen (e. g. hexane, heptane), cyclic hydrocarbons (e. g. cyclohexane, turpentine), esters (ethyl acetate, isopropylacetate), aromatic hydrocarbons (e. g. benzene, toluene, xylene), alcohols (e. g. ethanol, isopropanol), ketones (e. g. acetone, methyl ethyl ketone), halogenated hydrocarbons (e. g. carbon tetrachloride, chloroform), aldehydes (e. g. acetaldehyde, formaldehyde), ethers (e. g. diethyl ether, isopropyl ether), glycols (e. g. ethylene glycol, hexylene glycol) and nitro-hydrocarbons (e. g. nitroethane, nitromethane)

(2) Solvent Properties

Solvents from different chemical groups can differ markedly in their characteristics; however, within each group, chemical and solvent properties change only slightly as the molecular weight of the solvent increases. The main factors which influence the properties of organic solvents are: ①the number of carbon atoms present; ②the presence of only single bonds (saturated molecules) or double or triple bonds (unsaturated molecules) between adjacent carbon atoms; ③ the configuration of the solvent molecule, i. e. straight chain (aliphatic), branched chain or ring (i. e. cyclic and aromatic); ④the presence of functional groups, e. g. NH_2, NO_2, halogen, etc.

The solvent properties of organic solvents tend to increase with fewer numbers of carbon atoms in the molecule. Unsaturated molecules tend to be more reactive than their saturated counterparts.

(3) Solvent Characteristics

The following characteristics of organic solvents determine the type of hazards they present.

① Volatility: As organic solvents volatile (i. e. tend to evaporate), inhalational exposure is an important exposure pathway to be considered when assessing the health hazards that solvents may present. The greater the volatility of a solvent, the greater the vapor concentration in the air is. Two determinants of volatility are the vapor pressure and evaporation rate. Both indexes are temperature dependent and increase as the temperature increases.

The density of the solvent vapor may also need to be considered in emergency situations. As the density increases, the rate at which the solvent dissipates will decrease.

As a general rule, a vapor that is heavier than air (vapor density > 1) will tend to pool and spread near ground level in confined spaces, whereas a vapor which is lighter than air (vapor density < 1) will tend to rise and dissipate.

② Water and lipid solubility: The water and lipid solubility of a solvent will determine how readily it will be absorbed through the skin. Given that the skin can be described as a lipid-water bilayer, solvents such as dimethylsulfoxide and glycol ethers which are readily dissolved in both are well absorbed through the skin.

③ Chemical structure: The chemical structure of a solvent including any attached functional groups such as amino ($-NH_2$), nitro ($-NO_2$), methyl ($-CH_3$), and hydroxyl ($-OH$) will determine its toxicological properties, which tend to be similar within chemical groupings.

④ Flammability and explosiveness: The flammability and explosiveness of a solvent are clearly important determinants of hazard. Measures frequently used to give an indication of the flammability and explosiveness of solvents includes the flash and fire points, and the autoignition temperature. Explosive ranges or flammability limits of different solvents have been determined and refer to the concentrations over or above which a particular vapor will burn when ignited. Many organic solvents have low flash points and will burn if ignited. Chlorinated solvents have quite high flash points and are not usually flammable under conditions of normal use.

Some solvents may also be explosive, e. g. nitrocellulose. There may also be a risk of exothermic reactions of some solvents when mix with other materials, which may lead to fire or explosion.

(4) Uses and Occupational Exposure

Solvent chemistry is based on the principle that "like dissolves like". Therefore, for a solvent to be of any use it needs to have similar chemical characteristics to the substance it is trying to dissolve, thus solvents make it possible to process, apply, clean or separate materials.

Organic solvents are widely used to dissolve and disperse fats, oils, waxes, pigments, varnishes, rubber and many other substances. They are frequently used in paints, varnishes, lacquers, thinners, waxes, floor and shoe polishes, glues, fuels, antifreeze, degreasing, cleaning and dry cleaning agents, inks, pharmaceutical and pesticide products, preservatives, and laboratory processes.

Given the tendency for most organic solvents to evaporate at ambient temperatures and to be absorbed through the skin, the two most important exposure pathways for organic solvents in the workplace are through the lungs and skin.

For this reason, many countries promulgate exposure standards (e. g. TWA, STEL) for solvents in workplace air. In some circumstances, engineering controls and protective equipment/clothing may be required to ensure that worker safety is not compromised. Such requirements are generally detailed in the MSDS for the solvent.

(5) Health Effects

① Nervous system toxicity: Most organic solvents adversely affect the function of the central nervous system (CNS). The severity and type of effect depend on the vapor concentration, duration of exposure, and toxicity of the solvent. The effect observed may also depend on whether exposure to other materials at the same time and whether the individual is particularly sensitive to the solvent.

Signs and symptoms suggestive of CNS involvement range from headaches, tiredness, and dizziness to behavioral changes ("drunkenness"), unconsciousness, and death. The CNS effects generally wear off on cessation of exposure. However, prolonged repeated exposure to some solvents may impair perceptions and cause behavioral changes as well as other changes, and in some cases normal function may not return. Psychological tests can be used to assess CNS function. Such tests may include evaluation of language comprehension, logical and spatial thinking, and power of observation, coordination and memory tests.

Long-term exposure to high levels of n-hexane and methyl n-butyl ketone is associated with degeneration of nerve cells in the peripheral nervous system. Restless legs, muscle cramps, pain, weakness and loss of sensation in limbs are suggestive of such degeneration.

② Skin toxicity : Although solvents belong to a diverse range of chemical groups, their effects on skin are generally similar. Solvents will remove the fat (defatting). This makes the skin dry, scaly and eventually cracked. Deteriorated skin also allows greater absorption of solvent through the skin following direct skin contact.

Solvents like toluene, xylene, butanol and styrene cause skin irritation and irritant dermatitis. Wood turpentine, water-based paint preservatives (e. g. formaldehyde) and epoxy resins may cause allergic contact dermatitis.

③ Respiratory system toxicity: All organic solvents irritate the respiratory tract to some degree. Such irritation typically involves the upper respiratory tract (e. g. upper airways, nose, throat and trachea). Long-term exposure to the more potent irritants (e. g. aldehydes) may lead to chronic or persisting cough and increased sputum production.

④ Other system toxicity: Solvents may also affect other organs in the body. Chloroform and carbon tetrachloride are toxic to the liver. Glycol ethers and some chlorinated solvents may damage the kidneys. Benzene and some glycol ethers are harmful to bone marrow hematopoietic system, causing aplastic anemia. Some glycol ethers can also induce hemolytic anemia due to increasing osmotic fragility.

Chlorinated organic solvents, such as methylene chloride and trichloroethane are noted for their harmful effects on the heart. Chronic exposure to carbon disulphide is considered a contributory factor in coronary heart disease. Cardiac sensitization may occur following repeated exposure to solvents. It is due to increased sensitivity of the muscle of the heart to the effects of epinephrine on the rhythm of the heart. It can produce life threatening irregularities in the rhythm of the heart and should be considered as a possible cause of sudden death in healthy individuals who have been exposed to high levels of organic solvents.

Although organic solvents readily cross the placenta, most are not considered teratogenic. Notable exceptions are ethanol and some of the smaller chain glycol ethers.

⑤ Carcinogenicity: The IARC has classified a number of solvents in regard to their carcinogenicity.

Benzene has been classified as a Group 1 (carcinogenic to humans) carcinogen as it has been associated unequivocally with certain forms of leukemia in heavily exposed workers. However, it has not been associated with carcinogenic effects in any circumstances other than heavy occupational exposure. Dichloromethane, ethyl acrylate, tetrachloroethylene and styrene are classified as Group 2A (probably carcinogenic to humans). Other solvents including methyl acrylate, methyl chloride, methylmethacrylate monomer, petroleum solvents, toluene, 1,1,1-trichloroethane, 1,1,2-trichloroethane and xylene are in Group 3 (not classifiable as to its carcinogenicity to humans).

(6) Mixed Solvent Exposure

Given that more than one organic solvent may be present in a product (e. g. paint thinners may contain toluene, xylene, ethylbenzene, methylethylketone and acetone), it is important that not only are the effects of each solvent considered when determining the potential for the product to induce adverse effects, but the potential for additive or synergistic effects are also considered.

(7) Biological Monitoring

Occupational exposure to some organic solvents can be monitored by measuring the level of solvent or in some cases its metabolites in the urine.

For all solvents, biological monitoring may also include estimations of the unchanged compound in exhaled air or in blood, though such testing is not readily available and has logistical difficulties.

Interpretation of the results of biological monitoring need to take into account the duration since exposure, the distribution of the solvent or its metabolites in the body, and the rate at which the solvent or its metabolites are eliminated from the body. Other factors may also need to be considered. For instance, alcohol intake several hours or just before inhalation exposure to an organic solvent may inhibit its metabolism, thereby reducing the rate at which its metabolites are excreted. However, chronic alcohol consumption induces microsomal enzyme activity and may increase the metabolism of a solvent.

The American Conference of Governmental Industrial Hygienists has recommended biological exposure indices for the following solvents (n-hexane, benzene, toluene, xylenes, ethyl benzene, styrene, phenol, methyl ethyl ketone, perchloroethylene, trichloroethane, trichloroethylene, dimethylformamide, and carbon disulfide). For many solvents, significant levels may be present only in exhaled air. For solvents with relatively slow excretion, such as perchloroethylene and trichloroethane, analysis of blood is a reasonable alternative to exhaled air.

4. 2. 2. 1   Benzene

(1) Physical and Chemical Properties

Benzene is a clear, colorless aromatic hydrocarbon which has a characteristic sickly, sweet odor. Its boiling point is 80. 1℃ and freezing point is 5. 5℃. It is a volatile, highly flammable liquid, and its low boiling point and high vapor pressure cause rapid evaporation under ordinary atmospheric conditions. It is minimally soluble in water and is capable of mixing with polar solvents such as chloroform, acetone, alcohol, and carbon tetrachloride without separating into two phases.

Benzene is a highly stable aromatic hydrocarbon, but it does react with other compounds primarily by substitution of one or more hydrogen atoms. Some reactions occur which can rupture or cleave the molecule.

(2) Exposure Opportunities

Benzene is a ubiquitous agent. It is usually obtained through the distillation of coal tar or pyrolysis of petroleum. It is a component of motor fuel (gasoline or petrol) and is widely distributed in petroleum industries. Gasoline contains 1%—2% benzene in the U. S. , and higher levels ported elsewhere. Benzene is also an important starting agent and intermediate for chemical synthesis, and some relevant industries include plastic, rubbers, lubricants, dyes, detergents, drugs, and pesticides. Moreover, benzene is a valuable solvent, diluents, extracting, and is widely used in painting, organic synthesis, and adhesive materials.

Occupational exposure to benzene occurs in the chemical, printing, rubber, paint, and petroleum industries. Particularly heavy exposure occurs in maintenance, clean up, product sampling, and petroleum bulk transfer operations. Data from developing countries suggest that occupational exposures in those nations are widespread, especially in artisan work, shoe manufacturing, and small chemical industries. Benzene was previously used widely as a solvent, but this use has been decreasing in many countries, primarily because of health and safety concerns.

(3) Absorption, Distribution, Metabolism and Excretion

Benzene is readily absorbed by humans from inhalation, oral, and dermal exposures. The main route of exposure is inhalation. When a person is exposed to high levels of benzene in air, about half of the benzene passes through the lining of lungs and enters bloodstream. Benzene is also rapidly absorbed through the skin from both liquid and vapor phases. Dermal absorption is less than 1% of the applied dose due to rapid volatilization from non-occluded skin. Nearly complete absorption of orally administered benzene has been demonstrated in laboratory animal studies.

Once in the bloodstream, benzene is rapidly distributed throughout several body compartments. The parent compound can be stored mainly in lipid-rich tissues such as brain, liver, blood, kidney and adrenal gland after high doses acute exposure, and liver, abdominal cavity fat, and bone marrow, after low dose long term exposure. The concentration of benzene in fat, bone marrow and urine are about 20 times higher than that in the blood. Benzene is also found in the placenta and fetuses immediately following exposure.

In vivo, approximately 40% of absorbed benzene goes to metabolism, and 10% deposits in lipid-rich tissues and then releases slowly to participate in the metabolism of benzene. Initial biotransformation of benzene takes place primarily in the liver and cytochrome P450 2E1 (CYP2E1) is necessary for the expression of hematotoxicity.

The first step in benzene metabolism is the formation of the epoxide, benzene oxide, catalyzed by CYP2E1 (Figure 4.1). After formation of benzene oxide, the metabolism of benzene branches into several alternative metabolic pathways to produce several putative toxic metabolites. Benzene oxide rearranges nonenzymatically to form phenol, the major product of initial benzene metabolism. Alternatively, benzene oxide may react with glutathione (GSH) to form phenylmercapturic acid; undergo enzymatic conversion by epoxide hydrolase to benzene dihydrodiol with subsequent formation of catechol; or undergo an iron-catalyzed, ring-opening reaction to form trans, trans-muconaldehyde (MUC) with subsequent metabolism to trans, trans-muconic acid (MA). Phenol is further oxidized by CYP2E1 catalysis to hydroquinone. Further oxidation of hydroquinone to p-benzoquinone is catalyzed by myeloperoxidase (MPO). Most research has focused on the hypothesis that phenol, catechol, and hydroquinone are produced in the liver and transported to the bone marrow, where secondary metabolism are occurs and hydroquinone is activated to p-benzoquinone by the action of MPO. However, the fact that administration of phenol does not produce the same effects as benzene is a problem in the phenolic metabolite hypothesis. A combination of phenol and hydroquinone is required to reproduce the hematotoxic effects of benzene. All of the phenolic products may be conjugated with sulfate or glucuronic acid, and the conjugates of phenol and hydroquinone is the major benzene metabolites excreted in urine. Urinary phenol and MA concentrations are correlated with benzene exposure level and

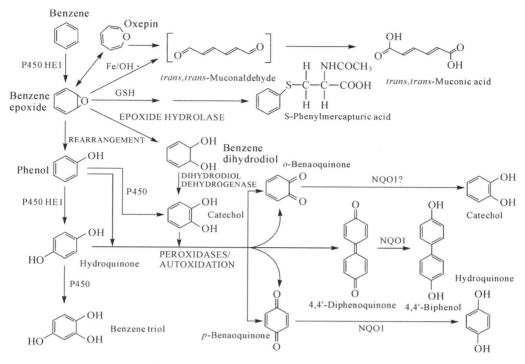

Figure 4. 1   Metabolic Pathways of Benzene

can be used to monitor benzene occupational exposure.

Acute benzene exposure causes central nervous system depression which is similar to the general anesthetic effects and is assumed to be a direct effect of benzene unrelated to its metabolites. The benzene can bind to nervous cells and inhibit the function.

Chronic exposure causes bone marrow depression leading to aplastic anemia and is also associated with an increased incidence of leukemia. Benzene metabolites are considered the toxic agents, not the parent compound.

There is evidence to support several different mechanisms by which benzene metabolites may cause hematotoxicity. Benzene metabolites form adducts with both proteins and DNA. Adduct formation with protein sulfhydryl groups inhibits tubulin polymerization during spindle formation and the activity of topoisomerase II in DNA plication and transcription. These effects may explain the clastogenic activity of benzene. Benzene itself is not mutagenic; however, mutagenicity of several of its metabolites is well established. Benzene metabolites may also induce oxidative stress by depleting GSH and by producing of reactive oxygen species that react with cellular macromolecules. Benzene also disrupts production of the cytokine IL-1, which is essential for hematopoiesis. Metabolite p-benzoquinone inhibits the activity of calpain, an enzyme that catalyzes the processing of pre-IL-1α to the mature cytokine. Metabolites may also inhibit stromal cells, which are necessary to support growth of differentiating and maturing bone marrow cells. All of these effects may be involved in causing the toxic effects of benzene.

(4) Clinical Findings

① Acute benzene poisoning: Human exposure to very high concentrations approximately 20,000 ppm, is fatal in 5 — 10 min. Concentrations of 7,500 ppm are dangerous to life within 30 min. Convulsive movements and paralysis followed by unconsciousness after severe exposures. Brief exposure to concentrations in excess of 3,000 ppm is irritating to the eyes and respiratory tract; continued exposure may cause euphoria, nausea, a staggering gait, and coma. Inhalation of lower concentrations (250—500 ppm) produces dizziness, drowsiness, headache, and nausea, whereas 25 ppm for 8 h has no clinical effect.

② Chronic benzene poisoning: The most significant toxic effect of benzene exposure is injury to the bone marrow. Chronic exposure to low concentrations may produce reversible decreases in blood cell numbers. Long-term exposures to higher concentrations lead to the onset of irreversible bone marrow depression. Clinically, an initial increase followed by a decrease in erythrocytes, leukocytes, or platelets is observed, with progression to anemia, leucopenia, and/or thrombocytopenia, respectively. If pancytopenia (i. e., the depression of all three cell types) occurs and is accompanied by bone marrow necrosis, the syndrome is termed aplastic anemia. The hypocellularity varies greatly from conditions in which the marrow is completely devoid of recognizable hematopoietic precursors to those in which the precursors of only one cell line are absent or arrested in their development. Typical symptoms may include light-headedness, headache, loss of appetite, and abdominal discomfort. With more severe intoxication, there may be weakness, blurring of vision, and dyspnea on exertion; the mucous membranes and skin may result in pale, and a hemorrhagic tendency may result in petechiae, easy bruising, epistaxis, bleeding from the gums, or menorrhagia.

Numerous case reports and epidemiological studies suggest a leukemogenic action of benzene in humans—the leukemia tending to be acute and myeloblastic in type, often following aplastic changes in the bone marrow. Acute myelocytic leukemia may be preceded by myelodysplastic syndrome, a preleukemic state characterized by abnormal marrow architecture, inadequate hematopoiesis, and many cells with chromosome damage. Benzene may also induce chronic types of leukemia.

The IARC has concluded that epidemiological studies have established the relationship between benzene exposure and the development of acute myelogenous leukemia. There is sufficient evidence that benzene is carcinogenic to humans (Group 1).

Direct contact with the liquid may cause erythema and vesiculation; prolonged or repeated contact has been associated with the development of a dry, scaly dermatitis or with secondary infections. Some skin absorption can occur with lengthy exposure to solvents containing benzene and may contribute more to toxicity than originally believed, but the dermal route is considered only a minor source of exposure for the general population.

(5) Diagnosis and Treatment

① Diagnosis: The diagnosis of acute benzene poisoning depends on a history of benzene exposure and associated neurological symptoms. Benzene has a sweet aromatic odor which may help in its detection. Laboratory testing for excess phenol in the urine will support the diagnosis. Benzene may also be detected in blood for a short period of time after exposure, and it may be measured in exhaled breath air. Hematological abnormalities, especially anemia, leukopenia, thrombocytopenia, pancytopenia, or acute myelogenous leukemia, associated with long-term benzene exposure suggest chronic benzene poisoning.

The laboratory evaluation of benzene-exposed persons should include the following: complete blood count with differential, Hematocrit (Hct), Hemoglobin (Hgb), erythrocyte count, erythrocyte indices (i. e., mean corpuscular volume, MCV; mean corpuscular hemoglobin, MCH; mean corpuscular hemoglobin concentration, MCHC), and platelet count. Plasma folate and vitamin B12 levels may be used to rule out megaloblastic anemia if the MCV is elevated. These laboratory tests will detect hematologic abnormalities that have been associated with relatively high levels of exposure to benzene. Persons with blood dyscrasias that persist after removal from exposure should be evaluated by a hematologist. Bone marrow aspiration and biopsy may be useful in narrowing the differential diagnosis in some cases.

② Treatment: There is no antidote for benzene poisoning; therefore, treatment for persons acutely exposed to benzene is generally supportive and symptomatic. Immediate removal of the patient from exposure, administration of oxygen, and monitoring and treatment of cardiopulmonary status are the first considerations. In cases of ingestion, respiratory distress may indicate pulmonary aspiration of gastric contents.

Contaminated clothing and shoes should be removed from an exposed person as soon as possible. If liquid benzene has contacted the skin or eyes, immediately wash the exposed skin with soap and copious water, and irrigate the eyes with running water for 3 to 5 min or until irritation ceases.

In cases of ingestion, do not induce emesis. Care must be taken to avoid aspiration of stomach contents during vomiting because benzene can produce a severe chemical pneumonitis. Ensure that the patient's airway is properly controlled and maintained before initiating orogastric lavage. Gastric lavage is indicated if large amounts of benzene have been ingested or if the patient is seen more than 1 hour after ingestion. Activated charcoal may be used; it decreases benzene absorption in experimental animals, and the benefits are likely to be similar in humans. Monitor the cardiac status of the patient: benzene is one of several solvents that may increase susceptibility of the myocardium to the dysrhythmogenic effects of catecholamines.

Epinephrine should be used only in the setting of cardiac arrest or severe refractory reactive airway disease because its use may lead to ventricular fibrillation secondary to the irritability of the myocardium.

In treating persons chronically exposed to benzene, the most important actions are to remove the patient from the source of benzene exposure and to prevent further exposure. Chronically exposed patients whose hematologic results do not return to normal despite removal from exposure should be managed in consultation with a hematologist or oncologist. Chemotherapy and bone marrow transplants are therapeutic options for leukemia and aplastic anemia, respectively.

(6) Prognosis and Prevention

① Prognosis: There is no specific antidote for benzene, but its effects can be treated, and most exposed persons recover fully. Persons who have experienced serious symptoms may need to be hospitalized. Recovery from moderate exposure to benzene may take 1 to 4 weeks. During this time, patients may continue to experience impaired gait, nervous irritability, and breathlessness for 2 weeks. Cardiac distress and yellow coloration of the skin may persist for up to a month.

② Prevention: Controlling exposures to benzene is the fundamental method of protecting workers. The other strategy of controlling is to promote the use of alternative solvents in industrial processes, glues and paints. Policies and legislation can be developed and implemented to remove benzene from consumer products.

Use stringent control measures such as process enclosure to prevent benzene release into the workplace. Use backup controls (e. g. double mechanical pump seals) to prevent the release of benzene due to equipment failure. Measurements to determine worker exposure to benzene should be taken to ensure that the average exposure level is lower than the workplace standards and limit the air concentrations that workers can be exposed to. Workers should be provided with and required to use chemical protective clothing, gloves, and other appropriate protective clothing necessary to prevent skin contact with benzene. Occupational health interviews and physical examinations should be performed at regular intervals. Additional examinations may be necessary if a worker reports symptom that may be attributed to exposure to benzene.

4.2.2.2 Toluene and Xylene

(1) Physical and Chemical Properties

The chemical formula for toluene is $C_6H_5CH_3$, and its molecular weight is 92.1. Toluene is a clear, colorless, flammable, volatile liquid with a sweet, pungent, benzene-like odor. Toluene mixes readily with many organic solvents, but is poorly soluble in water. The vapor pressure for toluene is 28.4 mmHg at 25℃. There are three forms of xylene in which the methyl groups vary on the benzene ring: meta-xylene, ortho-xylene, and para-xylene (m-, o-, and p-xylene). These different forms are referred to as isomers. Xylene is a colorless, sweet-smelling liquid that catches on fire easily, and is practically insoluble in water. The chemical formula for mixed xylenes is $C_6H_4(CH_3)_2$, and the molecular weight is 106.2. The vapor pressure for mixed xylenes is 6.728 mmHg at 21℃.

(2) Exposure Opportunities

Toluene or xylene may be inexpensive, less-toxic replacements for benzene, because they have similar chemical properties and may work as effectively as benzene. The exposure opportunities of toluene and toluene are similar to benzene.

The major use of toluene is as a mixture added to gasoline to improve octane ratings. Toluene is also used to produce benzene and as a solvent in paints, coatings, synthetic fragrances, adhesives, inks, and cleaning agents. Xylene is used as a solvent and in the printing, rubber, and leather industries. Xylene is also used in the production of ethylbenzene, as solvents in products such as paints and coatings, and is blended into gasoline. Occupational exposure to xylene may occur at workplaces where xylene is produced and used as industrial solvents.

(3) Absorption, Distribution, Metabolism and Excretion

Toluene and xylene are readily absorbed by humans from inhalation, oral, and dermal exposures. The main route of exposure is inhalation. Once in the bloodstream, toluene and xylene are distributed widely throughout the body, specifically adipose tissue, brain, liver, and kidneys. The liver converts toluene into organic acids. Toluene is metabolized by the cytochrome P-450 system. The end products include benzoic acid and hippuric acid. Hippuric acid is excreted by the kidney. Some toluene is excreted unchanged in expired air and urine.

Xylene is mainly oxidized to methylbenzoic acid, which is conjugated with glycine to form methylhippuric acid. Then methylhippuric acid binds to glucuronic acid and is excreted by the kidney.

Inhalation of high concentration of toluene or xylene mainly caused the anesthetic effect of the central nervous system. It has irritating effect on skin and mucosa.

(4) Clinical Findings

① Acute poisoning: The CNS is the primary target organ for toluene toxicity in both humans and animals for acute and chronic exposures. CNS dysfunction (which is often reversible) and narcosis have been frequently observed in humans acutely exposed to low or moderate levels of toluene by inhalation; symptoms include fatigue, sleepiness, headaches, and nausea. CNS depression and death have occurred at higher levels of exposure.

Human and animal data show that all xylene isomers or xylene mixtures produce similar effects, although specific isomers may not be equally potent in producing the effects. Acute inhalation exposure to mixed xylenes in humans has been associated with dyspnea and irritation of the nose and throat; gastrointestinal effects such as nausea, vomiting, and gastric discomfort; mild transient eye irritation; and neurological effects such as impaired short-term memory, impaired reaction time, performance decrements in numerical ability, and alterations in equilibrium and body balance. Acute dermal exposure in humans results in transient skin irritation and dryness and scaling of the skin.

② Chronic poisoning: Neurobehavioral effects have been observed in occupationally exposed workers. Chronic inhalation exposure to toluene causes irritation of the upper respiratory tract and eyes, sore throat, dizziness, headache, and sleeping difficulty. Chronic exposure of humans to mixed xylenes, as seen in occupational settings, has resulted primarily in neurological effects such as headache, dizziness, fatigue, tremors, incoordination, anxiety, impaired short-term memory, and inability to concentrate.

(5) Diagnosis and Treatment

Diagnosis: The diagnosis was made according to the history of occupational exposure of toluene or xylene, workplace site investigation data and associated neurological symptoms.

Treatment: There is no specific antidote for toluene or xylene toxicity. When treating these patients, the following actions should be taken: Carefully carry or drag victims to safety. In cases of respiratory compromise secure airway and respiration via endotracheal intubation, provide supplemental oxygen and administer β_2-agonists, if wheezing. Treat hypotension with aggressive IV crystalloid fluid. Treat hydrocarbon induced dysrhythmias with propranolol, esmolol, or lidocaine. No benefit to gastric lavage or activated charcoal. Correct electrolyte abnormalities. Administer blood products as needed.

(6) Prognosis and Prevention

Patients with acute or chronic mild to moderate intoxication of toluene or xylene can resume their original work after being cured, but patients with severe chronic toluene or xylene poisoning after treatment should be removed from the work position exposed to toluene or xylene.

Use a local exhaust ventilation and enclosure, if necessary, to control amount in the air. Control the concentrations of toluene and xylene in the air below the national standard. Personal Protective Equipment (PPE) is needed when working with toluene and xylene. Strengthening the occupational health surveillance of working populations. Occupational health interviews and physical examinations should be performed at regular intervals.

4.2.3　Aromatic Amino and Nitro Compounds

The aromatic amino compounds are a class of chemical derived from aromatic hydrocarbons, such as benzene, toluene, naphthalene, anthracene and diphenyl by the replacement of at least one hydrogen atom by ammo($-NH_2$) group. It is thus possible to produce a considerable range of compounds and, in effect, the aromatic amines constitute a large class of chemicals of great technical and commercial value. Aniline is the simplest aromatic amino compound, consisting of one$-NH_2$ group attached to a benzene ring and its derivatives are most widely used in industry.

The aromatic nitro compounds are a group of organic chemicals headed by nitrobenzene ($C_6H_5NO_2$) and derived from benzene and its homologues (toluene and xylene), naphthalene and anthracene by replacement of one or more hydrogen atoms by a nitro-group ($-NO_2$). The nitro-group may be replaced along with halogen and certain alkyl radicals at almost any position in the ring. Nitrocompounds of major industrial importance include nitrobenzene, dinitrotoluenes, trinitrotoluene (TNT), dinitrochlorobenzenes, dichloronitrobenzenes, etc.

（1）Uses and Exposure

Aromatic amino compounds are primarily used as intermediates in the manufacture of dyes and pigments. The largest class of dyestuffs is that of the azo dyes, another important class of dyestuffs is the triphenylmethane colours. Both manufactured from aromatic amines. In addition to serving as chemical intermediates in the dyestuffs industry, several compounds are employed as dyes or intermediates in the pharmaceutical, fur, hairdressing, textile, and photography industries.

Aromatic nitro compounds have few direct uses other than in the formulation of explosives or as solvents. The major consumption involves reduction to aniline derivatives used in the manufacture of dyes, pigments, insecticides, textiles, plastics, resins, elastomers, pharmaceuticals, plant-growth regulators, fuel additives, and rubber accelerators and antioxidants.

（2）Absorption Pathways

The principal risk of absorption lies in skin contact: the aromatic amines are nearly all lipid-soluble. In addition to skin adsorption, there is also a considerable risk of absorption by inhalation. This may be the result of inhaling the vapours, even though most of these amines are of low volatility at normal temperatures; or it may result from breathing in dust from the solid products handling. This applies particularly in the case of the amine salts such as sulphates and chlorohydrates, which have a very low volatility and lipid solubility: the occupational hazard from the practical point of view is less but their over-all toxicity is about the same as the corresponding amine, and thus the inhalation of their dust and even skin contact must be considered dangerous.

The fat-soluble nitro compounds are absorbed very easy through the skin. Dinitrophenol can penetrate the intact skin, however, as it is brilliant yellow, skin contamination is readily recognized.

Absorption by way of the digestive tract does represent a potential danger if workers do not exercise proper personal hygiene practices. Contamination of food and cigarette smoking with dirty hands are two examples of possible ingestion routes.

（3）Metabolism

The aromatic amino and nitro compounds undergo a process of metabolization within the organism (Figure 4. 2). Generally, the active agents are the metabolites, some of which induce methemoglobinemia, while others are carcinogenic. Metabolites of amines generally take the form of hydroxylamines (R—NHOH), changing to aminophenols (H_2N—R—OH) as a form of detoxification; a certain amount of nitro compounds is excreted unchanged through the kidneys, but the major portion is reduced to cyanogenic nitroso and hydroxylamine derivatives, which in turn are degraded to the ortho- and para-aminophenol analogues. Metabolites excreted in urine provide a means of estimating the degree of contamination when exposure levels reach detectable levels, and the amounts of which run parallel with the level of methemoglobinemia.

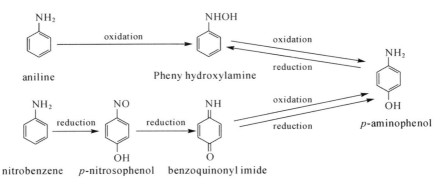

Figure 4. 2   Metabolic Pathways of Aniline and Nitrobenzene

(4) Health Effects

Aromatic amino or nitro compounds have various pathological effects, and each member of the family does not share the same toxicological properties. While each chemical must be evaluated independently, certain important characteristics are prominently shared by many of them.

① Hematotoxicity: Methemoglobinemia: Acute poisoning generally results from the inhibition of hemoglobin function through the formation of methemoglobin [the oxygen-carrying ferrous ion (Fe^{2+}) of the heme group of the hemoglobin molecule is oxidized to the ferric state (Fe^{3+})], resulting in the decreased oxygen-binding capacity of itself, as well as the increased oxygen-binding affinity of other subunits in the same hemoglobin molecule, which prevents them from releasing oxygen at normal tissue oxygen levels, leading to a hypoxia condition called methemoglobinemia. This can give the blood a bluish or chocolate-brown color. Aniline, nitrobenzene and trinitrotoluene are all methemoglobin inducers.

Methemoglobinemia is more often associated with nitro compounds and the single-ring aromatic amino compounds. Methemoglobin is normally present in the blood at a level of about 1% to 2% of the total hemoglobin. Cyanosis at the oral mucosa becomes apparent at levels of 10% to 15%, though subjective symptoms are normally not apparent until methemoglobin levels reach 30%. With increases of the level, the patient's skin colour deepens; subsequently, headache, weakness, malaise and anoxia, are to be succeeded. If absorption continues, it may results in coma, cardiac failure and death. Three out of four cases of cyanosis will exhibit the classical blue or ashen-grey appearance, but only one-third of the victims will complain of anoxia symptoms (headache, fatigue, nausea, vertigo, chest pain, numbness, abdominal pain, aching, palpitation, aphonia, nervousness, air hunger and irrational behavior). Blood and urine analyses are required for confirmation.

Most cases of acute poisoning react favourably to treatment and the methemoglobin disappears completely after two to three days.

Hemolysis: Hemolysis of the red blood cells can be detected after severe poisoning, and is followed by a process of regeneration demonstrated by the presence of reticulocytes. Under these circumstances, great amount of reductants, such as GSH, NADPH, which usually serve as essentials to eliminate the oxides within red blood cell and maintain its normal function, are consumed by much oxidative metabolites of aromatic amino and nitro compounds, and result in hemolysis, especially in whom with congenital glucose-6-phosphate dehydrogenase deficiency.

Heinz bodies: The presence of Heinz bodies (sedimentary paraglobin) in the red blood corpuscles may sometimes also be detected. This phenomenon of globin denaturation is often due to sulfhydryl combined with, and destroyed by oxidative metabolites of aromatic amino and nitro compounds.

② Carcinogenicity: Benzidine, β-naphthylamine and 4-aminodiphenyl were considered to be the "culprit" chemicals for bladder cancer of employees in some dye factories. Benzidine, β-naphthylamine and 4-aminodiphenyl have been classified as a Group 1 (carcinogenic to humans) by the IARC.

③ Dermatitis: Because of their alkaline nature, certain amines, particularly the primary ones, constitute a direct risk of dermatitis. Many aromatic amines, such as p-aminophenol and p-phenylenediamine, can cause allergic dermatitis. Dichloronitrobenzenes possess intermediate dermal toxicity. The mono- and di-nitrochlorobenzenes may also produce dermatitis due to primary irritation or sensitization in most people even after slight contact.

④ Liver injuries: Repeated exposure to nitro compounds (e. g. nitrobenzene, dinitrobenzene, trinitrotoluene) may be followed by severe liver impairment up to yellow atrophy. Certain diamines, such as toluenediamine and diaminodiphenylmethane, can result in toxic hepatitis after occupational exposure.

⑤ Urinary system damage: Hemorrhagic cystitis can result from heavy exposure to o- and p-toluidine, particularly the chlorine derivatives, of which chloro-5-o-toluidine is the best example. This hematuria appears to be short-lived and the relationship to development of bladder tumours is not established.

⑥ Toxic cataract: Long-term exposure to trinitrotoluene, dinitrophenol, dinitro-o-cresol may induce lens opacities of employees and further develop to toxic cataracts.

⑦ Nervous impairment: Nitrobenzene is a central nervous poison, causing in some cases, excitement and tremors followed by severe depression, unconsciousness and coma. In severe cases some compounds may induce optic neuritis and optic perineuritis.

⑧ Respiratory allergy: Cases of asthma due to sensitization to p-phenylenediamine, dinitrochlorobenzenes for example, have been reported.

(5) Treatment

① Prevent continuous absorption of toxicant: All casualties should be transferred from the toxic atmosphere to fresh air, disrobed all the contaminated clothing and footgear, and entire body surface should be carefully washed with soap and tepid water (never use hot water).

② Treatment of methemoglobinemia: Methemoglobinemia can be treated with supplemental oxygen, and 1% methylene blue solution 5—10 mL (1—2 mg/kg) is usually added into 20 mL 10%—25% glucose solution for intravenous injection. If necessary it can be administered repeatedly after 1—2 h until cyanosis disappears, or the level of methemoglobine is under 15%.

Methylene blue restores the iron in hemoglobin to its normal (reduced) oxygen-carrying state (Figure 4.3). This is achieved by providing an artificial electron acceptor (such as methylene blue, or flavin) for NADPH methemoglobin reductase (RBCs usually don't have one; the presence of methylene blue allows the enzyme to function at 5×normal levels). The NADPH is generated via the hexose monophosphate shunt. Large amount of vitamin C, coenzyme A and cytochrome C have synergistic therapeutic effects with methylene blue. If concentration of methemoglobin is less than 30%, the use methylene blue is not needed, and plenty of vitamin C and oral sugary drinks are recommended.

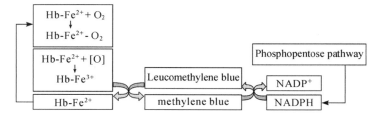

Figure 4.3   Detoxification Schematic of Drug for Methemoglobinemia

③ Symptomatic treatment: The therapeutic principles, measures and methods mentioned in general internal medicine for hepatic, nephritic, hematic and dermal diseases are applied equally to the same situations from aromatic amino and nitro compounds poisoning.

(6) Safety and Health Measures

The most important specific measure for the prevention of spillage or contamination of the work atmosphere by these compounds is proper plant design. Ventilation control of the contaminant should be designed as close to manufacturing location as possible. Work clothing should be changed daily and facilities for an obligatory bath or shower at the end of the working period should be provided. Any contamination of skin or clothing should be washed off immediately and the individual should be kept under medical supervision. Both workers and supervisors should be educated to be aware of the nature and extent of the hazard and to carry out the work in a clean, safe manner. Maintenance work should be preceded with sufficient attention to removal of possible sources of contact with the offending chemicals.

4.2.3.1 Aniline

(1) Physical and Chemical Properties

Aniline is also called aminobenzene or phenylamine. Pure aniline is a colourless liquid, but it darkens rapidly on exposure to light and air. It is normally a brown oily liquid. It is volatile, with unpleasant odor, and its melting point is −6.2℃ and boiling point is 184℃. Aniline is slightly soluble in water and is capable of mixing with some organic solvents like ether, alcohol, benzene, and chloroform.

(2) Exposure Opportunities

Aniline is widely used in the manufacture of synthetic dyestuffs. It is also used in printing and cloth marking inks and in the manufacture of resins, varnishes, perfumes, photographic chemicals, explosives, herbicides and fungicides. Aniline is used in the manufacture of rubber as a vulcanizing agent, as an antioxidant, and as an anti-ozone agent.

(3) Absorption, Distribution, Metabolism and Excretion

Aniline can be toxic if ingested, inhaled, or by skin contact. Rapid absorption through the intact skin is frequently the main route of entry from direct contact with either the liquid or the vapor.

(4) Clinical Findings

Anoxia caused by acute aniline poisoning is due to the formation of methemoglobin. The formation of methemoglobinemia is often insidious; the onset of symptoms may be delayed for up to 4 hours after skin absorption. Headache is commonly the first symptom and may become quite intense as the severity of methemoglobinemia progresses. Cyanosis occurs when the methemoglobin level is 15% or more. Blueness develops first in the lips, the nose, and the earlobes, and is usually recognized by fellow workers. The individual usually feels well, has no complaints, and is insistent that nothing is wrong until the methemoglobin concentration approaches approximately 40%. When methemoglobin concentration is elevated over 40% in red blood cells, weakness and dizziness may occur. When methemoglobin content increases to 70%, there may be ataxia, dyspnea on mile exertion, and tachycardia. Coma may ensue with methemoglobin levels of about 70%, and the lethal level is estimated to be 85%—90%. In general, higher ambient temperatures increase susceptibility to cyanosis from exposure to methemoglobin-forming agents.

The development of intravascular hemolysis and anemia due to aniline-induced methemoglobinemia has been postulated, but neither is observed often in industrial practice. In the severe cases, secondary jaundice, toxic hepatopathy, irritative symptoms of bladder and even acute renal failure may occur. Little myocardial damage may be observed. Occasional deaths from asphyxiation caused by severe aniline intoxication are said to occur.

The existence of chronic aniline poisoning is controversial, but some investigators have suggested that continuous exposure to small doses of aniline may produce anemia, loss of energy, digestive disturbance, and headache.

Peak methemoglobin levels may occur some hours after exposure, and it has been postulated that metabolic transformation of aniline to phenylhydroxylamine is necessary for the production of methemoglobin. Liquid aniline is mildly irritating to the eyes and may cause corneal damage.

(5) Diagnosis and Treatment

① Diagnosis: According to the occupational history of heavy exposure to aniline, the clinical manifestations of mainly methemoglobinemia, combined with laboratory test results (the elevated levels of methemoglobin in the blood, Heinz body phenomenon in erythrocytes, the increased levels of urinary p-aminophenol) and on-site occupational hygiene investigation, a comprehensive analysis was made to make the diagnosis.

② Treatment: Carefully carry or drag victims to safety. Victims should not be allowed to overexert themselves, as exposure to aniline can produce hypoxia (due to methemoglobinemia) which can be exacerbated by physical effort. Patients exposed only to aniline vapor who have no skin or eye irritation may be transferred immediately to the support zone. Other patients will require decontamination.

Immediate treatment for aniline overexposure consists of decontamination and cardiopulmonary support. Symptomatic individuals should be administered supplemental oxygen and the methemoglobin antidote, methylene blue, as soon as possible.

Patients with chronic intoxication of aniline after treatment should be removed from the work position exposed to aniline.

(6) Prognosis and Prevention

A solution of methylene blue may be given through a vein to patients who have been seriously exposed to aniline. Most patients recover within 24 hours, but they may need to be hospitalized for several days. The urine of a patient who has received methylene blue treatment may temporarily become blue to blue-green.

For specific prevention refer to the content of safety and health measures for amino and nitro compounds in this section.

The Occupational Safety and Health Administration (OSHA) sets a limit of 5 parts of aniline per million parts of air (5 ppm) in workplace air in any 8-hour shift, 40-hour workweek.

4.2.3.2 Trinitrotoluene

(1) Physical and Chemical Properties

2,4,6-trinitrotoluene, commonly known as TNT, is colorless, odorless, monoclinic prisms, crystals; commercial crystals are yellow. Its melting point is 80.1℃ and boiling point is 240℃. It is extremely difficult to dissolve in water, but is soluble in acetone, alcohol, ether and benzene. It can explode suddenly when being heated.

(2) Exposure Opportunities

TNT is used extensively in the manufacture of military and industrial explosives. Other industrial uses include chemical manufacturing as an intermediate in the production of dyestuffs and photographic chemicals.

(3) Absorption, Distribution, Metabolism and Excretion

Exposures to TNT both through inhalation and skin absorption can occur during its production, munitions manufacturing and loading, and blasting operations. TNT is absorbed by the bloodstream and travels to the organs. When it reaches the liver, it breaks down and changes into several different substances, such as 4-amino-2,6-dinitrotoluene (4-ADNT). Most of these substances travel through the blood to the kidneys and then leave the body in urine. Therefore, the concentration of 4-ADNT (the most content of metabolites) and prototype of TNT in urine can estimate the degree of exposure of the workers.

(4) Clinical Findings

TNT has multisystem toxicities involving hematic, hepatic, ocular, dermal and reproductive. Exposures exceeding 0.5 mg/m^3 cause destruction of red blood cells. Hemolysis is partially compensated for by enhanced regeneration of red blood cells in the bone marrow, which is manifest as an increased percentage of reticulocytes in peripheral blood. Among some groups of workers, there is a reduction in average hemoglobin and hematocrit values. Workers deficient in glucose-6-phosphate dehydrogenase may be particularly at risk of acute hemolytic disease. Above 1.0 mg/m^3, elevations of liver function enzymes may occur.

A characteristic TNT cataract is reportedly produced with exposures regularly exceeding 1.0 mg/m^3 for more than 5 years. The opacities did not interfere with visual acuity or visual fields. The induced cataracts may not regress once exposure ceases, although progression is arrested.

The vapor or dust can cause irritation of mucous membranes, resulting in sneezing, cough, and sore throat. Although intense or prolonged exposure to TNT may cause some cyanosis, it is not regarded as a strong producer of methemoglobin. Other occasional effects include leukocytosis or leucopenia, peripheral neuritis, muscular pains, cardiac irregularities, and renal irritation. The skin, hair, and nails of exposed workers may be stained yellow.

TNT is absorbed through skin rapidly, and reference to airborne levels of vapor or dust may underestimate total systemic exposure if skin exposure also occurs. Apparent differences in dose-response relationships based only on airborne levels may be explained by differences in dermal absorption. TNT causes sensitization dermatitis; the hands, wrist, and forearms are most commonly affected, but skin at frication points such as the collar line, belt line, and ankles is also often involved. Erythema, papules, and an itchy eczema can be severe.

Significantly lower semen volumes, a smaller percentage of motile spermatozoa, and a higher incidence of sperm malformation were reported in a case-control study in two TNT plants in China (Li et al., 1993). No studies found reproductive effects of TNT in females.

(5) Diagnosis and Treatment

The diagnosis of TNT poisoning depends on the occupational history of long-term exposure to TNT, the clinical manifestations damage to the liver, blood, and nervous system, and the workplace site investigation data. Laboratory testing for measure 2,4,6-trinitrotoluene or its breakdown products in the blood and urine will support the diagnosis.

Treatment: Patients are advised to eat a light, nutritious diet, and should not drink alcohol or take drugs that impair liver function. Use the medicines for liver protection and enzyme decrease. For severe patients with liver failure, it is recommended to carry out specialized symptomatic treatment. Other treatments are the same as internal medicine.

Patients with chronic intoxication of TNT after treatment should be removed from the work position exposed to aniline TNT.

(6) Prognosis and Prevention

For specific prevention refer to the content of safety and health measures for amino and nitro compounds in this section.

The Occupational Safety and Health Administration (OSHA) regulates levels of hazardous materials in the workplace. The maximum allowable amount of TNT in workroom air during an 8-hour workday, 40-hour workweek, is 0.5 mg/m^3.

4.2.4　Irritant Gases

4.2.4.1　Definition and Classification

Irritant gases are those which, when inhaled, or dissolve in the water of the respiratory tract mucosa, can cause an inflammatory response or provoke a physiologic response because of either their chemical reactivity or physical properties, usually caused by the release of acidic or alkaline radicals. Irritant gas exposures predominantly affect the airways, causing tracheitis, bronchitis, and bronchiolitis; and these exposures can also result in irritating to eyes and skin.

Irritant gases are mainly divided into the following categories:

Acids: inorganic acid, such as sulfuric acid, hydrochloric acid, nitric acid, chromic acid, chlorosulfonic acid; organic acids, such as formic acid, acetic acid, propionic acid, butyric acid.

Acid-forming oxides: sulfur dioxide, sulfur trioxide, nitrogen dioxide, dinitrogen pentoxide, chromic anhydride, etc.

Acid-forming hydrides: hydrogen chloride, hydrogen fluoride, hydrogen bromide and hydrogen sulfide, etc.

Halogen elements: fluorine, chlorine, bromine and iodine.

Inorganic chlorides: thionyl chloride, chlorine dioxide, phosphorus trichloride, boron trichloride, trichlorosilane, phosphorus oxychloride, arsenic trichloride, antimony trichloride, silicon tetrachloride, titanium tetrachloride, phosphorus pentachloride, phosgene, diphosgene, etc.

Halogenated hydrocarbons: methyl bromide, methyl iodide, chloropicrin.

Esters: dimethyl sulfate, toluene-2,4-diisocyanate, methyl chloroformate, methyl formate.

Aldehydes: formaldehyde, acetaldehyde, acrolein, chloral, etc.

Ketones: vinyl ketone, methacrylic ketone.

Aliphatic amines: monomethyl amine, dimethylamine, diethylamine, ethylenediamine.

Alkali-forming hydrides: ammonia.

Strong oxidizers: ozone.

Metal compounds: cadmium oxide, hydrogen selenide, nickel carbonyl, vanadium pentoxide.

Organic fluorides: monochlorodifluoromethane, tetrafluoroethylene, nitrogen trifluoride, oxygen difluoride, sulfur tetrafluoride, octafluoroisobutene, fluorophosgene, hexafluoropropylene, etc.

War gas: nitrogen mustard, phenarsazine hloride, lewisite.

Others: chloromethyl methyl ether, epichlorohydrin, carbon tetrachloride.

There are great different varieties of irritant gases, but more common are chlorine, ammonia, nitrogen oxides, phosgene, hydrogen fluoride, sulfur dioxide and sulfur trioxide, etc.

The irritant effects of these compounds above are most related to the action of acid or alkali. Although under normal conditions of temperature and pressure some substances may not exist as a gas, they can emit from the sources and finally change into vapors and gases by evaporation, sublimation and volatilization, which are easy to enter the body.

4.2.4.2   Exposure Opportunities

Irritant gases are commonly encountered as raw, ancillary materials, products or by-products and even wastes in chemical industrial areas. Most of them are corrosive, so they can erode many chemical storage facilities or pipeline, leading to leakage, dropping or effusing of these compounds slowly and slightly. On the other hand, these substances are usually stored in a tank, and accidental explosion caused by the sudden increasing pressure due to heating or violent collision of the gas tanks makes far-range spread of these toxicants. Because of noncompliance with the safety and health operating procedures or lack of good productive devices maintenance, the operating workers may expose to toxicants acutely or chronically, leading themselves to the risk of poisoning.

4.2.4.3   Toxicity

Based on water solubility, irritant gases can be divided into high, intermediate, or low water solubility. Common agents are grouped as follow: ①high water solubility: ammonia, hydrogen chloride, sulfur dioxide, chloramine; ②intermediate water solubility: chlorine, hydrogen sulfide, zinc oxide; ③low water solubility: phosgene, nitrogen dioxide. Among them, chlorine, phosgene, sulfur dioxide, hydrogen chloride or sulfide, nitrogen dioxide, ozone, and ammonia are the most common and important irritant gases.

The lung is highly vulnerable to the effects of respiratory irritants. The respiratory tract is protected by many layers of host defense, but they are primarily effective against infectious agents. Chemical hazards may bypass most of these host defenses in the upper airway and penetrate deeply to airways and alveoli. It is known that the respiratory tract is saturated with water in the upper section and is lined with a moist mucosa and comprises of a very large surface area. Therefore inhaled gases soluble in water to any appreciable extent tend to be dissolved readily and removed from the airway very efficiently, but gases that are less soluble in water penetrate the respiratory tract more deeply.

All lung irritant gases cause essentially the same type of pathological effect, in which the most pronounced one is located on the alveoli of the lungs and the smaller bronchial tubes. The great danger to be feared is the onset of acute pulmonary edema. The effect of inhaling irritant gases depends not only on the concentration and duration of exposure but also on the water solubility of specific agent. The pattern is that the severity is generally dose-related, or further from a response point of view, the atmospheric concentration is more important than the duration of exposure. In the case of very high dose or chronic exposure, the irritant gases can affect the entire respiratory tract, but in customary concentration exposure, the irritant gases can usually lead to local impairment. In the range of small to moderate doses, the following is typical: those with highly water soluble affect upper respiratory tract predominately, producing a stereotyped and acute pattern of damage with rapid onset of irritation, little or no potential for delayed symptoms, and recovery is often associated with major sequelae and sometimes significant respiratory impairment; those with intermediately water soluble affect all airways, some potential for delayed pulmonary injury/edema, combined with high or low water soluble symptoms; those with low water soluble affect lower respiratory tract predominately, to the terminal bronchiolar and alveolar regions, resulting in delayed symptoms that is known as "diffuse alveolar damage". Those relatively insoluble gases, such as phosgene, nitrogen dioxide, and ozone, are particularly dangerous because they can induce toxic pulmonary edema, an often-fatal outcome resembling ARDS.

Exposed to extreme high concentration of some irritant gases (e. g. more than 3,000 mg/m^3 of chlorine), "electric-shock-like death" may occur within a few minutes due to laryngospasm or cardiac arrest caused by vagus reflex.

4.2.4.4　Clinical Findings

(1) Acute Poisoning

Exposure to high concentration of irritant gases in the atmosphere causes immediate sensory irritation of the respiratory tract accompanied by smarting and watering of the eyes. This irritation of the respiratory tract causes catching of the breath, coughing and a sensation of tightness and constriction, and pain in the chest. After getting out of the poisonous atmosphere, the respiration remains rapid and shallow. Any attempt to drawing a deep breath gives rise to discomfort and provokes a fit of coughing. Nausea, retching, and vomiting are prominent features in the early stages of poisoning. There is slight or profuse expectoration. Headache, fatigue in all the limbs, often prostrate the patient.

The clinical presentation of toxic inhalation associated with the risk of pulmonary edema is stereotyped and varies little among the agents that can cause the syndrome. As edema develops in the lungs, the breathing becomes rapid and panting, but of a characteristically shallow type. The ears, lips and progressively the entire face assume a cyanotic, bluish-red tint which may deepen to the intense violet of fullest cyanosis, and there may be visible distension of the superficial veins of the face, neck or chest, especially in persons exposed with pure chlorine. In phosgene poisoning, this full cyanosis is often omitted, and the patient passes rapidly into a state of circulatory collapse, with a feeble, flickering pulse of over 120, a cold clammy skin, and a leaden hue in the face, in which only the lips and tips of the ears reveal the asphyxial cyanosis that underlies the failure of the man to win his fight for life. While in the stage of cyanosis, whether "blue" or "grey", the patient is always restless and very apprehensive of the seriousness of his condition. The expression is anxious and distressed, with the eyeballs staring and the lids half closed. At this stage casualties can be divided into three types: ① the milder case, with reddish flush in the face, with some hurry of respiration, and pain in the chest; ② the severe case, with "blue" cyanosed face, distended neck veins, and full, strong pulse over 100; ③ the severely collapsed case, with leaden "grey" cyanosis of the face, and rapid, thready pulse. The milder case is often drowsy and soon falls into sleep from which a person wakes refreshed. Coughing upon a deep breath, occasional vomiting after food or drink and a slight sense of rawness in the throat together with general debility, may persist for a few days, after which the patient becomes convalescent. During the early days of convalescence there is often a considerable slowing of the pulse from vagus action, which may bring it down to about 50 or even 45 in a minute. Such early bradycardia is also often seen at recovery stage in severe poisoning; it is also a sign that the patient is beginning to convalesce. Cases of severer cyanosis, if the depth of the reddish-blue color is well maintained and the pulse does not exceed 100, tend to recover in two or three days, and their recovery is generally similar to that of the milder cases. Provided that the circulation and the activity of the respiratory centre can be maintained, the edematous fluid in the lungs is soon absorbed, most of it vanishing by the fourth or fifth day. At any time however, particularly if subjected to much physical effort, those cases may rapidly pass into the most dangerous condition of "grey" cyanosis and collapse. The pulse becomes rapid, thready and irregular. The patient, though obviously weaker, becomes more restless and slightly wandering in mind, or semi-comatose. Even the worst of the "grey" cases may recover with proper treatment, but the mortality is always distressingly high. Recovery from this state of depressed circulation may be succeeded by severe and even fatal broncho-pneumonia. When this infective complication develops, the sputum becomes purulent and the temperature rises. Death usually follows rapidly. If the case lasts into the third week after gassing, one may justly be expected to survive the acute infection.

　　Some cases with insidious onset have been frequently reported in which men who have been exposed to gas can carry on their work for an hour or two with only trivial discomfort, and even to go home, then become rapidly worse, and passed into a condition of collapse with progressive edema of the lungs that may prove rapidly fatal. At other times men who have passed through a gas attack and have subsequently complained of only slight cough, nausea, and tightness of the chest whilst resting in some places, have collapsed and even died abruptly some hours later on attempting to perform some vigorous muscular effort. The percussion note may remain resonant over the chest, notwithstanding the existence of pulmonary edema. The breath sounds are weakened, especially over the back; they may also be harsh in character, but never tubular. Fine rales are heard, chiefly in the axillary region and at the back and sides of the chest, while rhonchi may be noted occasionally.

In the early acute stage, the physical signs give little indication of the gravity of the case or the extent of the damage to the lungs. The color, the pulse and the character of the respiration are the chief guides to prognosis. With the development of inflammatory complications and rising temperature, the physical signs become those of pleurisy, bronchitis or bronchopneumonia.

(2) Chronic Poisoning

Low-level continuous or intermittent exposure to irritant gases or chemical vapors may lead to chronic bronchitis, rhinitis, pharyngitis, conjunctivitis and even chronic obstructive pulmonary disease, although the role of such exposure is especially difficult to substantiate in smokers.

4.2.4.5　Diagnosis and Treatment

(1) Diagnosis

Diagnosis is usually obvious from the history of exposure to a special agent. Patients should have a chest X-ray and pulse oximetry. Chest X-ray findings of patchy or confluent alveolar consolidation usually indicate pulmonary edema. CT is used to evaluate patients with late-developing symptoms. Those with bronchiolitis obliterans that progresses to respiratory failure manifest a pattern of bronchiolar thickening and a patchy mosaic of hyperinflation. And the result of blood gas analysis shows hypoxemia.

(2) Treatment

Treatment does not differ by specific inhaled agent but rather by symptoms.

① Emergency symptomatic treatment at the scene: Evacuate all cases immediately, remove the victims lying down as soon as possible from the poisoning site to fresh air, ease their collars, belts and braces so as not to impede breathing, take off all the contaminated clothing, relieve all equipment avoiding physical effort as much as possible. Keeping patient warm should be directed especially when whose clothing is removed, and it is helpful in combating shock and diminishing the oxygen consumption that is entailed by the muscular movements of shivering. For eye or skin contamination, immediately rinse thoroughly with water or saline, for eyes burns, further administer with the 0.5% cortisone eye drops and antibiotic eye drops or ointment, for acid burns skin, use 2% to 3% sodium bicarbonate solution in the wet dressing, or for alkali burns skin, use 3% boric acid or 5% acetic acid water in the wet compress. Unroof significant skin blisters and treat with silver sulfadiazine. Those who show definite symptoms should not be allowed to leave their beds or stretchers for any purpose.

② General medical care: The essentials of treatment for acute poisoning by any pulmonary irritant gas are rest, warmth, oxygen, corticoids and medical monitoring. It is necessary to think of the lungs choked by an inflammatory edema which, none the less, may be absorbed in three or four days if the circulation can be maintained for so long. The diet should be fluid and sparingly given in the acute stage, but bland drinks should be allowed freely.

In clinical practice, cases of all degrees of severity may be met with, and it may be difficult at times to decide whether or not a man has really been gassed. The history of the case must be taken into account. Patients, regardless of severity, are required to stay in hospital for medical care. The length of observation period depends on the situation of exposure to gas (kinds, concentration, and duration) and, at least not less than 24 hours. It should be borne in mind that a delayed action may be exhibited by some pulmonary irritants, notably phosgene and the nitrogen oxides gases; but if no objective symptoms have a risen after the lapse of 48 hours the patient can be returned to duty with little delay.

During the observation period, the casualty should rest in bed absolutely, avoid physical load caused pulmonary capillary hydrostatic pressure as far as possible, keep warm, eliminate emotional tension and irritability, take sedatives if necessary, restrict the amount of intravenous fluids, and have chest X-ray examination as soon as possible. Medical monitoring indices including the changes of respiratory, pulse, blood pressure, dynamic blood-gas assay and chest X-ray should be taken into consideration.

If pulmonary complications develop (such as infective bronchitis, broncho-pneumonia), the patient should, if possible, be treated in a separate ward; otherwise, he should be separated by at least six feet from his nearest neighbor.

Expectoration should be encouraged by some postural device; vomiting is helpful in emptying the lungs, and often occurs spontaneously, but it is liable to produce exhaustion, and it should not be induced by powerful drugs such as apomorphine or ipecacuanha. Raise the foot of the bed or stretcher three or four feet for a few minutes at a time, with the idea of draining fluid from the chest, is sometimes effective in helping free expectoration. Expectorants should not be given to severe cases during the first two or three days for fear of increasing the tendency to cough and so augmenting the damage in the lungs. In mild cases, or when the acute symptoms have abated in the severe cases, ordinary expectorant mixtures containing ammonium carbonate and vinum ipecacuanha may be given with advantage and are helpful in checking the possible development of infective bronchitis.

The milder casualties are likely to recover after a short rest; those who have passed through a stage of severe cyanosis, however, or who have suffered from a complicating broncho-pneumonia require a prolonged period of convalescence. In convalescent stage, when definite cyanosis or severe symptoms have disappeared, all cases should be got up from bed as soon as possible; slight bronchitis or gastric disturbances, which usually are only temporary, do not contraindicate this, but cases of abnormally rapid or slow pulses should be rested a little longer.

A system of carefully graduated exercises, with full opportunities for lying down and resting in the intervals, should be instituted; the response to exercise of each individual, however, must be carefully studied, and exhaustion must be rigidly guarded against, as symptoms of effort syndrome may develop and add weeks or months to the period of convalescence.

③ Pulmonary edema treatment: Treatment is directed toward ensuring adequate oxygenation and alveolar ventilation.

• Oxygen therapy: Oxygen inhaling is an important therapeutic measure for pulmonary edema, especially for severe cases. It can elevate blood oxygen level, and promptly recovery from hypoxia. Because continuously inhalation of hyperbaric oxygen or hypertonic oxygen may cause oxidative damage in lung tissue, even induce pulmonary edema, and on the other hand, oxygen exchange is impeded by pulmonary edema, resulting in decreased blood oxygen levels. Therefore, the content of inhaled oxygen (called fraction of inspiration O_2, FiO_2) ranging from 40% to 60% is proper, thus the arterial partial pressure of oxygen (PaO_2) may maintain above 80 mmHg, or the arterial oxygen saturation (SaO_2) is more than 90%, which can basically meet the body's needs.

In order to tide the patients over the critical period of the first two or three days, oxygen should be administered continuously by means of some special apparatus, such as nasal catheter, oxygen mask, oxygen tent, that will ensure a suitable mixture with air. The common way of oxygen therapy is nasal catheter, and the oxygen flow rate is increased gradually from 2—3 L/min to 5 L/min. A sufficient current of oxygen ensure a change in the patient's color from livid blue or grey to a pink tint. This treatment must be maintained, day and night if necessary, with a progressive lessening of the oxygen supply, until the patient does not lapse into a cyanosis when the oxygen is withdrawn. Excessive oxygen flow can cause patients multiple excruciation as a result of local stimulus. Another apparatus is oxygen mask, the oxygen flow rate that with a simple mask should not be lower than 4 L/min. It is also available with a valve and the air bag mask ventilation. And oxygen tent can be used when conditions permit.

Positive end-expiratory pressure ventilation (PEEP) is the best oxygen therapeutic model. It can maintain a certain expansion of alveoli, increase the functional residual capacity, improve alveolar ventilation and arterial oxygen content, prevent intravascular fluid exudation, promote absorption of edema fluid in the alveoli, increase lung compliance, and improve the performance of hypoxia. But positive pressure ventilation increases venous pressure cutting down blood flow back to heart, reduces ejection of left ventricle. So it should be cautious. If the supply permits, oxygen should also be given to the milder cases of edema in order to prevent their lapsing into a more serious state of asphyxia.

The application of hyperbaric oxygen (HBO) for pulmonary edema due to irritant gases remains controversial. High concentrations of oxygen may cause peroxide damage in the lungs, decrease pulmonary surfactant; high tension oxygen may also exacerbate the bronchioles and alveolar damage, leading to alveolar rupture, pneumothorax, and pneumomediastinum.

• Corticosteroids therapy: The key for controlling progression of pulmonary edema is that early, sufficient, short-term applying of glucocorticoid. Dexamethasone dose for mild case is $40-80$ mg/day, moderate, $80-160$ mg/day, and in severe cases, $160-300$ mg/day, divided into $4-6$ time intravenously. Thereafter, the daily dose may be reduced according to the condition of the patients, and the total course should be no more than five days. Medication for the first time should have a larger dose pulse therapy.

• Improve alveolar ventilation: Bronchospasm easily caused by soluble strong irritant gases, can be relieved by aminophylline and glucose solution intravenous, or intramuscular injection, or aerosol inhalation which can ease local spasm, alleviate airway mucosal edema, and wet, dilute and promote mucus discharge. In the situation of much frothy sputum blocking the airway, patients should breathe in aerosol dimethicone which can unevenly reduce alveolar surface tension and make the bubble quickly burst into a liquid easy coughing out. Compared with inhalation of ethanol aerosol, its features are rapid, reliable, repeatable, and short duration of action.

Endotracheal intubation and tracheotomy are invasive. Tracheotomy surgical indications include some emergency: laryngeal edema, glottis spasm, and suffocation caused by blocking of hunk airway mucosal shedding, severe pulmonary infection, purulent and frothy sputum difficult to expectorate, incessant hypoxia difficult to improve, hypercapnia and pulmonary encephalopathy. Endotracheal intubation must be prudent because that aggravate airway damage could lead to mucosal shedding and airway obstruction.

Bronchodilators and O_2 therapy may suffice in less severe cases. Severe airflow obstruction is managed with inhaled racemic epinephrine, endotracheal intubation or tracheostomy, and mechanical ventilation. Endotracheal intubation must be considered early if upper airway is swelling. If intubated, patient may need to be added significant PEEP ventilation.

• Other auxiliary treatments: During the processing of acute lung injury, all the circumstance including blood condensed, viscosity, stasis, increased right heart load, dehydration and removal of moisture from the alveoli while filling the circulating with hypertonic saline results in the original viscosity of pulmonary circulation reaching to a unbearable degree. So diuresis should be limited. Appropriate diuretic maintains the balance or the PAWP (pulmonary arterial wedge pressure) under 18 cm H_2O so as to reduce blood viscosity and burden on the heart, promote intrapulmonary circulation, and fundamentally improve systemic hypoxia.

If necrotic mucosa sheds, the patient should be encouraged to cough up or, if necessary, perform tracheotomy to suck off the mucosa and prevent suffocation; for pneumothorax, stop positive pressure ventilation, apply antitussive, conventional exhaust or closed drainage. Correction of acid-base abnormalities and prophylactic antibiotics may be necessary. In addition, it should be supplemented with the energy mixture drugs to protect the myocardium, and reasonable nutritional support can promote patients recovery.

④ ARDS treatment: Traditional therapy for ARDS focus more on damage endpoint, namely severe pulmonary edema, ventilation or ventilatory dysfunction, and hypoxemia during processing. So the main treatment strategy are oxygen inhalation, anti-inflammatory, and anti-pulmonary edema, but with little success. Newly treatment strategy of ARDS pays close attention to special early intervention.

Studies on early radical scavenging have shown that the lungs can quickly gather considerable active oxygen radicals produced by the activation of inflammatory cells, and further initiate the steps of ARDS. These tremendous amount of reactive oxygen species can cause vascular endothelial injury, and leads to a series of pathophysiological reactions: moisture extravasation, pachyemia, increasing viscosity, blood stasis, microthrombus forming, disturbance of pulmonary circulation, and ultimately formation of a serious and difficult to retrieve hypoxemia. So the application of antioxidant and oxygen free radicals scavenger in early and timely manner, can effectively prevent or mitigate damage to the lung tissue, improve hypoxemia, and play an important role in the course of prevention and treatment of ARDS. Commonly used drugs are glucocorticoids, anisodamine, vitamin E, vitamin C, reduced glutathione, superoxide dismutase (SOD), chlorpromazine, promethazine, coenzyme Q_{10} (CoQ_{10}), etc. The most widely used drug in clinical for free radical scavenging is still glucocorticoids, and the application should be made sooner, the dosage should be large and 4 to 5 days to withdrawal.

Studies have shown that the key of ARDS hypoxemia is pulmonary blood flow stasis and micro-thrombosis. It suggests that the problem is not the "lungs" but the "blood". So anticoagulant, thrombolytic therapy can improve pulmonary circulation, ameliorate hypoxic condition of ARDS. Commonly used drugs are the same or similar to that mentioned in medicine, such as sodium nitroprusside, isosorbide dinitrate, phentolamine, anisodamine, heparin, ahylysantinfarctase, streptokinase.

The above measures combined with the aforementioned anti-pulmonary edema, can be effective in improving the condition of ARDS.

⑤ Obliterative bronchiolitis treatment: After the acute phase has been managed, physicians must remain alert to the development of reactive airways dysfunction syndrome (RADS), bronchiolitis obliterans with or without organized pneumonia, pulmonary fibrosis, and delayed-onset ARDS. And there is no effective treatment for obliterative bronchiolitis once it is established. During its development, the process may be arrested with steroids, which are sometimes required for prolonged periods. Bronchodilators help some patients with mixed airways disease to maintain function of the airways and comfort. Despite best efforts, some patients with obliterative bronchiolitis become progressively disabled, and even die from their complication.

4. 2. 4. 6 Prognosis and Prevention

The pulmonary edema due to any irritant gas is treated with supportive measures and corticosteroids. Most people recover fully; however, some with pre-existing emphysema or lung disease were handicapped in their struggle against pulmonary edema since the margin available for respiration was correspondingly less. Someone may have persistent lung injury with reversible airway obstruction (reactive airways dysfunction syndrome, RADS), bronchiolitis obliterans or pulmonary fibrosis; smokers may be at greater risk. There was evidence show that this invalidism was increased if the men were pressed to physical effort too early and too fast at the beginning of convalescence.

Since the irritant gas exposure causes pulmonary edema, which may be life-threatening. Action need to be taken to prevent the occurrence of pulmonary edema

(1) Inhalation of Atomizing Neutralizer

Inhale atomizing of 5% sodium bicarbonate in the situation of exposure to chlorine, nitrogen oxide, dimethyl sulfate, phosgene and other acidic compounds; or, 3% to 5% boric acid or 5% acetic acid solution in the circumstance of exposure to ammonia, amines, and other alkaline compounds. The basic formulation of the inhalation solution is composed of gentamicin 8 to 16 million units, dexamethasone 5 mg, and aminophylline 0.25 g, and then add 5% sodium bicarbonate or 3% to 5% boric acid to 20 mL, and finally add saline to 50 mL. Aerosol inhalation should be given 10—15 mL every 4 hours at the dosage of 10—15 mL.

(2) Use Glucocorticoids Early

Glucocorticoids should be administered early, sufficient and short in severe cases who may develop to pulmonary edema. It has many physiological effects in this issue: reducing the permeability and leakage of pulmonary alveolar capillary, relieving bronchial spasm, improving ventilation, maintaining the stability of lysosomal membrane to reduce the damage of the lung tissue, promoting alveolar epithelial type Ⅱ cells to secrete surfactant which decreasing surface tension and keeping alveoli expand; it can act as a powerful scavenger of oxygen free radicals; and it shows strong effects on detoxification, anti-allergic and anti-inflammatory. So it is essential for prevention and therapy of pulmonary edema.

Although the efficacy of corticosteroid therapy is unproved, it is frequently used. Usually in this stage, dexamethasone is given 30—60 mg/d intramuscularly for 1 to 2 days, and in severe cases the dose can be reached to 60—120 mg/d, divided 5 to 6 intravenous or intramuscular injection, and then halved daily, and continuous medication for 3 to 5 days.

(3) Intravenous Fluid Volume Restriction

Based on the gross volume of all fluid between in and out of the body within 24-hour, a negative balance about 500 to 1,000 mL should be sustained. The amount of intravenous fluid must be limited by not aggravating the degree of pulmonary edema. Appropriate diuretic, such as furosemide, may be used for this purpose.

4. 2. 4. 7 Chlorine

(1) Physical and Chemical Properties

Chlorine (Cl_2) is a yellowish-green gas with odorous and strong irritant, which is readily soluble in water and alkaline solutions as well as in organic solvents (e. g. carbon disulfide, carbon tetrachloride). Chlorine gas dissolves in water and form hypochlorous acid and hydrochloric acid. Chlorine reacts with carbon monoxide at high temperature to form more toxic phosgene ($COCl_2$), which burns and explodes when mixed with flammable gases in sunlight.

(2) Exposure Opportunities

Electrolysis of salt in industrial production can produce chlorine, and the application of chlorine gas can produce various chlorine-containing compounds (e. g. carbon tetrachloride, bleach powder). Chlorine is used as a strong oxidizer and bleaching agent in pharmaceutical, leather and paper industries. Chlorine can also be used for disinfection of hospitals and tap water.

(3) Absorption, Distribution, Metabolism and Excretion

Due to its water solubility, chlorine mainly acts on the trachea, bronchus, bronchioles and alveoli. After chlorine gas is inhaled, it reacts with the water of respiratory mucosa, produce hypochlorite and hydrochloric acid. However, human body does not have the ability to decompose hypochlorite into hydrogen chloride and new ecological oxygen, thus causing damage to the body. Hydrogen chloride can cause edema, congestion and necrosis of upper respiratory mucosa; hypochlorite can penetrate the cell membrane and destroy the integrity and permeability of the membrane as well as the gas-blood barrier and gas-liquid barrier of the alveolar wall, causing congestion of the mucosa in the eyes and respiratory tract, inflammatory edema and necrosis also can be found. High concentration of hypochlorite can cause deep lesions of respiratory tract and induce pulmonary edema, it may also cause vagal reflex cardiac arrest or laryngeal spasm, resulting in electroshock-like death.

(4) Clinical Findings

① Acute poisoning.

• Stimulus response: Symptoms of eye and respiratory irritation.

• Mild intoxication: Acute tracheobronchitis or peribronchitis.

• Moderate intoxication: Bronchopneumonia, interstitial pulmonary edema, localized alveolar edema, asthma-like episodes.

• Severe intoxication: Alveolar or central pulmonary edema; ARDS; Asphyxia or sudden death from cardiac arrest.

• Others: Acute dermatitis or burns of the eyes and skin.

② Chronic poisoning: Symptoms developed from prolonged exposure to low concentrations of chlorine: Symptoms irritation of upper respiratory tract, conjunctiva and skin irritation; Increased incidence of non-specific respiratory diseases (e. g. Bronchial asthma, emphysema, etc.); Neurasthenia and gastrointestinal disorders, rashes, sores and dental acidosis.

(5) Diagnosis and Treatment

① Diagnosis: According to the short-term inhalation of a large amount of chlorine gas after the rapid onset, combined with clinical symptoms, signs, chest X-ray performance, and referring to the results of labor hygiene survey for comprehensive analysis to make a diagnosis.

② Treatment.

Site disposal: Move patients immediately out of chlorine exposure sites and expose to the fresh air; Give symptomatic treatment when irritation inflammation appears.

Reasonable oxygen inhalation therapy.

Application of glucocorticoid: The purpose is to prevent and treat pulmonary edema.

Maintain airway opened.

Control the amount of fluid entering the body.

Prevent secondary infection: Rational use of antibiotics.

Supplement: Chlorine burns of the skin are usually treated as acid burns; Eye irritation symptoms should be thoroughly cleaned with clean water or subconjunctival injection with weak alkaline solution (e. g. sodium bicarbonate).

(6) Prognosis and Prevention

① Prognosis: Patients with chlorine poisoning can resume their original work after being cured, but patients with asthma-like symptoms after treatment should be removed from the work position exposed to irritating gases.

② Prevention.

• Strictly control the concentration of chlorine in the workplace.

• Strictly observe the safe operation rules and keep the workplace ventilated.

• Waste gas containing chlorine should be purified by lime before being discharged.

• When staff repairing equipment or rescuing chlorine poisoning patients on site, they must wear protective facial mask of oxygen mask.

4. 2. 4. 8   Nitrogen Dioxide

(1) Physical and Chemical Properties

Nitrogen Dioxide (NO_2) is reddish brown at 21. 1 ℃, with a pungent smell gas, and which present as dark brown liquid under 21. 1℃ degrees. It is colorless solid in -11℃. The chemical property of NO_2 is stable, and its molecular weight is 46. 01, the boiling point is 21. 2 ℃, soluble in alkaline, carbon disulfide and chloroform, but poorly soluble in water.

(2) Exposure Opportunities

① The chemical industry: Nitric acid production and nitric acid leaching metal can release a lot of smoke; some nitro compounds such as nitro explosives and nitrocellulose fibers can produce Nitrogen Dioxide.

② Fuel emissions: Satellite launches, rocket propulsion, automobile and internal combustion engine emissions, small explosives used in mines and tunnels are known to contain or produce Nitrogen Dioxide.

③ Welding industry: The high temperature produced by electric welding, gas welding and gas cutting can combine oxygen and nitrogen in the air to form Nitrogen Dioxide.

(3) Absorption, Distribution, Metabolism and Excretion

Nitrogen Dioxide is difficult to dissolve in water, which has little stimulation on the mucosa of the eyes and upper respiratory tract. Nitrogen Dioxide mainly enters the deep part of the respiratory tract, generating nitric acid and nitrite to stimulate and corrode the lung tissue. The increased permeability of alveoli and capillaries that leads to pulmonary edema. Nitrogen Dioxide is absorbed into the blood to form nitrates and nitrites. Nitrate can cause vasodilation and decrease blood pressure, while nitrite can oxidize hemoglobin to methemoglobin, which leads to tissue hypoxia.

(4) Clinical Findings

① Acute poisoning: Acute nitrogen dioxide intoxication rarely cause irritation symptoms of the conjunctiva and oropharyngeal mucosa. In severe cases, extreme dyspnea, marked cyanosis, white or bloody sputum, massive wet rales in both lungs, confusion of consciousness, agitation, convulsions, coma, decreased blood pressure, shock, and often life-threatening. Acute poisoning is easy to be complicated with severe pneumothorax, mediastinal emphysema or severe myocardial damage, etc.

② Chronic poisoning: Long-term inhalation of low concentration of Nitrogen Dioxide can lead to chronic bronchitis, pulmonary fibrosis, which manifest as dry pharynx, pharyngeal pain, cough, shortness of breath and other symptoms. In addition, varying degrees of neurological symptoms can be seen in chronic intoxication.

③ Delayed obstructive bronchiolitis: A small number of patients with nitrogen dioxide poisoning had no obvious acute poisoning symptoms at the beginning, but sudden cough, chest tightness, progressive respiratory distress and other symptoms can be found two weeks later.

(5) Diagnosis and Treatment

① Diagnosis: According to the occupational history of heavy exposure to nitrogen dioxide in a short period of time, the clinical manifestations of respiratory system damage and chest X-ray signs, combined with blood gas analysis and on-site occupational hygiene investigation to diagnose.

② Treatment.

• Site disposal: Make patients immediately out of nitrogen dioxide exposure, place in the fresh air repose rest and give symptomatic treatment.

• Active prevention and treatment of pulmonary edema and delayed obstructive bronchiolitis.

• Reasonable oxygen inhalation therapy.

• Prevention and control of infection and complications, paying attention to maintaining water electrolyte and acid-base balance.

　　● Nitrogen dioxide poisoning patients with methemoglobin can be treated with Methylene Blue, Vitamin C, glucose solution, etc.

　　(6) Prognosis and Prevention

　　① Prognosis

Patients with acute mild to moderate intoxication of nitrogen dioxide can resume their original work after being cured, but Patients with severe nitrogen dioxide poisoning after treatment should be removed from the work position exposed to irritating gases.

　　② Prevention

Strictly control the concentration of nitrogen dioxide in the workplace: Time-weighted average allowable concentration is 5 mg/m^3 and the allowable concentration for short time exposure is 100 mg/m^3 (in China). Staffs with obvious cardiovascular and respiratory diseases (e. g Asthma, Pulmonary Heart Disease, etc.) should not be exposed to nitrogen dioxide.

4.2.5   Asphyxiating Gases

4.2.5.1   Definition and Classification

The air we breathe mainly contains by volume about 78% nitrogen and 21% oxygen (O_2). Mammalian cells depend on O_2 so that their mitochondria can perform the energy-producing process of respiration. Asphyxiation, which is synonymous with respiratory failure, can be defined as insufficient oxygenation at the cellular level. And according to the difference of toxicological mechanisms, asphyxiating gases can be divided into simple asphyxiants and chemical asphyxiants.

Simple asphyxiants have, in themselves, no effects on the body system. They do not suppress cardiac output or alter the function of hemoglobin. Rather, they cause asphyxiation only when present in high enough concentrations to lower the concentration of O_2 in the inspired air to levels at which SaO_2 [saturation of O_2 in arterial blood (in percent)] and PaO_2 [partial pressure of O_2 in arterial blood (in mm Hg)] fall, resulting in inadequate O_2 delivery to tissues and lead to tissue hypoxia. As the concentration of oxygen decreases in the air that we breathe, the body becomes increasingly deprived of oxygen and a number of pathophysiological effects occur. Human beings are asymptomatic while breathing air containing 16.5% to 21% O_2 by volume. Concentrations of O_2 in the inspired air of 12% to 16% cause tachypnea, tachycardia, and slight incoordination. At O_2 levels of 10% to 14%, emotional lability and exhaustion with minimal exertion can be expected. Breathing air containing 6% to 10% O_2 results in nausea, vomiting, lethargic movements, and perhaps unconsciousness. Breathing less than 6% O_2 produces convulsions, thereafter apnea, and followed by cardiac standstill. The aforementioned symptoms occur immediately on breathing an O_2-deficient atmosphere. Since exercise increases the tissue need for O_2, symptoms occur more quickly during exertion in an O_2-deficient environment. Should the victim survive the hypoxic insult, some or all organs may show evidence of hypoxic damage, which may or may not be reversible with time, depending on the degree and duration of the hypoxia and the extent of the tissue injury.

The so-called inert gases such as helium, neon and argon and materials such as hydrogen, nitrogen, methane and carbon dioxide are all simple asphyxiants (although some data are available which indicate that carbon dioxide may have other chronic effects). Because of the immediate lethality of these gases, only air-supplying respiratory protective devices and self-contained breathing apparatuses are recommended for use during escape from exposure to these gases.

On the other hand, chemical asphyxiants prevent the normal uptake of oxygen by tissues by interfering with specific elements in oxygen delivery and body's metabolic processes, thereby causing significant health risk and death, even in situation where the oxygen concentration is still able to maintain life. The representative chemical asphyxiants are carbon monoxide, hydrogen sulphide, cyanides and aniline. Hydrogen sulfide (H_2S) has a warning smell of rotten eggs. However, usual olfactory adaptive changes and toxic inactivation of the olfactory nerve may render the exposed individual unable to smell the gas at higher concentrations. Fatal exposures to H_2S occur in a variety of industries including petroleum and natural gas extraction and processing, underground coal mines, livestock raising (the agitation of manure in storage and treatment), sewers and human sewage treatment facilities (sewer gas), and where decomposition of fish may occur such as in fish product processing and in the fish-storage holds of fishing vessels. H_2S binds to and inactivates cytochrome oxidase in mitochondria, preventing the cellular metabolism of oxygen. In addition to its asphyxiant effects with initial compensatory tachycardia, hyperpnea, and subsequently respiratory depression, survivors of initial exposures may have delayed noncardiogenic pulmonary edema [adult respiratory distress syndrome (ARDS)] due to the direct irritant effects on the lungs. This material is extremely fast-acting and a concentration as low as 700 ppm can be rapidly fatal. Aniline liquid is readily absorbed through the intact skin and vaporizes at room temperatures and can, therefore, be readily inhaled. Once absorbed aniline combines to form methaemoglobin and thus reduces the oxygen uptake.

4. 2. 5. 2　Common Chemical Asphyxiants

(1) Carbon Monoxide (CO)

① Physical and chemical properties: CO is a colorless, nonirritating, tasteless and odorless gas. It is sparingly soluble in water, but is soluble in aqueous ammonia, ethanol, and benzene, respectively. CO is flammable and explosive. It burns in air to give carbon dioxide, and is widely used as an important industrial fuel. It has reducibility and is also used as an important reducing agent in the chemical industry.

② Exposure opportunities: CO is the product of incomplete combustion of carbon in oxygen—incomplete burning of wood, furnace oil, kerosene, gasoline, natural gas, propane, or any other carbon-containing material and is thus frequently produced in industrial processes when ventilation is inadequate or equipment malfunctions so as to burn material less completely. CO is also manufactured for use in industrial chemical processes and stored and shipped as a nonliquefied or liquefied compressed gas. Highly toxic or fatal exposures frequently occur when motor vehicle exhaust is concentrated in an enclosed space; when gas appliances, including gas clothes dryers, malfunction and are improperly vented; when fireplaces or furnaces with faulty flues release their combustion products into the breathing air of the home or workplace; and when propane-powered equipment such as tow-motors and fork lifts incompletely combust their fuel. Unvented kerosene heaters burning improperly are an important source of hazard. Firefighters are frequently exposed to CO in their work and should wear air-supplying respirators when in or near an area of combustion, including the smoldering remains of fires.

③ Absorption, distribution, metabolism and excretion: Predominant route of exposure is inhalation of contaminated air. Following this, CO rapidly enters all parts of the body including the blood, brain, heart, and muscles. In blood, CO quickly distributes into erythrocytes where is exists primarily as a complex with hemoglobin (Hb) to form carboxyhemoglobin (COHb); in muscle, as a complex with myoblobin forming carboxymyoglobin (COMb); and in the maternal system, CO distributes to fetal tissues and binds to fetal Hb and other heme proteins. CO is eliminated from the body predominantly through exhalation and $< 10\%$ by oxidative metabolism. Exercise decreases the CO elimination half-time. The precise mechanisms by which the effects of CO are induced upon bodily systems, are complex and has not been fully understood. Known mechanisms mainly include CO binding to hemoglobin, as well as to myoglobin and mitochondrial cytochrome oxidase, and CO causing brain lipid peroxidation.

When CO is not ventilated it binds to hemoglobin, which is the principal oxygen-carrying compound in blood; this produces a compound known as COHb. The traditional belief is that CO toxicity arises from the formation of COHb, which decreases the oxygen-carrying capacity of the blood and inhibits the transport, delivery, and utilization of oxygen by the body. The affinity between hemoglobin and CO is approximately 230 times stronger than the affinity between hemoglobin and oxygen so hemoglobin binds to CO in preference to oxygen; and the rate of dissociation of CO from hemoglobin is about 3600 times slower (with a half-life of about 4 hours breathing ambient air at rest) than that of O_2 from hemoglobin.

In addition, hemoglobin is a tetramer with four oxygen binding sites. The binding of CO at one of these sites increases the oxygen affinity of the remaining three sites, which causes the hemoglobin molecule to retain oxygen that would otherwise be delivered to the tissue. This situation is described as CO shifting the oxygen dissociation curve to the left. Because of the increased affinity between hemoglobin and oxygen during CO poisoning, the blood oxygen content is increased. But because all the oxygen stays in the hemoglobin, none is delivered to the tissues. This causes hypoxic tissue injury. Hemoglobin acquires a bright red color when converted into COHb, so poisoned cadavers and even commercial meats treated with CO acquire an unnatural reddish hue.

④ Clinical findings: CO is a highly toxic to all aerobic forms of life, and has no warning properties to the exposed. Exposures at 100 ppm or greater can be dangerous to human health. Health effects of CO are determined by the dose (how much), the duration (how long), and the route of exposure. Although CO poisoning represents a multisystem insult, the highest oxygen requirements—the brain, heart and cardiovascular system, and the fetus and neonate—are particularly sensitive to the effects of hypoxia and affected first. Most clinical manifestations are referable to the central nervous system, but it is likely that myocardial ischemia is responsible for many CO-induced deaths.

• Acute CO poisoning: The initial symptoms of acute CO poisoning include headache, nausea, malaise, and fatigue. These symptoms are often mistaken for a virus such as influenza or other illnesses such as food poisoning or gastroenteritis. Headache is the most common symptom of acute CO poisoning; it is often described as dull, frontal, and continuous. Increasing exposure produces cardiac abnormalities including fast heart rate, low blood pressure, and cardiac arrhythmia; central nervous system symptoms include delirium, hallucinations, dizziness, unsteady gait, confusion, seizures, central nervous system depression, unconsciousness, respiratory arrest, and death. Less common symptoms of acute CO poisoning include myocardial ischemia, atrial fibrillation, pneumonia, pulmonary edema, high blood sugar, lactic acidosis, muscle necrosis, acute kidney failure, skin lesions, and visual and auditory problems.

One of the major concerns following acute CO poisoning is the severe delayed neurological manifestations that may occur. Problems may include difficulty with higher intellectual functions, short-term memory loss, dementia, amnesia, psychosis, irritability, a strange gait, speech disturbances, Parkinson's-like syndromes, cortical blindness, and a depressed mood. Depression may even occur in those who did not have pre-existing depression. These delayed neurological sequelae may occur in up to 50% of poisoned people after 2 to 40 days. It is difficult to predict who will develop delayed sequelae; however, advanced age, loss of consciousness while poisoned, and initial neurological abnormalities may increase the chance of developing delayed symptoms.

One classic sign of CO poisoning is more often seen in the dead rather than the living-people have been described as looking pink-cheeked and healthy. However, since this "cherry-red" appearance is common only in the deceased, and is unusual in living people, it is not considered a useful diagnostic sign in clinical medicine. In pathological (autopsy) examination the ruddy appearance of CO poisoning is notable because unembalmed dead persons are normally bluish and pale, whereas dead CO poisoned persons may simply appear unusually lifelike in coloration. The colorant effect of CO in such postmortem circumstances is thus analogous to its use as a red colorant in the commercial meat-packing industry.

• Chronic CO poisoning: Chronic exposure to relatively low levels of CO may cause persistent headaches, lightheadedness, depression, confusion, memory loss, nausea and vomiting. It is unknown whether low-level chronic exposure may cause permanent neurological damage. Typically, upon removal from exposure to CO, symptoms usually resolve themselves, unless there has been an episode of severe acute poisoning. However, one case noted permanent memory loss and learning problems after a 3-year exposure to relatively low levels of CO from a faulty furnace. Chronic exposure may worsen cardiovascular symptoms in some people. Chronic CO exposure might increase the risk of developing atherosclerosis. Long-term exposures to CO present the greatest risk to persons with coronary heart disease and in females who are pregnant.

⑤ Diagnosis and treatment: The diagnosis can be confirmed by finding a source and monitoring the level of CO in the home (e. g. defective furnaces), workplace, or vehicle; negative screenings for other illnesses; abnormal CO or COHb levels in biological specimens; and abatement of symptoms when the CO source has been eliminated.

CO may be quantitated in blood using spectrophotometric methods or chromatographic techniques in order to confirm a diagnosis of poisoning in a person or to assist in the forensic investigation of a case of fatal exposure. A CO-oximeter is used to determine COHb levels. Typical COHb level in nonsmokers is 0. 5%—1. 5%. Blood COHb is the principle biomarker for identifying exposure to CO. The relationship between COHb levels and exposure is complicated by physiological factors that influence CO uptake and elimination. COHb blood saturations may range up to 8%—10% in heavy smokers or persons extensively exposed to automotive exhaust gases. In symptomatic poisoned people, they are often in the 10%—30% range, while persons who succumb may have postmortem blood levels of 30%—90%.

Therapy in acute CO poisoning is directed to general supportive measures while speeding the dissociation of CO from hemoglobin so that oxygen may once again be delivered to organs. Once the patient has been removed from exposure, inhaling of oxygen should be taken as soon as possible. In the preintensive care setting, the mainstays of therapy are to sustain ventilation if necessary by assisted ventilation (such as with an inflatable bag and oral airway or endotracheal tube) and the administration of 100% oxygen. Administration of 100% oxygen can shorten the half-time for reduction of blood COHb from approximately 320 minutes to 80 minutes. Those who are unconscious may require cardiopulmonary resuscitation (CPR) on site.

Hyperbaric oxygen (HBO) is also used in the treatment of CO poisoning, as it may hasten dissociation of CO from COHb and cytochrome oxidase to a greater extent than normal oxygen. HBO at three times atmospheric pressure reduces the half-life of CO to 23 minutes, compared to 80 minutes for regular oxygen. It may also enhance oxygen transport to the tissues by plasma, partially bypassing the normal transfer through hemoglobin. However it is controversial whether HBO actually offers any extra benefits over normal high flow oxygen, in terms of increased survival or improved long-term outcomes. Circumstances in which HBO has been most convincingly advocated are those in which the patient is believed to be at risk of permanent neurologic damage or death. COHb levels greater than 25% to 40%, transient loss of consciousness, lethargy, stupor, and coma are believed to be indicators of this risk. Exchange transfusion has recently been suggested as a means to increase oxygen delivery more rapidly than 100% oxygen therapy but has not been systematically evaluated.

Further treatment for other complications such as seizure, hypotension, cardiac abnormalities, pulmonary edema, acidosis and delayed neuropsychiatric impairment may be required.

(2) Hydrogen Cyanide (HCN)

Cyanides are a family of compounds containing the highly reactive cyanide anion. The common inorganic compounds include hydrogen cyanide (HCN) and two cyanide salts—sodium cyanide and potassium cyanide; and the common organic compounds include cyanohydrins, acrylonitrile. All that release the cyanide ion in the air or in the body have similar toxicities.

① Physical and chemical properties: At room temperature, HCN is a colorless or pale-blue liquid (hydrocyanic acid); at higher temperatures, it is a colorless gas (boiling point 26℃, freezing point − 13.4℃). It is very volatile, producing potentially lethal concentrations. The vapor is flammable and potentially explosive. HCN has a faint, bitter, almond-like odor and a bitter, burning taste. It is miscible with water and alcohol, and slightly soluble in ether, and partially ionizes in water solution to give the cyanide anion, CN^-.

② Exposure opportunities: Cyanide salts and hydrogen cyanide are used or produced in various occupational settings where activities include electroplating, some metal mining processes, metallurgy, metal cleaning, organic chemicals production, tanning, photography and photoengraving, firefighting, fumigation of ships, gas works operations, and as reagents in analytical chemistry. It also is employed in the preparation of acrylonitrile, which is used in the production of acrylic fibres, synthetic fibers, synthetic rubber, various plastics, dyes, pigments, nylon, and insecticides and fumigants.

③ Absorption, distribution, metabolism and excretion: Cyanide gas and salts are rapidly absorbed following inhalation or oral exposure. Liquid hydrogen cyanide, hydrogen cyanide in aqueous, and the concentrated vapor are all absorbed rapidly through the intact skin and may cause systemic poisoning with little or no irritant effect on the skin itself. The liquid in contact with the eye may cause only local irritation; however, the attendant absorption may be hazardous. Absorbed cyanide is rapidly distributed throughout the body. Some of the cyanide is transformed to thiocyanate, which is less harmful and expelled from the body during urination. A small amount of cyanide is converted in the body to carbon dioxide, which expelled through breath. It can also bind cobalt ions, being chemically similar to iron ions; and bind vitamin B_{12} to form the harmless cyanocobalamin form of vitamin B_{12}. Cyanide metabolites are excreted in the urine, with small amounts excreted through the lungs. At low levels of exposure to cyanide compounds, most of the cyanide and its products leave the body within the first 24 hours after exposure.

HCN is an extremely poisonous. It can cause rapid death due to metabolic asphyxiation. Cyanide has a high affinity for certain sulfur compounds (sulfanes, which contain two covalently bonded but unequally charged sulfur atoms) and for certain metallic complexes, particularly those containing cobalt and the trivalent form of iron (Fe^{3+}). The cyanide ion can rapidly combine with iron in cytochrome a_3 (a component of the cytochrome or cytochrome oxidase complex in mitochrondria) to inhibit this enzyme, thus preventing aerobic metabolisms in the affected cells and causes cell death and organ dysfunction, particularly in organs most sensitive to anoxia. The venous blood of a patient dying from cyanide poisoning is bright red and resembles arterial blood because the tissues have not been able to utilize the oxygen brought to them. The cell then utilizes anaerobic metabolism, creating excess lactic acid and a metabolic acidosis. Because cytochrome oxidase is present in practically all cells that function under aerobic conditions, and because the cyanide ion diffuses easily to all parts of the body, cyanide quickly halts practically all cellular respiration. Exposure appears to affect both aortic and carotid chemoreceptors directly, causing increased firing (and hyperpnea as an early symptom). Death may occur within seconds or minutes of the inhalation of high concentrations of hydrogen cyanide gas.

Cyanide also has a high affinity for the ferric iron of methemoglobin and one therapeutic stratagem induces the formation of methemoglobin to which cyanide preferentially binds. And although thiocyanates are less harmful than cyanide in humans, they are known to affect the thyroid glands, reducing the ability of the gland to produce hormones that are necessary for the normal function of the body.

④ Clinical findings.

• Acute poisoning: The organs most susceptible to cyanide are the central nervous system (CNS) and the heart. Most clinical effects are of CNS origin and nonspecific.

About 15 seconds after inhalation of a high concentration of cyanide vapor, there is a transient hyperpnea followed in 15—30 seconds by the onset of convulsions. Respiratory activity stops two to three minutes later, and cardiac activity ceases several minutes later, or at about six to eight minutes after exposure.

The onset and progression of signs and symptoms after inhalation of a sublethal concentration of vapor are slower. The first effects may not occur until several minutes after exposure, and the time course of these effects depends on the amount absorbed and the rate of absorption. The initial transient hyperpnea may be followed by a feeling of anxiety or apprehension, agitation, headache, confusion, vertigo, fatigue, a feeling of weakness, dyspnea, nausea with or without vomiting, and muscular trembling. Thereafter, loss of consciousness, respiration decreases in rate and depth, convulsions, apnea, and followed by cardiac dysrhythmias and standstill. Because this cascade of events is prolonged, diagnosis and successful treatment are possible.

Physical findings are few and non-specific. There are two characteristic findings, nevertheless they are not always observed. The first is severe respiratory distress in an acyanotic individual. The evidence of "cherry-red" skin suggests either circulating carboxyhemoglobin from carbon monoxide poisoning or a high venous oxygen content from failure of extraction of oxygen by tissues poisoned by cyanide or hydrogen sulfide. However, cyanide victims may have normal appearing skin and may be cyanotic, although cyanosis is not classically associated with cyanide poisoning. The second classic sign is the bitter almonds odor or taste in the nose and mouth. However, about 50% of the population is genetically unable to detect the odor of cyanide. The casualty may be diaphoretic with normal sized or large pupils. An initial hypertension and compensatory bradycardia are followed by a declining blood pressure and tachycardia. Terminal hypotension is accompanied by bradyarrhythmias before asystole. In survivors of an acute poisoning, a delayed neurologic syndrome associated with leukoencephalopathy has been described.

● Chronic poisoning: Workers chronically exposed to hydrogen cyanide at low concentrations showed an increase in symptoms such as headaches, weakness, changes in taste and smell, irritation of the throat, nausea, vomiting, vertigo, effort dyspnea, lacrimation, abdominal colic, precordial pain, and nervous instability. Industrial exposure to hydrogen cyanide solutions has caused dermatitis, itching, scarlet rash, papules, and nose irritation and bleeding.

⑤ Diagnosis and treatment: The diagnosis of cyanide poisoning is based on an exposure history of cyanide, clinical features, and laboratory findings.

Laboratory findings in a poisoned person as follow:

● Cyanide and thiocyanate in blood or urine can be used as biomarkers of recent exposure. For blood cyanide concentration, mild effects may be apparent at concentrations of 0.5—1.0 fg/mL, and concentrations of 2.5 fg/mL and higher are associated with coma, convulsions and death. An elevated concentration of thiocyanate in either blood or urine is evidence of cyanide exposure.

● Acidosis: Metabolic acidosis with a high concentration of lactic acid (lactic acidosis), or a metabolic acidosis with an unexplained high anion gap (if the means to measure lactic acid are not available) may be present. Because oxygen cannot be utilized, anaerobic metabolism with the production of lactic acid replaces aerobic metabolism. Lactic acidosis, however, may reflect other disease states and is not specific for cyanide poisoning.

● Oxygen content of venous blood greater than normal. This is also because of poisoning of the intramitochondrial respiratory chain and the resulting failure of cells to extract oxygen from arterial blood. This finding is also not specific for cyanide poisoning.

It should be differential with other diseases having similar manifestations, for example, inhalational exposure to either cyanide or a nerve agent may precipitate the sudden onset of loss of consciousness followed by convulsions and apnea. The nerve agent casualty has miosis (until shortly before death), copious oral and nasal secretions, and muscular fasciculations. The cyanide casualty has normal sized or dilated pupils, few secretions, and muscular twitching but no fasciculations. In addition, the nerve agent casualty may be cyanotic, and the cyanide casualty usually is not cyanotic.

The primary goal of therapy is to remove the cyanide from the enzyme cytochrome a_3 in the cytochrome oxidase complex. A secondary goal is to detoxify or bind the cyanide so that it cannot reenter the cell to reinhibit the enzyme.

Rapid treatment is essential. Antidotes must be administered without delay to have a beneficial effect. If exposure has occurred by ingestion, gastric lavage while protecting the airway and administering antidotes may remove residual cyanide from the stomach. Skin decontamination may be needed. If ventilation is reduced, mechanical ventilation should be administered; 100% oxygen is generally recommended as supportive therapy but would not be expected to alter the poisoning of cytochrome oxidase in cells.

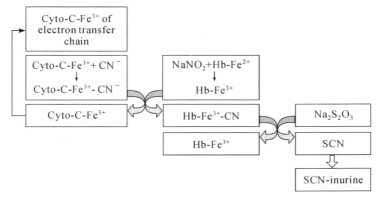

Figure 4.4   Detoxification Schematic of Drug for Cyanide Poisoning

Two antidotes are used (Figure 4.4). The commercially available cyanide antidote preparation contains amyl nitrite, sodium nitrite, and sodium thiosulfate. If the patient is breathing spontaneously, amyl nitrite ampoules may be administered by inhalation until an intravenous line can be placed and the intravenous regimen begun. The protocol is to rapidly administer sodium nitrite by the intravenous route to generate methemoglobin from hemoglobin. Methemoglobin has a high affinity for cyanide, and cyanide will preferentially bind to methemoglobin rather than to the cytochrome. Most methemoglobin formers have clinically significant side effects. The nitrites, which were first used to antagonize the effects of cyanide over a century ago, cause orthostatic hypotension, but this is relatively insignificant in a supine casualty or placing the patient with the head tilted down (Trendelenburg position) and administering intravenous fluid. Amyl nitrite, historically the first nitrite used, is a volatile substance formulated in a perle that is crushed or broken for the victim to inhale. In an apneic patient a means of ventilation is necessary. Another methemoglobin former, sodium nitrite, is formulated for intravenous use. The standard ampule contains 300 mg of the drug in 10 mL of diluent, and this is injected intravenously over a two-to four-minute period. The next step of the protocol is to give a slow intravenous infusion of thiosulfate, which converts cyanmethemoglobin to thiocyanate. The thiocyanate, which is less toxic than cyanide, is excreted in urine. The hepatic enzyme rhodanese catalyzes the one-way reaction of cyanide and a sulfane to thiocyanate. Sodium thiosulfate is packaged in a 50-mL ampule containing 12.5 g of the drug. Intravenous injection of all 12.5g follows successful completion of the intravenous injection of sodium nitrite. Half of the original dosage of each drug may be repeated if symptoms persist.

An alternate treatment regimen that has been used more extensively is to give an intravenous infusion of hydroxocobalamin (vitamin B_{12}), which is meant to form a cyanocobalamin complex that can be excreted in urine.

4.2.6　Pesticides

Pesticide is a generic term for any substance or mixture of substances intended for preventing, destroying, repelling, or mitigating any pest. Pests are living organisms which occur where they are not wanted or that cause damage to crops, humans or other animals.

4.2.6.1　Classification

(1) Classification by the Targets

Pesticides can be classified into insecticides, herbicides, fungicides, growth regulators, and rodenticides.

(2) Classification by the Way of Organism Killed

Pesticides can be classified into contact poison, stomach poison, fumigant poison, systematic poison, etc.

(3) Classification by Chemical Structure

Pesticides can be classified into organochlorine, organophosphorus, pyrethroid, carbamate, organic nitrogen, organic sulfur, phenolic acid, ether, phenoxycarboxylic acid, urea, sulfonylurea, triazobenzene, amidine, organic metal and heterocyclic compounds.

(4) Classification by Component

Pesticides can be classified into original drugs and preparations. Preparations refer to solvents, auxiliaries and other components except active ingredients, such as pigment emetic agents and impurities.

(5) Classification by Degree of Hazard

According to the WHO, pesticides can be classified into four categories by degree of hazard: Extremely, highly, moderately, and slightly hazardous.

Insecticides, herbicides, fungicides, and rodenticides are the most widely used pesticides. The most prominent classes of insecticides are organochlorines, organophosphates, carbamates and pyrethroids. All the chemical insecticides used today are neurotoxicants. Given the fact that insecticides are not selective and affect nontarget species as readily as target organisms, it is not surprising that a chemical that works on the nervous system of insects could elicit similar effects in human.

4. 2. 6. 2   Organochlorines

The chemical structure of organochlorines is diverse, but they all contain chlorine, which places them in a larger class of compounds called chlorinated hydrocarbons.

Organochlorines were used extensively from the mid-1940s to the mid-1960s to control a wide variety of insect pests due to the properties of lipid solubility, low volatility, chemical stability, and slow rate of biotransformation and degradation. These properties also led to their demise because of their persistence in the environment, bioaccumulation and biomagnification through the food chains.

4. 2. 6. 3   Organophosphates

The first organophosphorus compounds were first synthesized by a group of German chemists in 1937. These very potent compounds were kept secret during World War II and were originally developed as potential chemical warfare agents. After the war, these organophosphorus compounds were re-purposed as insecticides, and many organophosphate insecticides continue to be used today. Today, there are some 200 different organophosphate insecticides in the marketplace, formulated into literally thousands of products. At present, organophosphates are responsible for the majority of occupational poisonings and deaths from pesticides in the United States and throughout the world.

(1) Physical and Chemical Properties

The basic structure of organophosphorus pesticides is the central pentavalent phosphorus (P), which binds to sulphur (S) or oxygen (O) through a double bond, to two methoxy or ethoxy groups (R_1 and R_2), and to one leaving group that is highly variable (X) (Figure 4. 5).

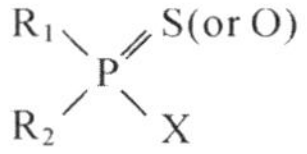

$$R_1 \diagdown \ \diagup S(\text{or O})$$
$$P$$
$$R_2 \diagup \diagdown X$$

Figure 4. 5   Basic Structure of Organophosphorus Pesticides

Organophosphorus pesticides are usually white crystals, and industrial products are light yellow or brown oily liquids. Except for a few varieties such as dichlorvos, most of them have a special odor, which is similar to garlic or leek. The boiling point of them is high. The organophosphorus pesticides are not heat-resistant because they will decompose or even explode when heated below 200℃.

Organophosphorus pesticides have a high refractive index and their relative density is more than 1. The vapor pressure of them at room temperature is low, so their vapor will escape either in liquid or solid form and cause poisoning. Generally, they are insoluble in water, and soluble in aromatic hydrocarbons, ethanol, acetone, chloroform and other organic solvents, except for petroleum ethers and aliphatic hydrocarbons.

(2) Exposure Opportunities

① Occupational exposure: Opportunities of occupational exposures to pesticides include manufacturing, preparing and application processes of pesticides, examination and repair of the equipment, and harvesting and handling of crops.

　② Environmental and living exposure: Oral pesticide poisoning is the main cause of organophosphorus pesticide poisoning in daily lives. Acute poisoning can be caused by mistaking pesticides accidentally, attempting suicides or eating contaminated vegetables or fruits. Using organophosphorus pesticides to treat skin diseases can also lead to poisoning.

　(3) Absorption, Distribution, Metabolism and Excretion

　① Absorption: Organophosphorus pesticides can be absorbed by respiratory tract, gastrointestinal tract, and skin. The absorptions via inhalation and ingestion are relatively rapid and complete. In typical work situations, the absorption via the skin contact is the most common route of acute poisoning. The dermal absorption depends on the pesticide formulation, the site of contamination, and the duration of the exposure. In general, pesticides formulated as powders, dusts or granules are not absorbed as readily as liquid formulations. Also, for each part of the body, the rate at which dermal absorption occurs is quite different. The genital areas have the highest absorption rate, followed by the head (including the ear canal and the scalp), followed by abdomen, feet and hands. Absorption from a cut or abraded skin increases greatly.

　② Distribution: When the pesticides were absorbed, it can be quickly distributed to all tissues in the body with blood flow. The content of pesticides was the highest in the liver, followed by kidney, lung and spleen, while the concentrations of pesticides in muscle, skeleton and brain were relatively low. Organophosphorus pesticides containing fluorine, oxygen and other groups can enter brain tissue through blood-brain barrier, and some pesticides can reach fetus through placental barrier. In view of the inherent instability of the organophosphorus pesticides, storage in human tissue is not expected to be prolonged. However, some organophosphorus pesticides are very lipophilic and may be taken into, and then released from, fat depots over a period of many days.

　③ Metabolism: Organophosphorus pesticides are metabolized mainly in the liver, and generally undergo both phase Ⅰ and phase Ⅱ metabolisms. Phase Ⅰ metabolisms are mainly manifested as oxidation reaction and hydrolysis reaction. Usually oxidation reactions increase the toxicity of parent compounds. One typical activation reaction is oxidative desulphuration, in which thion group containing parent compounds are activated to their corresponding oxon compounds with the catalysis of cytochrome P450 enzymes, resulting in a significant increase in toxicity. Hydrolysis of phosphoric and phosphorothioic acid ester occurs via a number of different tissue hydrolases, for example, carboxylesterases, arylesterases, phosphorylphosphatases, phosphotriesteraes, and carboxyamidases. Hydrolysis reactions generally are detoxification processes. Genetic factors, especially paraoxonase (PON) activity levels, can affect metabolism and detoxification of organophosphates and may account for differing susceptibility to poisoning.

　④ Excretion: The organophosphates are readily metabolized and excreted. The metabolites are mainly excreted by the kidney with urine and a small part with feces.

Alkylphosphate metabolites of organophosphates are excreted in the urine and can be useful as a measure of recent absorption in exposure assessment and biomonitoring.

⑤ Mechanism of toxicity: In response to nerve stimulation, acetylcholine (ACh) is released from the pre-synapse into the synapse and travels across the synaptic cleft where it binds transiently to acetylcholine receptor on the post-synapse, starting a new action potential in the receiving cell. Once the signal triggered, acetylcholine is released back into the synapse and then rapidly bound and hydrolyzed by acetylcholinesterase (AChE), which can inactivate acetylcholine by hydrolyzing acetylcholine to acetate and choline.

Similar to acetylcholine, organophosphorus pesticides can enter the active site of acetylcholinesterase. If the phosphorylated enzyme contains methyl or ethyl groups, the enzyme is regenerated in several hours by hydrolysis. On the other hand, virtually no hydrolysis occurs with an isopropyl group and the return of acetylcholinesterase is dependent upon synthesis of a new enzyme.

Inhibition of acetylcholinesterase results in the accumulation of free, unbound acetylcholine at the nerve endings of all cholinergic nerves, there is continual stimulation of electrical activity. Excess acetylcholine initially causes excitation, and then paralysis, of cholinergic transmission, resulting in some or all of the cholinergic symptoms, depending on the dosage, frequency of exposure, duration of exposure, and route of exposure, as well as other factors such as combined exposure to other chemicals and individual sensitivity and susceptibility.

It is generally believed that a prolonged action resulted from a persistent excess of acetylcholine at the neuromuscular junction is associated with the occurrence of intermediate syndrome (IMS), however, the exact underlying mechanisms are not clearly defined. It was reported that IMS could be attributed to muscle fiber necrosis following acute cholinergic crisis. There was also a notion that IMS could be due to a conformational change in acetylcholine receptor.

A single or repeated exposure to organophosphorus pesticides may cause the neurodegenerative disorder termed organophosphate induced delayed neurotoxicity (OPIDN). The neuropathological lesion is characterized with myelin degeneration of distal portions of the long and large diameter tracts of the CNS and PNS following the distal axonopathy caused by a chemical transection of the axon. Studies on mechanisms eliminated the acetylcholinesterase as targets of OPIDN. It was proposed that neuropathy target esterase (NTE), which is present in neuronal and non-neuronal tissues, is the target of OPIDN. Since the introduction of NTE hypothesis, numerous studies have been carried out, however, controversial evidence has been obtained and the exact mechanisms remain unrevealed.

(4) Clinical Findings

① Acute poisoning: Acute organophosphorus pesticides poisoning can manifest different phases of toxic effects, namely, acute cholinergic crisis, intermediate syndrome

(IMS), delayed neuropathy, and chronic neurotoxicity.

• Acute cholinergic crisis: Acute cholinergic crisis develops within a few minutes to several hours after exposure. Inhibition of acetylcholinesterase results in the accumulation of acetylcholine at both the muscarinic and nicotinic receptors in the central nervous system (CNS) and the peripheral nervous system (PNS). Therefore, typical manifestations of cholinergic crisis include muscarinic symptoms, nicotinic symptoms and the CNS symptoms.

Signs resulting from stimulation of the muscarinic receptors of the parasympathetic autonomic nervous system include manifestations of increased secretion of glands, excitation of smooth muscles, and inhibition of cardiovascular activity. Details of the clinical signs include sweating, salivation, nausea, vomit, abdominal cramps, diarrhea, bronchorrhea, bronchospasm, dyspnea, blurred vision, contracted pupil, miosis, bradycardia, hypotension and arrhythmia. The mnemonic DUMBELS (diarrhea, urination, miosis, bronchospasm, emesis, lacrimation, salivation) describes the signs of muscarinic excess seen with organophosphate poisoning. Signs resulting from the stimulation of the nicotinic receptors of the parasympathetic divisions of the autonomic nervous system as well as the junctions between nerves and muscles include tachycardia, hypertension, muscle fasciculation, tremors, muscle weakness, and flaccid paralysis. Signs resulting from effects on the central nervous system include restlessness, emotional liability, lethargy, generalized weakness, loss of memory, mental confusion, ataxia, convulsion, coma, and inhibition of respiration and circulation center. Death can occur within a very short period of time if life threatening conditions, such as respiratory failure, are not treated promptly and appropriately.

• Intermediate syndrome (IMS): Intermediate syndrome was termed because it arose in the interval between the end of the acute cholinergic crisis and the onset of organophosphate induced delayed neurotoxicity (OPIDN). Typically, IMS occurs within 24 to 96 hours following exposure to various organophosphorus pesticides, such as fenthion, dimethoate, monocrotophos and methamidophos. Intermediate syndrome was mainly characterized by significant weakness of proximal limb muscles, ocular muscle, neck flexors, respiratory muscles, and muscles innervated by motor cranial nerves. The syndrome progresses over time and may result in respiratory failure amongst the most severe cases. Intermediate syndrome has been considered as a major contributing factor of organophosphate-related morbidity and mortality because of its frequent occurrence and probable consequence of respiratory failure. The prognosis of IMS, however, is likely to be favorable if respiratory failure can be promptly recognized and treated accordingly. With appropriate therapy, full recovery from IMS could be made 5 to 18 days after the onset of muscle weakness.

• Organophosphate induced delayed neurotoxicity (OPIDN): A number of organophosphorus pesticides, including omethoate, trichloronate, trichlorfon, parathion, methamidophos, fenthion and chlorpyrifos, have been implicated in causing OPIDN in human.

OPIDN is a neurodegenerative disorder characterized by a delayed onset of prolonged ataxia and motor neuron spasticity, usually OPIDN occurs 2 to 3 weeks after acute exposure to excessively high levels of certain organophosphorus pesticides. The clinical features are predominantly motor neuropathy and primarily manifest as numbness and weakness of the lower extremities, followed by progressive ascending weakness of limb muscles.

• Organophosphate induced chronic neurotoxicity (OPICN): After exposure to a single large toxic dose or to small subclinical doses of organophosphorus pesticides for a long period of time, persistent neurodegenerative disorder can be developed and continued for a prolonged time ranging from weeks to years after exposure, which is defined as organophosphate induced chronic neurotoxicity (OPICN).

Organophosphate induced chronic neurotoxicity (OPICN) may be caused by an acute exposure that results in cholinergic toxicity, or by exposure to subclinical doses that do not produce acute poisoning. The symptoms of OPICN are a consequence of damage to both the PNS and CNS, which are related primarily to CNS injury and resultant neurological and neurobehavioral abnormalities. Clinical signs include headache, drowsiness, dizziness, anxiety, apathy, mental confusion, restlessness, labile emotions, anorexia, insomnia, lethargy, fatigue, inability to concentrate, memory deficits, depression, irritability, confusion, generalized weakness and tremors. Respiratory, circulatory, and skin problems may be present as well in cases of chronic toxicity. Because CNS injury predominates, improvement is slow and complete recovery is unlikely.

② Chronic poisoning: An individual may experience progressive ChE inhibition but remain no symptoms. Epidemiological studies in populations with occupational exposure to pesticides show increased risk of cancer, birth defects, adverse effects on reproduction and fertility, and neurological damage. The increased risk can occur without any evidence of past acute health effects or poisoning and from long-term exposure to low levels not considered toxicologically significant.

(5) Diagnosis and Treatment

① Diagnosis: The diagnosis of organophosphorus pesticides posioning depends on a history of pesticide exposure. In the absence of a reliable history, the diagnosis of organophosphorus pesticides poisoning may be based on the clinical features. Cholinesterase levels are helpful in diagnosing organophosphorus pesticide poisoning, but not in managing the illness. The red cell (acetyl) cholinesterase level is a more accurate assessment of poisoning. Blood should be drawn in a heparinised tube before treatment is begun. In cases of unknown organophosphorus poisoning, the first aspirate or the formulation of the pesticide if available, may be used to identify the type of organophosphorus pesticide.

② Treatment.

• Prevention of continuous absorption of the poison.

The patient should be immediately removed from the poisoning environment to the place with windy or fresh air in order to keep the airway open. If the patient is wearing clothes, and the skin is exposed to toxic pollution, there is a need to remove the contaminated clothing first, and then rinse thoroughly with fresh water to remove pollution from the skin (use warm water in the winter). If the contaminant reacts with water, dry paper towel should be used to remove the contaminant before rising with water. In the case of gas or vapor inhalation poisoning, patient should be given high pressure oxygen as soon as possible. For oral poisoning, immediate induce vomiting, gastric lavage, catharsis and other measures should be taken.

● Detoxification.

a. Antagonist of acetylcholine. Atropine is a tropane alkaloid extracted from deadly nightshade (Atropa belladonna). Atropine prevents acetylcholine from stimulating the receptor site and thus acts as an antagonist.

Atropine competes with acetylcholine for the muscarinic acetylcholine receptor sites. In detail, atropine itself does not produce an excitant effect but rather limits the excitant effects of acetylcholine. Through the above process, atropine lowers the parasympathetic activity of all muscles and glands regulated by the parasympathetic nervous system. Therefore, atropine is used to counteract the initial muscarinic effects of the accumulating neurotransmitter.

However, atropine is a highly toxic antidote and great care must be taken. Frequent small doses of atropine (subcutaneously or intravenously) are indicated for mild signs and symptoms following a brief but intense exposure. Large cumulative doses of atropine, up to 50 mg daily, may be essential to control severe muscarinic symptoms. The status of the patient must be monitored continuously by examining for the disappearance of secretions (dry mouth and nose) and sweating, facial flushing, and mydriasis (dilatation of pupils).

b. Regenerator of cholinesterase. Pralidoxime chloride, or 2-pyridine aldoxime methyl chloride (2-PAM), belongs to a family of compounds called oximes that bind to organophosphate inactivated acetylcholinesterase. It is used to combat poisoning by organophosphates or acetylcholinesterase inhibitors, in conjunction with atropine and diazepam. When the antidote, 2-PAM, is administered, the partially positively charged quaternary nitrogen on 2-PAM is attracted to the electronegative anionic site of acetylcholinesterase. Then 2-PAM's strongly negative oxygen attacks the organophosphate's phosphorus, displacing the enzyme-organophosphate bond. After which 2-PAM attaches to the organophosphate and the 2-PAM-organophosphate conjugate moves out of the site and acetylcholinesterase activity is restored. This is sometimes referred to as regeneration of cholinesterase.

The use of 2-PAM may not be necessary for cases of mild intoxication and should be reserved for moderate to severe poisonings. For patients with moderate to severe nicotinic and CNS signs and symptoms, treatment by slow intravenous infusion should be initiated as soon as possible, because the longer the interval between exposure and treatment, the less effective the 2-PAM will be. If given within 24 to 48 hours of exposure, 2-PAM can reactivate acetylcholinesterase and restore enzyme function. Once aging occurs, 2-PAM is less effective.

● Symptomatic treatment.

Treatment options currently focus on alleviating the symptoms. During the treatment, initial management is directed at protecting and maintaining an open airway with respiratory support, and it is of important effect to provide proper nutrition therapy on the recovery of the patients.

(6) Prognosis and Prevention

The most effective means to prevent the occurrence of pesticides poisoning is to minimize the exposure. Firstly, wear proper protective clothing and equipment, such as long-sleeved shirt and pants, chemical-resistant gloves and boots, and eye ware whenever handling pesticides. Avoid wearing soft contact lenses when working with pesticides. Soft contact lenses may absorb pesticide vapors from the air and hold them against the eyes. Secondly, use all pesticides in well-ventilated areas to avoid inhalation of fumes. Thirdly, do not eat, drink, or tobacco smoking while working with pesticides, since trace amounts of chemicals may be transferred from hand to mouth. Wash the hands thoroughly with soap and water after handling pesticides. Finally, pesticides should be stored in their original container along with their label.

4. 2. 6. 4　Other Pesticides

(1) Pyrethroids

Pyrethroids pesticides are synthetic pesticides that mimic the chemical structure of natural pyrethroids. Based on function or clinical effects of toxicity, they can be divided into two classes, which are type Ⅰ and type Ⅱ. They are widely used because of their high efficiency, lower toxicity to human and livestock, shorter residue time in the environment and wide range of insecticidal effect. Pyrethroids are oily liquid, yellow or brown, and a small number of ducts are white crystals such as deltamethrin. They are soluble in a variety of organic solvents, insoluble in water, volatile little, stable in acidic solution, easy to decompose in alkali.

Pyrethroids affect nerve excitability by delaying throid causing repetitive nerve discharge. The type Ⅱ pyrethroids produce an even longer delay in sodium channel closure, resulting in persistent nerve depolarization and eventual blockage of axonal conduction. The type Ⅱ pyrethroids may also alter and bind Y-aminobu tyric acid (GABA) receptor-mediated chloride channels. Clinically, massive type Ⅰ pyrethroid exposures have produced pronounced salivation, coarse whole bod tremors, and choreoathetosis with terminal seizures. In humans, large absorbed doses of these pyrethroids are thought to cause incoordination, tremor, salivation, vomiting, and diarrhea, however rarely cause death. The type Ⅱ pyrethroids have produced a unique cutaneous paresthesia several hours after cutaneous exposure.

There is no known effective medical treatment, therefore prevention is considerably important. Symptomatic treatment and supportive therapy are the main pyrethroids poisoning treatment.

(2) Carbamates

The carbamates, like the organophosphates, are used in commercial farrming, home gardening, and control of domestic animal ectoparasites. Aldicarb, oxamyl, and methomyl are highly toxic carbamate insecticides; dioxacarb, carbaryl, and isoprocarb are less toxic. Most carbamates are white crystals, odorless, and soluble in organic solvents.

The N-methyl carbamate esters cause reversible inhibition of acetylcholinesterase. As in the case of organophoshates, postsynaptic cholinergic receptors are flooded with acetylcholine, resulting in a characteristic clinical manifestations. Unlike the phosphorylated enzyme, the carbamylated acetylcholinesterase enzyme can undergo spontaneous hydrolysis *in vivo*, which reactivates the enzyme. Less severe toxidrome of shorter duration can be expected from carbamate poisoning because of this hydrolysis. The clinical manifestations of carbamate poisoning is similar to that of organophosphates. Poisoning usually develop within 10－30 minutes through ingestion, and 2－4 hours after occupational exposure.

Symptomatic treatment of the patient poisoned by carbamate insecticide includes aggressive respiratory support and atropine to reverse severe muscarinic manifestations. Because of the shorter duration of effect from *in vivo* hydrolysis, atropine treatment is usually required for less than 24 hours. The most important difference in treatment for carbamate and organophosphate poisoning involves 2-PAM. It is reasonable to administer 2-PAM cautiously, when the patients are exposures to pesticides mixed with Carbamate and organophosphates.

4.2.6.5　Regulatory Standards

In most countries, pesticides must be approved for sale and use by a government agency. China is the world's largest producer and consumer of pesticides. Pesticide use in China accounts for over one-third of total world pesticide usage. The Ministry of Agriculture (MOA) of China issued revisions to the country's pesticide registration requirements, which officially came into effect on November 1, 2017. In the United States, the Environmental Protection Agency (EPA) is responsible for regulating pesticides under the Federal Insecticide, Fungicide, and Rodenticide Act (FIFRA) and the Food Quality Protection Act (FQPA). The EPA regulates pesticides to ensure that these products do not pose adverse effects to humans or the environment. Only certified applicators who have passed the exam can purchase or supervise the application of restricted usage of pesticides. The EPA regulates pesticides under two main acts, both of which were amended by the Food Quality Protection Act of 1996. In addition to the EPA, the United States Department of Agriculture (USDA), the United States Food and Drug Administration (FDA) also set standards for the level of pesticide residue that is allowed on or in crops.

4.2.7   Prevention and Control of Occupational Poisoning

4.2.7.1   Principles of Prevention and Control

Numerous people are suffering from occupational poisoning, which also caused economic burdens. Prevention is the guiding principle for occupational safety and health (OSH) legislation in the world. Occupational poisoning can be prevented by traditional occupational hygiene measures based on the hierarchy of controls. Occupational poisoning is caused by productive poisons, the integrated management measures including eliminate exposure and reduce exposure to the productive poisons should be taken to prevent it. The prevention and control of occupational poisoning also followed the principle of tertiary prevention.

4.2.7.2   Prevention and Control Measures

(1) Elimination of Hazards in the Workplace

The ideal way to prevent occupational poisoning is to eliminate the poisons in the work environment. It is thus appropriate not to adopt work processes that will generate poisons.

(2) Substitution by Alternative Materials, Tools or Machines

If it is not possible to avoid work processes with health hazards, use safer alternative materials, tools or machines as far as practicable to minimize adverse health effects on the employees.

(3) Engineering Control Measures

If the poisons in the work environment cannot be completely eliminated or substituted by using safer alternative materials, tools, or machines, other control measures should be used to reduce employees' exposure to poisons. Controlling the poisons at source by engineering methods is an effective measure widely adopted. Engineering control measures include: enclosure, isolation, and good ventilation system.

(4) Administrative Measures

① Formulation, provision and monitoring of safety management system and guidelines: Employers from different industries should formulate a safety management system and a set of guidelines having regard the nature of work in their respective industries. Regular monitoring should also be carried out to ensure employees strict implementation of the guidelines to safeguard their safety and health.

② Regular repair and maintenance: Regular repair and maintenance of machines can ensure their proper function in order to protect the occupational health of employees.

③ Job rotation and appropriate rest breaks: Rotating employees to different work positions as far as practicable can reduce their prolonged contact with work hazards in a particular work position.

(5) Personal Protective Equipment

Although controlling poisons at source is an ideal way to prevent occupational diseases, the use of appropriate PPE will be the last resort if the control measures cannot eliminate or reduce poisons to meet relevant standards. PPE should be used to combine with other control measures since PPE alone is not sufficient for protecting the health of employees. While using PPE, one should pay attention to the correct way of wearing such equipment, regular checking of its effectiveness and cleanliness as well as proper storage after use.

(6) Health Surveillance

Health surveillance is of considerable importance for early detection of any deviance in employees' health due to work, so that they can seek appropriate treatment as early as possible and take corresponding preventive measures at the workplace.

4.3　Occupational Dust Exposure and Pneumoconiosis

Dusts are finely divided solids that may become airborne from the original state without any chemical or physical change except for fracture. Dusts are solid particles, ranging in size from below 1 μm up to at least 100 μm, which may be airborne, depending on their origin, physical characteristics and ambient conditions. Occupational dust, also named productive dust or industrial dust, is a kind of solid particles suspending in the workplace. They are produced in the production process and can be suspended in the air of the production environment for a long time. Occupational dust can cause a variety of occupational lung diseases, which is an important occupational harmful factor threatening the health of the occupational population.

4.3.1　Occupational Dust Exposure

4.3.1.1　Sources of Dust

Dust in the workplace is released from any form of mechanical breakdown and the movement of dusty materials. Dust exposure is linked to occupations and workplaces both in the industrial and agricultural settings.

(1) Mechanical Breakdown

Specific dust-producing operations include sandblasting, rock drilling, jack hammering, stone cutting, sawing, chipping, grinding, polishing, cleaning foundry castings and use of abrasives. The most common occupations are associated with mining, quarrying, tunneling, construction, drilling and foundry work.

(2) Movement of Dusty Materials

The powder and granule handling operations include weighing, mixing and transferring dusty raw materials and products such as bag filling, conveyor belts and transfering from one container to the other. The transportation of bags or any containers with dusty materials may constitute a moving dust source, particularly when the bags have holes, or containers are not properly closed.

（3）Recirculation of Previously Emitted Dust Particulates

The previously generated dusts can be recirculated by mechanical vibration and air flow change.

4.3.1.2   Classification of Dust

The dust is divided into three types including inorganic, organic and mixed dusts by chemical component.

（1）Inorganic Dusts

The dusts are found in the work environment, including mineral dusts such as those containing free crystalline silica (e. g. , as quartz), coal and asbestos, metallic dusts such as lead, cadmium and nickel, and man-made dusts such as cement and corundum.

（2）Organic Dusts

The dusts come from plants and animals, including animal dusts such as hairs, leather, bone and horny dusts, plant dusts such as cotton, linen, wood, pollen and tea dusts, and man-made dusts such as synthetic fibre, dyes, rubber, and synthetic resin dusts.

（3）Mixed Dusts

In the production environment, most of the dust exists in the form of two or more kinds of dust, which is called mixed dust. For example, coal miners exposed to coal silica dust, and fur processing contains fur and soil dust.

4.3.1.3   Factors Influencing the Adverse Effects of Dust on Human Body

The adverse health effects on the workers induced by productive dusts are affected by their source, classification and physical and chemical properties. From the perspective of hygiene, the main physical and chemical characteristics of dust should be considered as follows:

（1）Chemical Composition

The chemical compositions of dusts in the workplace air determine their toxicological hazard to the body. Dusts with different chemical compositions can cause symptoms of respiratory or skin irritation, poisoning, sensitization and fibrosis. For example, free silica dust can cause silicosis, asbestos dust can cause asbestosis, and manganese dust can cause manganese poisoning.

（2）Dust Dispersity

Dispersion refers to the degree of the composition of dust particle size, and is always expressed as the diameter or the percentage of mass of dust particles. The former is called particle dispersion, where the smaller the particle size is, the higher the dispersion is. The latter is called mass dispersion, where the more particles with small mass, the higher the dispersion is. The small particles fall slowly in the air and have the greater chance being inhaled. The particles with higher dispersion have the larger surface area, and are easier to participate in the physiological and biochemical reactions and are more harmful to human body.

The particle dispersion is also important in determining its ability to penetrate deeply into the lung. Dust is classified by size into three primary categories including inhalable dust, respirable dust and total dust. The aerodynamic equivalent diameter (AED) of particle less than 15 μm is called inhalable dust, wherein dust with a larger particle size (10 − 15 μm) is mainly retained in the nose, throat, and upper respiratory tract. The dust particles with particle size below 5μm can reach the deep respiratory tract and alveoli, which is called respirable dust. Total dust includes all airborne particles, regardless of their size or composition.

(3) Dust Concentration and Exposure Time

Dust concentration refers to the mass of dust in air per unit volume (mg/m^3). There is a dose-response relationship between dust dose and the prevalence of pneumoconiosis. The higher dust concentration in the working environment with a long-term exposure may result in greater harmful effects on human body.

(4) Others

The hardness, solubility, charge, explosion and health protection facilities of dust particles are also factors that affect the harmful effects of dust on human body. Irregular hard shape of dust is easy to cause mechanical damage to the respiratory tract. Quartz dust is difficult to dissolve and can continue to cause harmful effects in the body. Charged dust particles tend to be trapped in the lung, affecting the phagocytosis speed of macrophages and increasing the hazards of dust.

4.3.1.4　Major Hazards of Dust on Human Body

Dust is particularly concerned because it is well known to be associated with classical occupational lung diseases, such as pneumoconiosis. At the same time, the respiratory tracts have defense mechanism that protects respiratory health by removing dust from the respiratory system.

(1) Defense Mechanisms of Respiratory System

The bodies can protect the workers against some dusts. Not all the dust that the workers breathe in can enter the lungs. Once inhaled, the particles first pass through the upper airways from the nose, then through the trachea and the bronchi to the bronchioles. The defense mechanisms of the respiratory system include the following three aspects.

① Blocking of nasal cavity, larynx and tracheobronchial tree: When a large number of dust particles are inhaled with the air flow, most particles may be exhaled. Some dusts deposit in the upper respiratory tract by the impact and interception and then are removed to reduce the entry into respiratory bronchioles and alveoli.

② Discharge of mucus-cilia system: Mucus is a secretion produced by mucous membranes, which protects epithelial cells by coating foreign particles so that they can be coughed out of the body. Cilia are microscopic hairs that line the airways and attempt to brush foreign particles out of the lungs.

③ Phagocytosis of macrophages: They are special cells that attempt to engulf and digest particles and can signal lymphocytes and other immune system cells to respond to specific pathogens. Human macrophage cells are capable of digesting a number of particles but they cannot digest asbestos fibers which can cause the cell to burst.

(2) Major Hazards of Dust on Human Health

Different chemical composition and physical properties of dust can lead to different diseases, including the following aspects:

① Pneumoconiosis: Pneumoconiosis is a systemic disease caused by long-term inhalation of occupational dust and retention in the lungs during occupational activities, which characterized by a diffuse fibrotic reaction (microscopic scarring) around the small airways and alveolus of the lung. Pneumoconiosis is a general name for a number of dust-related lung diseases. Pneumoconiosis remains the most prevalent occupational lung disease worldwide, especially in the developing countries. According to the etiology, pneumoconiosis can be divided into silicosis, asbestosis, carbon pneumoconiosis, mixed dust pneumoconiosis and metallic pneumoconiosis. Because pneumoconiosis usually takes 20 or 30 years to develop, workers often do not notice symptoms until they are over 50 years old. The main symptoms are coughing and difficulty in breathing, which gradually increase. Complications include emphysema and increased risk of tuberculosis. Asbestosis patients are more likely to develop lung cancer, especially if they smoke cigarettes. Damaged lungs cause the heart work harder, and heart problems can accompany severe cases of pneumoconiosis.

A total of 13 types of pneumoconiosis were included in the "Classification and Catalogue of Occupational Diseases" revised in 2013 in China. The 13 types of pneumoconiosis are namely, silicosis, coal worker's pneumoconiosis, graphite pneumoconiosis, carbon black pneumoconiosis, asbestosis, talc pneumoconiosis, cement pneumoconiosis, mica pneumoconiosis, pottery worker's pneumoconiosis, aluminosis, welder's pneumoconiosis and foundry pneumoconiosis, and other pneumoconiosis that can be diagnosed according to "diagnosis of occupational pneumoconiosis" and "pathological diagnosis of occupational pneumoconiosis". Among them, silicosis and coal worker's pneumoconiosis are the most common, accounting for nearly 90% of the total cases of pneumoconiosis in China.

② Other respiratory system diseases: Some dusts can cause allergic reactions in the respiratory system. The effect of most sensitizers is gradual and will appear a few weeks or even years after exposure. The sensitizers can cause certain cellular changes, so further exposure after a period of incubation can lead to acute allergic reactions. The two main respiratory diseases of allergic type caused by occupational exposure to dusts are occupational asthma and extrinsic allergic alveolitis. Occupational asthma may be caused by certain grain dust, flour and sawdust, as well as metals. Extrinsic allergic alveolitis is caused by molds (and their spores) that grow on other materials, especially in humid environments. The cases of extrinsic allergic alveolitis include farmer's lung, bagassosis and suberosis.

Excessive exposure to dusts from cotton (mainly in cotton, carding and spinning operations), flax, sisal and soft hemp may cause byssinosis (also known as "brown lung"). Byssinosis is an obstructive lung disease, which is usually characterized in the initial stages by shortness of breath, chest tightness and wheezing on the first day after returning to work, but with the development of the disease, the symptoms will become more serious and more permanent. The increase in dyspnea leads to varying degrees of weakness.

③ Local irritation and inflammatory injuries: The irritation to the respiratory system may be caused by particles. The response of the respiratory system to inhalable particles depends, to a large extent, on the location of particles. Some dusts have an irritating effect on the upper respiratory tract. Irritant dusts that settle in the nose may lead to rhinitis, which is a mucosal inflammation. Exposure to stimuli can also lead to bronchitis and bronchitis.

④ Systemic poisoning: Some chemical dusts can enter the organism and pass to the bloodstream, thus exerting toxic action on one or more organs or systems. Systemic poisoning can be acute, or chronic, depending on the type of chemical and degree of exposure. Toxic metal dusts such as lead, cadmium, beryllium and manganese may cause systemic poisoning, thus affecting blood, kidneys or the central nervous system.

⑤ Carcinogenesity: Many dusts are confirmed carcinogens. For example, asbestos, particularly crocidolite, may cause lung cancer and mesothelioma. Usingasbestos-containing products in building materials could pose a risk for developing asbestos cancer. Free silica, hexavalent chromium and certain chromates, arsenic, particles containing polycyclic aromatic hydrocarbons (PAHs), and certain nickel-containing dusts may be associated with some cancers. Certain wood dusts have been recognized as the cause of nasal cancer. Exposed to significant doses of ionizing radioactive particles may cause lung cancer, or may metastasize from the lungs and damage other organs. Soluble carcinogens may pose a risk to both lungs and other organs.

4.3.2　Silicosis

Silicosis is a common type of pneumoconiosis, which is caused by long-term inhalation of dust with high content of free silicon dioxide (SiO_2) and characterized by inflammation and scarring in the formation of nodular lesions in the lungs. Silicosis is a kind of potentially fatal, irreversible, progressive and untreatable fibrotic lung disease. Although silicosis is an ancient occupational disease, new cases are still reported both in the developed and developing countries. Silicosis continues to progress even when the workers stop exposing dust. Extremely high exposures are associated with much shorter latency and more rapid disease progression. Exposure to respirable crystalline silica occurs in a number of industries and can result in a variety of diseases.

4.3.2.1　Causes of Silicosis

The pathogenic substance of silicosis is crystalline silica or free silicon dioxide (SiO_2).

Silicon is the second most common element in the earth's crust, making up approximately 28%. Because silicon is easy to combine with oxygen, there is no free silicon in nature, and silicon exists as free SiO_2 and silicates. Free SiO_2 is widely distributed in nature. 95% of ores contain free SiO_2, quartz contains free SiO_2 up to 99%, sandstone contains 80%, and granite contains more than 65%. Silica can exist in three forms, including crystalline, crypto crystalline and amorphous (non-crystalline silica) silica. In crystalline silica, the atoms and molecules are arranged in a three-dimensional repeating pattern. Crystalline silica exists as at least eight different polymorphs (same chemical composition but different structure), while the most common polymorphs are quartz, cristobalite, and tridymite. In crypto crystalline silica, the silicon oxygen tetrahedron arranges irregularly, mainly contain agate and flint. Amorphous silica mainly exists in diatomite, silica gel and silica vapor produced by quartz smelting. The fibrogenic effects is greater in crystalline, followed bycrypto crystalline and amorphous.

Free SiO_2 dust is commonly known as silica dust. Dust operations containing more than 10% free SiO_2 are called silica dust operations. Exposure to free SiO_2 occurs in a wide variety of occupations, in which the most common industries are mining and mining-related occupations. Workers engaged in these specific occupations may have the potential for exposures to free SiO_2 dust. Free SiO_2 particles are produced during many work tasks, including sandblasting, mining, rock drilling, quarrying, jewelry making, brick cutting, glass manufacturing, tunneling, foundry work, stone working, ceramic manufacturing and construction activities.

4.3.2.2 Types of Silicosis

Free SiO_2 content, dust concentration, exposure time and individual factors are the main factors affecting silicosis. Higher free SiO_2 content will lead to shorter onset time and more serious progress. Age, health status, nutrition status, personal hygiene habits and respiratory diseases of workers have certain effects on the occurrence of silicosis, especially active tuberculosis and other chronic respiratory diseases during dust exposure are prone to silicosis. Silicosis usually develops after exposure to silica dust for 5—10 years. Exposure to low concentration free SiO_2 dust may cause disease for 15—20 years.

(1) Acute Silicosis

Individuals with acute silicosis will start to develop symptoms within several weeks to up to 2 years, and it is often caused by exposure to very high levels of silica dust. This type of silicosis develops the fastest symptoms include severe shortness of breath, cough, weakness, and weight loss. In severe cases, acute silicosis can cause death. Acute silicosis occurs frequently in gold mining, quartz sand crushing and tunnel construction.

(2) Delayed Silicosis

Delayed silicosis is the most common form of silicosis. It is developed over a long period of time about 15—20 years and is caused by low levels of exposure to silica dust. Some workers, although exposed to high concentration of silicon dust, have no obvious abnormality in X-ray chest radiographs, or abnormality was found but not yet diagnosed as silicosis. They were diagnosed as silicosis years after being separated from silica dust. Sufferers may not be aware that they have this form of silicosis in the early stages of the disease and may not have any clear symptoms other than coughing or lack of breath.

4.3.2.3 Mechanism of Silicosis

Normally, 97%—99% of the dust entering the respiratory tract can be discharged by the body within 24 hours. However, if the dust concentration in the production environment is too high, the workers are exposed to it for long time, and the dust entering the respiratory tract exceeds the body's ability to remove it, the dust will accumulate in the lungs. The more dust accumulated in the lungs, the more harmful to health.

Silicosis has a definite cause, but its pathogenesis is complex. So far, many theories such as mechanical stimulation, chemical poisoning, surface activity, immune response and silicic acid polymerization have been put forward by scholars all over the world, but it is still difficult to explain the whole process of silicosis. With the development of biological science and technology, the study on the pathogenesis of silicosis is deepening. In recent years, some new progress has been acquired in the process of exploring the complex mechanism of silicosis. It is believed that silicosis is initiated when alveolar macrophages phagocytize silica particles in an attempt to clear them from the lung. When alveolar macrophages containing silica die, they release silica particles that are then re-engulfed by other alveolar macrophages, thus inducing a cycle of injure.

(1) Damage and Death of Macrophage

When the free silica particles reach the alveolar macrophage, they are engulfed by the alveolar macrophage which may lead to damage of the lysosomal membranes. The macrophages engulfed particles called dust cell. Silica dust can make the macrophages disintegrate to death, the mechanism is mainly through the following aspects. The activity of hydroxyl groups on the surface of quartz dust (silanol group) can interact with hydrogen ions in alveolar macrophages and multi-core white cell membranes to form hydrogen bond, generate hydrogen exchange and electron transfer. This reaction will increase the cell membrane permeability, reduce liquidity and change the function of cells, eventually lead to cell rupture.

Quartz particles can directly damage the macrophage cell membrane, destroy the integrity of the cell membrane and increase the permeability of the membrane, which then lead to a large number of extracellular calcium ions into the cell and form "calcium overload", and cause the breakdown of macrophages and death. Lipid peroxidation of cell membrane induced by quartz dust is also involved in the damage process of macrophage. The peroxidation of the phospholipids and unsaturated fatty acids in the membranes of the cellular and intracellular structures, results in damage of the membranes. The changes of the membrane structures of the cells make the lysosomals release the hydrolytic enzymes and kill the macrophage.

(2) Production of Collagen Fibers and Formation of Silicotic Nodules

The production of collagen fibers and the formation of silicotic nodules are very slow process, and its pathogenesis can be summarized as these aspects. The structure and function damage of macrophages, lymphocytes, epithelial cells and fibroblasts by quartz particles can lead to the production and release of various cytokines, such as tumor necrosis factor (TNF-α), interleukin-1 (IL-1), interleukin-6 (IL-6) and transforming growth factor-β1 (TGF-β1). These cytokines constitute a complex cytokine network, which activates intracellular transcription factors through a variety of signal transduction pathways. Silica dust can activate the inflammatory body NLRP3 directly or indirectly, and then activate caspase-1 and downstream LI-1β and LI-18 to play a pro-inflammatory role. In the process of silica dust leading to apoptosis of macrophages, chemokines can be released to recruit new inflammatory cells and further expand the inflammatory response. These processes stimulate fibroblasts to proliferate and produce collagen around the silica particle, thus resulting in fibrosis.

The silica particles can damage the alveolar type I epithelial cells and make the modified swelling and disintegration. Type II epithelial cells will act as stem cells to repair injured type I epithelial cells. However, when the impairment exceeds the repaired ability of type II epithelial cells, basement membrane will be damaged leading to pulmonary interstitial bared and fibroblasts recruit activated to produce large amounts of fibronectin and collagen. The production of collagen fibers provides the material basis for the formation of silica nodules.

The activation of alveolar macrophages leads to an alteration and impairment in macrophage function. The release of certain inflammatory cytokines such as IL-1 leads to activation of humoral and cellular immunity responses. This stimulates production of antibodies against collagen. The antigen-antibody complexes are formed to stimulate the fibroblasts to produce more collagen and deposit on the collagen fibers to form transparency changes, which eventually leads to nodule formation.

Th1 cytokines can activate lymphocytes in the early stage of lung injury and participate in tissue inflammation. Th2 cytokines promote fibroblast proliferation, activation and initiate fibrosis process. Silica dust promotes the polarization of regulatory T lymphocytes from Th1 to Th2, induces increased TGF-β1 secretion, and further promotes fibroblast proliferation and the synthesis and secretion of collagen. In addition, silica dust can induce stress on alveolar macrophage lysosomes, leading to the increase of autophagosomes, inhibition of autophagy degradation. This promote the induction of death receptors, mitochondria and endoplasmic reticulum signaling pathways to mediate the apoptosis of various lung effector cells, thereby promoting the process of pulmonary fibrosis.

4. 3. 2. 4   Pathological Feature

The primary feature that develops in the lungs of workers exposed to silica dust is silicotic nodule in the upper zones of the lung. The postmortem examination of silicosis patient showed that the lung volume increased and the gas content decreased. The lung became stiffer and heavier, and will sink into the water. The discrete, pale and gritty nodules can be seen on the surface of the lung, and the fused masses are hard and rubbery with loss of elasticity of lung tissue. There is extensive pleural thickening and adhesion. The dark gray lymph nodes can be seen at the lung hilum and bronchus bifurcation.

The basic pathological changes of silicosis are silicotic nodule formation and diffuse interstitial fibrosis (Figure 4.6). Silicotic nodules are typical pathological feature of silicosis. The pathological changes of silicosis can be classified into nodular silicosis, diffuse interstitial fibrosis silicosis, silicosis protein deposition and mass silicosis.

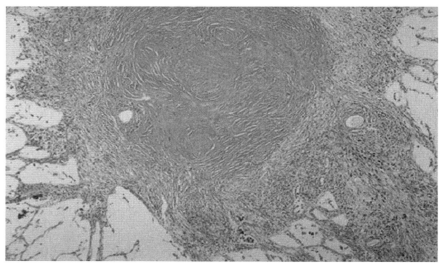

Figure 4. 6   Microscopic Image of A Typical Silicotic Nodule Containing Collage Fibers

(1) Nodular Silicosis

Macroscopically, silicotic nodules are slightly domed on the surface of the lung and usually seen in subpleural and intrapulmonary sections with scattered silicotic nodules 1—5 mm in diameter. Under microscope various stages and types of nodules are seen. A typical silicotic nodule is composed of multiple concentric rings of collagenous fibers with a central or lateral occlusion of small blood vessels or bronchi. The macrophages that contain the silica particles are present at the periphery of the nodule. Early silicotic nodule collagen fibers are thin and loosely arranged, interspersed with numerous dust cells and fibroblasts. In mature silicotic nodules, the collagen fibers become thick and dense, and the collagen fibers may become transparent. Because lack of blood supply and therefore also oxygen delivery, the tissue in the center of the nodule is caused necrosis. With further development, the number and density of silicotic nodules is increased, their size is enlarged, and then they fused into a mass. Exposure to higher dose of free SiO_2 dust, the formation time of silicotic nodules is longer, and the nodules were more mature and typical. Although the diameter of some silicotic nodule is small, but it is very mature and appear central calcium salt deposition. This is always cause by the long-term inhalation of free SiO_2 dust with low dose.

(2) Diffuse Interstitial Fibrosis Silicosis

Diffuse interstitial fibrosis silicosis is caused by exposure to the dust with low content of free SiO_2 for a long time, or inhalation a small amount of dust with high content of free SiO_2. This silicosis progresses slowly, and the lesions are mostly diffuse interstitial fibrosis. The pathological features were diffuse hyperplasia of fibrous tissue around alveolar septum, pulmonary interlobular septum, respiratory bronchus and small blood vessels, which connected radially and stellate. This is the pathological basis of the "ground-glass" changes seen on chest X-rays. Sometimes large masses of fibrosis form, interspersed with dust particles and dust cells.

(3) Silicosis Protein Deposition

The pathological features are that the alveolar cavities have a large amount of protein secretion, known as silicotic protein. Subsequently, it may be accompanied by fibrous hyperplasia, forming small fibrous foci and even silicotic nodules. Most of them are found in young workers exposed to high concentration and high dispersion of free SiO_2 dust in a short period of time, also known as acute silicosis.

(4) Mass Silicosis

When the above types of silicosis further develop, focal fusion occurs and mass lesions may form. This type is more common in the posterior segment of the upper lobe and the dorsal segment of the lower lobe. Macroscopically, the clumps are black or gray-black, cordlike, conical or irregular. Under the microscope, nodular and diffuse interstitial fibrotic lesions, collagen fibrosis and hyaline degeneration can be observed, as well as extruded vessels, nerves and dystrophic necrosis, thin wall cavities and calcification lesions. Atrophic alveolar cavities are filled with dust cells and dust particles, and compensatory emphysema occurs in the alveolar tissue around the mass. Close to the chest wall can form lung vesicles, pleural thickening and extensive adhesion. Sometimes amalgamative tuberculosis can form silicosis tuberculosis foci.

4.3.2.5　Clinical Findings

(1) Symptoms and Signs

Damaged lung tissue means that the lungs cannot perform their function of supplying oxygen to the blood. These symptoms of silicosis develop over time, and the lung tissue becomes irreversibly damaged by fibrosis and is replaced by solid nodular scar tissue. Because chronic silicosis develops slowly, signs and symptoms may not appear until many years after exposure.

The symptoms of silicosis include shortness of breath after physical activity, cough, expectoration, fatigue, chest tightness and chest pain. Shortness of breath is the first symptom. It usually begins some years after the beginning of exposure to dust. At first, the shortness of breath may occur only during exercise, but eventually it occurs also during rest. In the late stages of silicosis, pulmonary function dysfunction are the most common form, including decreased lung volumes and diffusing capacity, obstructed airways, frequently with pulmonary hypertension, and occasionally with mild hypoxemia.

(2) Chest X-ray (Radiograph)

The detection of silicosis in dust exposed workers is based on the chest X-ray. Abnormalities are usually bilateral, symmetric, and predominant in the inner mid-lung fields. The chest X-ray showed increased lung texture, thickening, even distortion and disorder fracture. Small rounded or irregular opacities appear, and large mass shadows appear on the later radiographs. Small opacities (shadows) and large opacities are the main basis of X-ray diagnosis of silicosis. The opacities caused by dust inhalation can be classified into two types according to whether they are round or irregular in shape. The round opacities seen on the X-ray represent the summation of pathologic silicotic nodules. They are usually found predominantly in the upper zones of the lung tissue and may later spread to other zones. The small opacities are less than 10 mm in diameter. The round opacities measuring less than 1.5 mm are designated as p, those measuring 1.5 to 3 mm are designated as q, and those measuring 3 to 10 mm are designated as r.

The irregular opacities are a group of dense shadows with different thickness, length and shape, which are unconnected or interwoven together in disorder, showing a network or honeycomb shape. In the early stage, it is more common in the middle and lower regions of both lungs, interwoven between the lung textures. When the mesh shadow is dense, the lung field is "ground-glass" turbidity. The pathological basis of the irregular opacities is pulmonary interstitial fibrosis. The irregular opacities are termed s (up to 1.5 mm), t (1.5—3 mm), or u (3 — 10 mm) by width. For small opacities, the term profusion (intensity) is used to describe the concentration of small opacities in the affected zones of the lungs. There are four main categories and twelve subcategories of profusion, ranging from 0/0 (no small opacities present) to 3/+ (a high concentration of small opacities present). The large opacities are defined as the opacities with the diameter or width of more than 10mm in the lung field, which is an important X-ray manifestation of advanced silicosis. It is in the shape of a long strip, oval or round shape, mostly in the upper and middle part of the lungs, and is in the shape of an octagon. The pathological basis of the large opacities is mass fibrosis.

Egg shell calcification is strongly suggestive of silicosis, although this feature is seen infrequently. Pleural abnormalities may occur but are not a frequent radiographic feature in silicosis.

(3) Complications of Silicosis

Silicosis can make an individual susceptible to infections. The common complications of silicosis include pulmonary tuberculosis (TB), pulmonary and bronchial infection, spontaneous pneumothorax and pulmonary heart disease. Tuberculosis is the most common complication of silicosis. Silicosis once concomitant tuberculosis, can make silicosis accelerates aggravate. Tuberculosis is hard to control, and silicosis concomitant tuberculosis is the common reason that the patient dies.

4.3.2.6   Diagnosis of Silicosis

The diagnosis of silicosis base on some key elements, including reliable silica dust exposure history of patient, the labor hygiene survey data (especially the dust concentration in working environment, dispersion and dust free SiO_2 content, operation mode and protection measures, etc.), the reference dynamic observations and epidemiological investigation of pneumoconiosis. The technical quality qualified high-kilometer post-front X-ray film is the main basis that reveals findings consistent with silicosis. There are no underlying illnesses that are more likely to be causing the abnormalities. Pulmonary function testing may reveal airflow limitation, restrictive defects, reduced diffusion capacity, mixed defects, or may be normal (especially without complicated disease). Most cases of silicosis do not require tissue biopsy for diagnosis, but this may be necessary in some cases, primarily to exclude other conditions.

According to the diagnostic criteria for pneumoconiosis disease (GBZ 70—2015), the pneumoconiosis diagnosis expert group discuss to make a diagnosis and X-ray stage. The main basis of staging is: small opacities (shape, size, density, distribution range) and large opacities. The patient's chest radiographs were compared with the standard pneumoconiosis radiographs to determine the staging, and other similar lung diseases were excluded. If necessary, diagnosis can also be made according to the "pneumoconiosis pathological diagnostic standard" (GBZ 25—2014).

(1) Stage 1 Pneumoconiosis

The pneumoconiosis is one of the following circumstances:

① The small shadows with class 1 level overall intensity exit, and the distribution is at least 2 lung zones.

② Exposure to asbestos dust, the small shadows with class 1 level overall intensity exit, and the distribution is only 1 lung zone and with pleural plaques.

③ Exposed to asbestos dust, the small shadows with class 0 level overall intensity exit, but at least 2 lung zones had small shadows of 0/1 and with pleural plaques.

(2) Stage 2 Pneumoconiosis

The pneumoconiosis is one of the following circumstances:

① The small shadows with class 2 level overall intensity exit, and the distribution is over 4 lung zones.

② The small shadows with class 3 level overall intensity exit, and the distribution is up to 4 lung zones.

③ Exposure to asbestos dust, the small shadows with class 1 level overall intensity exit, and the distribution is over 4 lung zones, accompanied by pleural plaques and involving part of the heart or diaphragmatic surface.

④ Exposure to asbestos dust, the small shadows with class 2 level overall intensity exit, and the distribution is over 4 lung zones, accompanied by pleural plaques and involving part of the heart or diaphragmatic surface.

(3) Stage 3 Pneumoconiosis

The pneumoconiosis is one of the following circumstances:

① A large shadow appeared, and its long diameter is not less than 20 mm, short diameter not less than 10 mm.

② The small shadows with class 3 level overall intensity exit, and the distribution is more than 4 lung zones and with aggregation of small shadows.

③ The small shadows with class 3 level overall intensity exit, and the distribution is more than 4 lung zones and with large shadows.

④ Exposure to asbestos dust, the small shadows with class 3 level overall intensity exit, and the distribution is over 4 lung zones, and the length of a single or multiple pleural plaques on both sides added up to more than half of the length of the unilateral chest wall or involved the cardiac margin so that some of them showed unkiness.

4.3.2.7　Treatment of Silicosis

There is no known medical treatment to reverse silicosis, therefore treatment options currently focus on alleviating the symptoms and preventing complications. Removal from exposure may decrease the rate of disease progression. Individuals who develop silicosis should be given the option of transfer to silica-free jobs. The purpose of medical management is to prevent and treat pulmonary TB or other complications, relieve symptom, delay the process of the disease, lengthen the life span of patients and raise their quality life. Appropriate treatment for heart failure and TB should begin if these complications exist. All individuals should be strongly advised to stop smoking and offered smoking cessation information and support. Regular follow-up examinations to assess progression and possible screen for lung cancer should be scheduled.

4.3.3　Coal Worker's Pneumoconiosis

Coal is one of the main energy and chemical raw materials, which can be divided into lignite, bituminous coal and anthracite. As the mechanization of coal mining and the increasing degree of coal pulverization, the amount and dispersion of coal dust also increases. After silica dust, coal dust and coal silicon dust are the second hazardous dust to workers' health in coal mine. Coal worker's pneumoconiosis also known as black lung disease is caused by workers' long-term inhalation of coal dust in the production environment. It is a common health hazardous of coal miners and others who expose to coal dust.

4.3.3.1　Causes of Coal Worker's Pneumoconiosis

(1) Occupational Exposure to Coal Dust

Coal dust may be inhaled by workers in the process of coalfield geological exploration, coal mine construction, coal production, coal washing, coal transportation, loading and unloading, etc. The influence factors affecting the pathogenicity of coal mine dust are the content of free SiO_2. The content of free SiO_2 in coal dust is below 10%. If the content of free SiO_2 in coal dust is less than 5%, it is called pure coal dust. The concentration and dispersion determine the pathogenicity of coal mine dust.

(2) Causes of Coal Worker's Pneumoconiosis

① In the production environment, there is rarely pure coal dust, which is usually mixed dust. It should be considered that mixed dust can have a combined effect.

② Individual factors and health status of workers also play a role in the occurrence of coal worker's pneumoconiosis, especially rheumatoid pneumoconiosis, which is a manifestation of pneumoconiosis peculiar to coal workers.

③ The higher the content of free SiO_2 in coal dust, the shorter the onset time and the more serious the lesion.

④ The occurrence and lesion degree of coal worker's pneumoconiosis are related to the accumulation of coal dust in the lung, which mainly depends on dust concentration, dispersion, exposure time and protective measures. Exposure to the higher concentration and the greater dispersion of dust for longer time will increase the inhaled and accumulated of dust in the lung, which lead to the higher likelihood of development and severity of pneumoconiosis.

4.3.3.2　Types of Coal Worker's Pneumoconiosis

(1) Silicosis

The rock drillers, rock loaders and support workers worked in tunneling working face are exposed to rock dust. Pneumoconiosis occurred in these occupations shows a typical silicotic nodule change in the lung pathology, so it is called silicosis. The characteristics of silicosis are high incidence, short working life (10 to 15 years) and rapid disease progression.

(2) Anthracosis

Pneumoconiosis is caused by long-term inhalation of coal dust during the production process. It occurs in the simple coal mining, coal preparation, loading and unloading of coal. The free SiO_2 in coal dust is less than 5%. The characteristics of anthracosis are low incidence (generally less than 5%), long working life (20 to 30 years), mild lesions and slow progress.

(3) Anthracosilicosis

Most of the coal miners in China have worked in both rock roadway and coal mining face. They are exposed to coal dust and silica dust. These coal miners suffer from pneumoconiosis with pathological changes of both silicosis and anthracosis. It is called anthracosilicosis, which is the most common type of pneumoconiosis in coal mines. The characteristics of anthracosilicosis are long working life (15 to 20 years) and rapid disease progression.

4.3.3.3 Mechanism of Coal Worker's Pneumoconiosis

The mechanisms of coal worker's pneumoconiosis are not fully understood. Currently, there are focused on mechanical damage, cytotoxicity, generation of reactive oxygen species and production of collagen fibers. The structure and function damage of macrophages, epithelial cells and fibroblasts also can release cytokines, such as tumor necrosis factor (TNF-α), interleukin-1 (IL-1) and transforming growth factor-β1 (TGF-β1). These cytokines can activate the inflammatory response through a variety of signal transduction pathways. The particles damage the alveolar epithelial cells and basement membrane, activate fibroblasts recruit to produce large amounts of fibronectin and collagen. In addition, coal dusts induce stress on alveolar macrophage lysosomes, leading to the increase of autophagosomes, inhibition of autophagy degradation. These promote the induction of death receptors to mediate the apoptosis of various lung effector cells, thereby promoting the process of pulmonary fibrosis.

4.3.3.4 Pathological Feature

The pathological changes of coal worker's pneumoconiosis vary with the proportion of inhaled silica dust and coal dust. Except for silicosis suffered by rock drillers, it is mainly a mixed type with the characteristics of interstitial diffuse fibrosis and nodule. The main pathological changes are as follows:

(1) Coal Macule

Coal macule also known as coal dust focus, it is the most common characteristic lesion of coal worker's pneumoconiosis and the basic indicator of pathological diagnosis. Macroscopically, there have coal spots with different diameters on the surface of lung pleura, ranging from 0.5 to 1 cm, which are star-shaped, unshaped, polygonal and elongated. Some coal spots are fused into thin sheets, with a diameter up to 2 cm. The lung parenchyma is soft and dark. The slices showed scattered black spots or focal lesions, often accompanied by emphysema around the coal dust lesions. Microscopically, coal macule is composed by coal dust cell foci and coal dust fiber foci. A number of coal dust and coal dust cells can be observed in the alveolar space, alveolar wall, and peribronchial and perivascular tissues to form coal dust cell foci. The size of coal dust cell foci is different, and the fibrosis appeared following coal dust cell foci. The early stage is reticular fibers, and the late stage is characterized by a small amount or medium amount of fibrous tissue, which is cordlike or irregularly arrange to form the coal dust fiber foci.

(2) Perifocal Emphysema

Perifocal emphysema is another pathological feature of coal worker's pneumoconiosis, which is more common around coal dust fibrous lesions. The enlarged air cavity scatters around the coal plaque and coexists with the coal macule, which is called perifocal emphysema. Because of coal dust and dust cells accumulation around the II respiratory bronchus, it makes the smooth muscle and other structures of the wall damage to form lobular centricity emphysema. It is called lobular central emphysema. If the lesion develops further, it expands into the alveolar tract, alveolar duct, and alveoli, that is, the whole lobular area to form the whole lobular emphysema.

(3) Coal Silicon Nodules

Coal silica nodules are round or irregularly shape and protrude to the surface on the cut surface of the lung. Typical coal silica nodules have collagen fiber arranged in a swirl pattern in the center and a large number of coal dust cells and fibroblasts around them. Atypical coal silica nodules have no collagen fiber core. Collagen fiber bundles are irregular and loose, and dust cells are scattered among the collagen fibers.

(4) Interstitial Fibrosis

In the alveolar septum, interlobular septum, small blood vessels, bronchioles and subpleural, there are different degrees of interstitial cells and fiber hyperplasia, accompanied by coal dust and dust cell deposition, interstitial widening and thickening. In the late stage, it forms thick and thin strands and diffuse fiber grid, which is called lung interstitial fiber hyperplasia.

(5) Massive Fibrosis

Massive fibrosis, also known as progressive massive fibrosis (PMF), is a manifestation of advanced coal worker's pneumoconiosis, but it is not an inevitable result of advanced coal worker's pneumoconiosis. The lung tissue shows dense and black mass lesions, which mostly distributed in the upper and posterior parts of both lungs with long fusiform and non-plastic lesions. There are two types of microscopically observed tissue structures. One is diffuse fibrosis, in which there are many coal dust and coal dust cells in fibrous tissues and around lesions, but nodule changes are not observed. The other is a massive fibrotic lesion with coal-silica nodules, but interstitial fibrosis and coal dust are still the main lesions. The massive fibrosis of coal worker's pneumoconiosis is different from silicosis fused masses. There are more nodules and less interstitial fibrosis in silicosis fused masses.

4.3.3.5   Clinical Findings

(1) Symptoms and Signs

The patients are generally asymptomatic at an early stage. Respiratory symptoms and signs, such as shortness of breath, chest pain, chest tightness, and cough, occur when the lesion progresses, especially when it develops into massive fibrosis or a bronchial or pulmonary infection. When engaged in slightly heavy work or climbing, the shortness of breath is aggravated. When combined with pulmonary infection and bronchitis, the corresponding signs can be observed.

(2) Pulmonary Function Changes

In coal worker's pneumoconiosis patients with extensive pulmonary fibrosis, airway stenosis, and especially the massive destruction of alveoli due to emphysema, the lung function tests showed decreased or impaired ventilation, diffusion, and gas exchange function.

(3) X-ray Characteristics of Coal Lung

Small and medium-sized nodules are the most common, and some cases show needle-like nodules (p, q), which are often irregular and star-shaped. The density of nodules is lower than that of silicon nodules, and the edges of nodules are generally fuzzier than that of silicon nodules. Early distribution is in the middle and lower lung areas, late distribution will go to be the whole lung field.

Pulmonary interstitial fibrosis is the pathological basis of reticulum. Because interstitial fibrosis occurs around small blood vessels, bronchioles, and alveolar spaces, it is very fine on X-ray chest radiography, which is difficult to display clearly. It is often blurred and become "ground-glass" changes. The hilum of lung is slight enlargement, slight increase in density, few hilar morphologic changes and lymph node enlargement. The lung texture is obviously increased, thickened and distorted.

(4) X-ray Characteristics of Coal Silicosis

Small round shadows are more common, mostly p and q small shadows. The pathological basis of small round shadow is silica nodule, coal silica nodule and coal dust fiber focus. Irregular small shadows are less common than small round shadows. Most of them are reticular, some are densely honeycombed, and their pathological basis is coal dust focus, diffuse interstitial fibrosis, bronchiectasis and lobular central emphysema. Large shadows can be seen on chest radiographs of silicosis and coal silicosis patients, mostly formed by dense and fused small shadows. It can also be fused by a small number of patches and cable-like shadows.

Peripheral emphysema is more obvious, forming a large shadow with clear edges, dense density and uniformity. Coal lung patients rarely have large shadows. The hilar shadow is enlarged, the density is increased, sometimes can also be seen lymph nodes egg-like calcification or mulberry calcification shadow. The lung texture is increased, thickened, distorted, and beaded. The texture is disordered and staggered in a honeycomb shape. Diffuse, localized and vesicular emphysema are common. The vesicular emphysema is characterized by a small pile of small shadows with a diameter of 1 to 5 mm, known as "white circles and black spots", with large pulmonary vesicles in later stages. Intercostal phrenic angle atresia and adhesion are often observed.

4.3.3.6 Diagnosis of Coal Worker's Pneumoconiosis

The diagnosis of coal worker's pneumoconiosis also needs to collect the following materials, which is in accordance with the diagnosis of silicosis.

(1) Detailed and Reliable Career History

(2) The Labor Hygiene Survey Data

(3) High Kilovolt Post-front X-ray Film with Qualified Technical Quality

(4) Refer to the Necessary Dynamic Observations and Epidemiological Data

(5) Excluding Other Underlying Diseases

At present, the occupational pneumoconiosis diagnostic criterion (GBZ 70 — 2015) is performed for diagnosis and stage.

4. 3. 3. 7　Treatment of Coal Worker's Pneumoconiosis

There is no known medical treatment to cure coal worker's pneumoconiosis. Removal from exposure can decrease the rate of disease progression. The purpose is to prevent and treat the complications, relieve symptoms, delay the process of the disease, lengthen the life span of patients and improve their quality life.

4. 3. 4　Asbestosis

Asbestosis is mainly caused by long-term inhalation of excessive amounts of asbestos fibers during the production process. It is a typical representative of diffuse fibrotic pneumoconiosis, which is defined as a chronic inflammatory and diffuse pulmonary fibrosis with no or minimal nodular damage. The disease is the most prevalent among workers who had an extensive exposure to mining, manufacturing, handling or removal of asbestos.

4. 3. 4. 1　Causes of Asbestosis

Asbestos is a general term that refers to a group of minerals made of long, crystalline fibres, and is divided into two types, serpentine and amphibole. Serpentine is mainly composed by chrysotile asbestos, which is white asbestos and has a hollow tubular filament with a soft, bendable and woven property. Chrysotile asbestos mainly comes from Canada, Russia and China, and widely used worldwide. Amphibole is a kind of silicate with chain structure and mainly exists in the form of crocidolite – blue asbestos, amosite – brown asbestos, amphibole, tremolite and amphibole. Among them, the crocidolite and amosite are widely used and mainly produced in Africa, Australia and Finland. All types of asbestos are hazardous, but blue and brown asbestos are much more dangerous than white asbestos. While the most common type of asbestos for industrial use was white asbestos. In the United States, white asbestos has been the most commonly used type of asbestos, and accounts for approximately 95% of asbestos found in buildings in the United States.

Asbestos fibres are very strong and resistant to heat, electricity and chemicals. It was widely used in industries such as insulation, shipbuilding and railways, electricity generation, building and construction. In 2017, 1. 3 million tonnes of asbestos was mined worldwide. Russia was the largest producer with 53% of the world total, followed by Kazakhstan (16%), China (15%), and Brazil (11. 5%). Asia consumes some 70% of the asbestos produced in the world with China, India and Indonesia the largest consumers.

Several factors are involved in how asbestos exposure affects an individual. These include the type, size, shape and chemical makeup of the asbestos fibers, dust concentration and exposure time. The higher content of asbestos fiber in the dust, the longer the contact time, and the more fibers inhaled into the lung. The smaller the particle size and the more deposition in the lung, the more likely it is to cause pulmonary fibrosis. Due to the straight and hard property of blue asbestos, it can penetrate the lungs and reach the pleura. So its ability inducing pulmonary fibrosis and carcinogenesis are the strongest, the lesions appear early and the more amount of asbestos bodies forming. However, chrysotile is soft, flexible and rich in magnesium oxide, which lead to chrysotile dust easily blocked and dissolved in the bronchioles, and result in faster clearing and less cytotoxicity than blue asbestos in the lungs. Unfortunately, asbestos lung can still occur and develop after dust-free operation. In addition, the occurrence of asbestosis can also be affected by individual differences and lifestyle habits such as smoking and drinking.

4.3.4.2   Occupational Exposure to Asbestos

There are many operations with a particularly high risk of asbestos exposure, such as the process of mining and blasting the silicate ore, and during the use of asbestos products including construction, shipbuilding, electric welding, refractory materials, insulation materials manufacturing.

4.3.4.3   Mechanisms of Asbestosis

The mechanisms by which asbestos causes asbestosis are not fully understood. Currently, there are three hypotheses to account for the mechanisms including mechanical damage, cytotoxicity and generation of reactive oxygen species. The asbestos fibers have been shown to interfere physically and penetrate through the walls of the respiratory bronchioles and alveolar ducts to pulmonary interstitial. The diffusive fibrosis of pulmonary interstitial takes place. The physical stimulation of asbestos fibers also can cause pleura damages. The magnesian ion on the membranes of asbestos fibers may interact with membranes of the macrophage to form ionic channels. Then the membrane permeability will increase and the hydrolytic enzymes in the lysosomes will be released to result in cell breakage. When alveolar macrophages attempt to engulf and digest an asbestos fiber, they release reactive oxygen species (ROS) including $O2^-$, H_2O_2 and $\cdot OH$. Excessive ROS can cause biofilm oxidative damaged, and lead to the damage of substrate membrane and the release of oxides, growth factors and cytokines, which in turn promote myofibroblast proliferation and collagen deposition, and ultimately lead to fibrosis of lung tissue.

4.3.4.4   Pathological Feature

The histological diagnosis of asbestosis requires an appropriate pattern of diffuse pulmonary interstitial fibrosis plus the finding of asbestos bodies and asbestos-related pleural disease.

In early asbestosis, the pulmonary interstitial fibrosing process is limited to the walls of alveoli immediately around the respiratory bronchioles. From this centriacinar position, pulmonary interstitial fibrosis extends outward until it ultimately links adjacent bronchioles. At this time, the initial, predominantly peri-bronchiolar pattern of fibrosis may no longer be evident. Asbestosis is characterized as having a lower lobe and peripheral distribution.

The second feature necessary for a histologic diagnosis is the finding of asbestos bodies. Asbestos bodies are golden-brown, beaded, or dumbbell-shaped structures with a thin, translucent core. They form from the deposition of an iron-protein-mucopolysaccharide coating on the surface of an inhaled asbestos fiber by alveolar macrophages. The finding of asbestos bodies alone is insufficient for a histologic diagnosis of asbestosis and indicates only asbestos exposure.

The pleura appear to be more sensitive than the lung parenchyma to the effects of asbestos fibres. Asbestos exposure can lead to a number of asbestos-related pleural diseases including pleural plaques, pleural effusions and diffuse pleural thickening. Pleural plaques are the commonest manifestation of asbestos exposure. Pleural plaques usually affect the parietal pleura. Pleural plaques are patches of thickening pleura, which consist of mature hyaline collagen fibers. Pleural plaques have a white or pale yellow shaggy appearance. Peural effusions are relatively uncommon and the earliest manifestation of disease following asbestos exposure, usually occurring within 10 years from exposure. Effusions usually last for $3-4$ months and then resolve completely. They can also progress to diffuse pleural thickening. Diffuse pleural thickening is non-circumscribed fibrous thickening of the visceral pleura with areas of adherence to the parietal pleura and obliteration of the pleural space. It often extends over the area of an entire lobe or lung, with fibrotic areas involving costophrenic angles, apices, lung bases, and interlobar fissures.

4. 3. 4. 5　Clinical Findings

(1) Symptoms and Signs

The clinical symptoms usually include slowly progressing shortness of breath and dry, persistent cough. The symptoms usually begin many years after the initial exposure to asbestos. In most cases, the symptoms do not become apparent until 15 to 30 years after exposure. At first, the shortness of breath may occur only during exercise, but eventually it occurs even during rest. As asbestosis symptoms progress, the victim may experience chest pain that tends to worsen when they inhale. In addition to the above, other asbestosis symptoms that may occur include chronic fatigue, unexplained weight loss and tightness in the chest.

Asbestosis patients exhibit dry inspiratory crackles, which are clicking or rattling noises made by the lungs during inhalation. Other indications of asbestosis include clubbing of the fingers and failure of the right side of the heart will.

(2) Chest X-ray (Radiograph)

The abnormal chest X-ray and its interpretation remain the most important factors in establishing the presence of pulmonary fibrosis. The findings usually appear as small, irregular parenchymal opacities, primarily in the lung bases. X-rays often show pleural changes in people who have been exposed to asbestos. These changes include pleural plaques, diffuse pleural thickening and pleural effusions. Pleural plaques are the most frequent lesions as discrete, elevated, opaque, shiny fibrosis lesions that are currently common in exposed persons. Diffuse pleural thickening and pleural effusions are early manifestations of inhalation exposure to high concentrations of asbestos. Pleural effusions can be an early indication of mesothelioma and warrant further evaluation.

(3) Complications of Asbestosis

Complications of asbestosis include lung infection, emphysema and pulmonary heart disease, emphysema and cancer.

4.3.4.6　Diagnosis of Asbestosis

The general diagnostic criteria for asbestosis include history of asbestos exposure, chest X-ray or chest CT scan, and pulmonary function tests. Diagnosis of asbestosis depends on new diagnostic criteria of pneumoconiosis (GBZ 70—2015).

4.3.4.7　Treatment of Asbestosis

There is no known medical treatment to reverse silicosis, therefore prevention is critically important. Removal from exposure may decrease the rate of disease progression. The purpose is to prevent and treat the complications, relieve symptoms, delay the process of the disease, lengthen the life span of patients and raise their quality life. Individuals who develop silicosis should be given the option of transfer to silica-free jobs.

4.3.5　Other Pneumoconiosis

4.3.5.1　Graphite Pneumoconiosis

The pneumoconiosis is caused by excessive inhalation of graphite with diffuse fibrosis and emphysema lesions. Cases are rare and severity can vary depending on the level of exposure. There are two types of graphite including natural graphite and synthetic graphite. Natural graphite ores contain different proportions of silicate and free silica. The graphite ore accounted for 5% to 15% free silica content. Graphite is a very versatile non-metallic mineral with excellent properties such as acid and alkali resistance, high temperature, electrical conductivity, lubrication, strong adhesion and corrosion resistance. There are high levels of graphite dusts during the processes of mining, crushing, flotation, drying, screening and packaging graphite ore. In addition, the process of synthetic graphite production also can generate a large amount of graphite dusts. Especially in the graphite packaging process, the particle size is very thin and light, and almost all the dust suspended in the air can be inhaled, which is extremely harmful to the human body. Graphite is widely used as raw material to manufacture various graphite products, such as crucibles, electrodes, brushes, and corrosion-resistant pipes. Graphite pneumoconiosis can be divided into graphite pneumoconiosis caused by graphite dust with a SiO_2 content of less than 5% and graphite silicosis caused by graphite dust with a SiO_2 content of more than 5%. The workers will develop graphite pneumoconiosis after they being exposed to graphite for about 15—20 years. Most patients had no obvious symptoms, some patients may have mild dry cough, cough black sticky sputum, chest tightness, shortness of breath and other symptoms. Some p or q small shadows can be seen on the chest X-ray.

4.3.5.2   Carbon Black Pneumoconiosis

The pneumoconiosis is characterized by the accumulation of carbon in the lungs caused by inhaled coal black dust. Carbon black is a gaseous or liquid hydrocarbon, obtained by incomplete combustion and thermal cracking mostly based on petroleum, coke, natural gas, and turpentine as raw materials. The carbon component accounts for 90% to 95%, and free silica contains 0.5% to 1.5%. The exposure time is 15 years up to 25 years or more, with an average of 24 years. Patients are with clinical symptoms of cough, slightly rash, shortness of breath, but not obvious. The majority of patients can still participate in normal productive labor with no positive signs. The course of the disease is extremely slow, and the prognosis is good. On the chest X-ray, in early significantly increased lung markings is visible more obvious to middle and lower lung area. With lesions progress to lung field, p small shadow can be seen, sometimes to see a little s small shadow. Whole lung area is frosted glass sense. Sometimes, emphysema and mild pleural thickening and adhesions can be found. 4.3.5.3 Talc Pneumoconiosis

The pneumoconiosis is a type of silicatosis caused by long-term inhalation of talc dust. Talc is a trioctahedral mineral composed of hydrated magnesiumsilicate with the structural formula $[Mg_6Si_8O_{20}(OH)_4)]$, which often contain impurities such as a certain amount of the amphibole asbestos, free silica, aluminum oxide, iron oxide and magnesium oxide. The incidence of talc pneumoconiosis is slow, which will occur after exposure to talc dust for about from 10 to 25 years. In an early phase, no obvious symptoms are seen. The dry cough or sputum production, chest pain, shortness of breath and other symptoms are developed. Chest X-ray shows irregular-shaped small shadows and pleural changes. Round small nodular shadows are more obvious than asbestosis. The large shadows can be seen in terminal stage. Talc plaques are visible at the place of diaphragm on side of the chest wall and pericardium.

4.3.5.3   Cement Pneumoconiosis

The pneumoconiosis is also a kind of the silicate pneumoconiosis and mainly caused by the long-term inhalation of dust generated by the high concentration of the cement production process. Cement is a synthetic cement silicate, any of various mixtures of limestone, clay, slag, gypsum, iron powder, and coal dust, used as a building material. Free silica content is of 2% to 5%, and there are elements such as calcium, aluminum, magnesium, chromium, cobalt, nickel. The raw materials of cement dust can cause mixed pneumoconiosis. This will occur when a person has been exposed to the dust over a period of time of an approximately 8 — 34 years. Cement pneumoconiosis has a long latency period. The clinical symptoms mainly are shortness of breath and respiratory symptoms including dry cough and little sputum. Irregular small shadows are visible in the middle and lower lung fields in the chest X-ray.

4.3.5.4   Mica Pneumoconiosis

The pneumoconiosis belonging to the silicate pneumoconiosis is due to the long-term inhalation of dust generated by the high concentration of mica dust. Mica is natural aluminum-containing silicate minerals. Its crystal structure contains silicon oxide layer. Mica is widely distributed in nature with complex component and various kinds containing aluminum, iron, magnesium, potassium and other ingredients. The progress of the disease is slow. The symptoms are similar to other silicate pneumoconiosis including shortness of breath and cough. The main chest X-ray findings are irregular small shadows. Round small p shadows with blurred edges can be seen. The pleural changes are not obvious.

4.3.5.5　Kaolin Pneumoconiosis

The pneumoconiosis also called pottery worker's pneumoconiosis is caused by long-term inhalation of a large number of clay dusts in ceramic manufacturing workers and china clay mining workers. Pottery is a variety of containers or materials made of by crushing quartz, clay, feldspar and gypsum, through batching process, blank making, finished products, drying, blank repair, glazing, firing and other process. There are mostly mixed dusts including quartz and silicate in workplaces. The raw material is inconsistent, and the formulations may also be different. Therefore, free silica content is usually in between 8.7% to 65%. The dispersion of the mixed dust less than 5 μm account about from 70% to 90%. As the particles less than 5 μm belong to respirable dusts, which is easily inhaled and deposited in the lung. The smaller the particle size is, the longer the suspension time, the more likely to cause pulmonary fibrosis. The potter in the production process can be exposed to the dust. The average incidence age is more than 25 years. The clinical symptoms are mild including early mild cough, a small amount of expectoration, chest tightness and shortness of breath when manual labor or climbing. The pneumoconiosis is easily complicated by tuberculosis. Many small irregular shadows are seen in the chest X-ray. Irregular shadows gradually thicken as the disease progresses to form large shadow.

4.3.5.6　Aluminum Pneumoconiosis

The pneumoconiosis is caused by long-term inhalation of higher concentrations of aluminum dust or alumina dust. Aluminium is a silvery white, soft and ductile metal. Aluminium is the third most abundant element after oxygen and in the Earth's crust (about 8%). Aluminium is the most widely used due to its excellent physical and chemical property, such as ductility, low gravity, malleability, reflectivity, corrosion resistance, and high electrical conductivity. It often exists in the bauxite rock, silicates, cryolite and other aluminum salts, in the presence of Aluminium salts combining with oxygen, sulfur, fluorine, silicon, and other species.

Release of great amount of dusts and fumes containing Aluminium and its compounds may occur in workshop, such as potrooms, exploration, mining, smelting welding, manufacturing, and polishing. The components of dust is different in different workplaces. For example, Al(OH)$_3$ and AlF$_3$ are the key source in the Aluminium fluoride plant; Aluminium oxides and low level of AlF$_3$ are found in the smelter potroom, Aluminium oxides are main source in the foundry; Aluminium oxides and Na_3AlF_6 are exposed in Aluminium potrooms, foundries, smelters, welding and remelting plants.

It is widely used in transportation, construction and electric-power transmission and other areas. Inhalation of dust or fumes containing Aluminium is the main route of occupational exposure. The average incidence age is 24 years from 10 to 32 years. The patients may have a cough, chest pain, chest tightness, shortness of breath, fatigue and other symptoms. Chest X-ray shows smaller irregular shadow, often in the middle and lower lung areas. Low density of small round shadows most of the p-shaped shadows also can be seen, and the realm is not very clear. As the disease progresses, small shadows increase to distribute to total lung, but no fusion shadows are formed.

4.3.5.7 Welder's Pneumoconiosis

The pneumoconiosis is caused by long-term inhalation of high concentrations of welding fumes. The welding technology is indispensable in modern industrial process. The dusts or fumes generated by electric welding depend on the type of welding rod, base material and the metal to be welded. The welding rod is composed by core wires and coverings. A large amount of iron powder, carbon, manganese, silicon, nickel, sulfur and phosphorus consist of core wires. And coverings are mainly composed of marble, quartz, ferromanganese, ferrosilicon, and mica. So the core wires, coverings and base materials are welded in the arc under high temperature including melting, evaporation and oxidation to produce a large number of metal oxides and other welding fumes in the air of working environment, such as iron oxide, SiO_2, manganese oxide, ozone and various trace metals and nitrogen oxides. Especially in a poorly ventilated and closed container such as boiler, oil tank and hull equipment, the concentration of welding fume is very high. The particle size of welding dust is very fine, mostly in the range of 0.4 to 0.5 μm. The incidence age ranges from 15 to 20 years, with the shortest onset for four years. The symptoms include chest tightness, chest pain, cough, expectoration, shortness of breath and others. The main chest X-ray findings are irregular small shadows often in the middle and lower lung areas. The widely distributed p-shaped shadows will appear sometimes with low intensity.

4.3.5.8 Founder Pneumoconiosis

The pneumoconiosis is caused by long-term inhalation of dusts with complex components, in which free SiO_2 content is not high in foundry casting operations and modeling jobs. The casting process, molding sand crushing, mixing, transport and use in the sand box apart, fettling and cleaning castings, can produce a lot of mixed dust, such as clay, kaolinite, graphite, pulverized coal, limestone and talc. The pneumoconiosis induced by foundry dusts mainly manifested as nodular and dusts spot type and pulmonary interstitial fibrosis damages, which has a slow onset and progress, and the incidence age is more than 20 years. No special symptoms are found in the early stage. As the disease progresses, it can cause chest tightness, chest pain, cough, expectoration, shortness of breath and others symptoms, which is not more serious. However, due to the bad operating environment and poor posture labor, the disease often can be complicated by chronic bronchitis and emphysema, and then lung function may have varying degrees of damage. The chest X-ray shows the lungs appear obvious irregular small shadows t in the middle and lower lung area. With the progress of the disease, the small shadows increase often accompanied by significant emphysema. Middle and lower lung area sometimes can appear small round shadows with lower density. Large shadows are extremely rare.

4.3.6　Prevention and Control of Pneumoconiosis

In most parts of the world, silicosis and other pneumoconiosis are widely spread and millions of workers continue to be exposed to dusts running an unacceptably high risk of developing the diseases. Occupational airborne particulates are important causes of death and disability worldwide. In the absence of effective specific treatment of pneumoconiosis, the only approach towards the protection of workers' health is the control of exposure to productive dusts. The effectiveness of prevention largely depends on a range of preventive measures.

China government has always paid great attention to the prevention and control of pneumoconiosis. Experiences of China have convincingly demonstrated that it is possible to significantly reduce the incidence rate of pneumoconiosis with well-organized pneumoconiosis prevention programs. The effective way to control the dust is to take comprehensive measures including legislation measures, organization measures, technical measures and health care measures.

In China, after many years of occupational health practice, the comprehensive measures for prevention and reduction of dust hazards have been summarized as an "eight-word" policy, namely, innovation, water, seal, wind, protection, management, inspection, and education.

① Innovation means to reform the production process and production equipment, such as replacing high-dust materials with low-dust and dust-free materials, and replacing high-dust-producing equipment with low-dust-producing equipment and non-dust-producing equipment. Innovation is the fundamental measures to reduce or eliminate the dust hazards.

② Water means to use wet production operation to prevent dust suspension and to reduce the dust concentration in the air.

③ Seal means to adopt air-tight production equipment or to convert an open production process to a closed one. This is an important measure to prevent dust from escaping and to control air pollution in the workplaces.

④ Wind means to strengthen ventilation. Especially when the production process cannot be sealed or there is still dust after sealing, the ventilation measures should be taken directly to remove the dusty air from the dust-producing point to ensure that the dust concentration in the air of the workplace meets the sanitary standards.

⑤ Protection means to offer personal protective facilities, such as respirator, masks and dust-proof clothing, and to ensure the protective facilities to be reasonably and correctly used.

⑥ Management means to strengthen regular maintenance and administration to ensure all dustproof facilities running properly.

⑦ Inspection means to carry out regular physical examination for the dust-exposure workers, and to monitor the dust concentration in the workplace regularly.

⑧ Education means to strengthen the publicity and dust prevention training, to popularize dust prevention knowledge, and to let all exposure workers know the dust hazards entirely.

4.3.6.1   Legislation Measures

The legislation measures mainly include occupational exposure limits and technical standards, laws and regulations for preventing and controlling the hazards of dust. In China, the State Council issued the Decision on Prevention of Hazards of Silica Dust in Factories and Mines in 1956. Since then, the State Council, the Health Ministry and the original Ministry of Labor have issued many laws and regulations. The Provision for Pneumoconiosis Control of the People's Republic of China was issued by the State Council in 1987. Law of the People's Republic of China on Prevention and Control of Occupational Diseases was implemented in 2002, which was revised in 2011 and 2016. The revised law and regulations provides a clear legal basis for preventing and controlling the hazards of pneumoconiosis.

4.3.6.2   Organization Measures

Employers should improve work environment and conditions to meet the national occupational health standards and health requirements, and take measures to ensure that employees receive occupational health protection. Employers should strengthen health education and training for workers to improve their awareness of dust hazards produced by themselves and capabilities of prevention and control of pneumoconioses. Furthermore, employers should also establish and improve a responsibility system for the prevention and control of pneumoconioses and strengthen the management of prevention and control of pneumoconioses.

4.3.6.3   Technical Measures

(1) Technical Innovation and Reform

The research, development, promotion, and application of new technologies, new processes, new equipment, and new materials are the most fundamental measures in the prevention and control of dust hazards, for example, using automation technology to avoid workers from contacting dust, if possible, replacing quartz raw materials with low quartz raw materials and artificial asbestos instead of natural asbestos.

(2) Wet Operation

Wet operation is using water sprays, wet methods for cutting, chipping, drilling, sawing and grinding, which is an economic, simple and practical method to prevent and control the hazards of dust. The wet sprayed concrete technique has good virtue of improving the working condition within the tunnel.

(3) Airtight Operation

Airtight refers sealing dust processes and discharging dusts through ventilation. Under the condition that wet operation is impossible, a closed air extraction and dust removal method should be used. It is effective to combine closed dust source with dust removal by local exhausting.

4.3.6.4 Health Care Measures

According to the provisions of the work safety administrative department of the State Council, the employer should conduct regular tests and evaluations of the occupational disease hazard factors at its work sites.

For employees conducting operations with exposure to productive dusts, the employer should organize pre-job, on-the-job, and off-the-job occupational health examination for employees according to the provisions of the work safety administrative department and health administrative department of the State Council. The employees should get paper file of the examination results. The expenses for the occupational health examination should be covered by the employer.

Personal protection is vital important because it is the last line of defense against dust hazards. Employers must adopt effective personal protective facilities against pneumoconioses. The protection items for personal use provided by employers for employees must meet the requirements for the prevention and control of occupational diseases. In addition, workers with dust exposure should also pay attention to personal healthcare, such as no smoking in the workplace.

4.4 Physical Hazards

4.4.1 High Temperature

Healthy human body maintains its core body temperature around 37℃ for the body to perform efficiently. Variations, usually of less than 1℃, occur with the time of the day, level of physical activity, or emotional state. The maintenance of core body temperature within the acceptable range of 36℃ to 38℃ requires a constant exchange of heat between the body and the environment. The amount of heat to be exchanged is a function of air temperature, air velocity, humidity, radiant temperature, physical activity, clothing, skin temperature, and evaporation of sweat, which can be expressed with the following basic heat balance equation.

$$S=(M-W)\pm C\pm R-E$$

S is the change in heat storage, M is the metabolic heat, W is work done in the environment, C is heat gained or lost by convection and conduction, R is heat gained or lost by radiation, E is evaporative heat loss. Each of the terms in the equation represents a rate of energy transfer. Positive values for any of the variables signify that the body is gaining heat in that manner, while negative values indicate a loss of heat.

The main source of heat gain is the metabolic heat of the body. Metabolic heat is generated within the body by the biochemical processes which vary with the level of activity. A high workload may lead to high heat production by the body, therefore, for those performing physically demanding work the metabolic rate must be considered even when environmental temperature feel cool to those performing less strenuous activities.

In most circumstances, there are four principal environmental determinants of heat stress. They are ambient air temperature, speed of air movement, relative humidity of air, and thermal radiation. Wet bulb globe temperature (WBGT) index is a simple approximation of the combined effects of all these four principal environmental determinants, and WBGT is the most widely used and accepted index for the assessment of heat stress in industrial settings. Operations involving high air temperatures, high humidity, radiant heat sources, direct physical contact with hot objects, WBGT index exceeding the specified limit, or strenuous physical activities have a high potential for inducing heat stress in employees engaged in such operations.

4.4.1.1　Classification and Exposure Opportunities

High temperature operation can be divided into the following three basic types according to the characteristics of its meteorological conditions.

(1) High-temperature, High-heat Radiation Operation

It is always found in the opportunities of coking, iron making, steel rolling and other workshops in the metallurgical industry; casting and heat treatment workshops in the machinery manufacturing industry; furnace and kiln workshops in ceramics, glass, enamel, brick and other industries; thermal power plants and boiler room and etc. The meteorological characteristics of these sites are high temperature, high thermal radiation intensity, and low relative humidity, forming a dry and hot environment.

(2) High-temperature, High-humidity Operation

The heat radiation intensity is not large, and the formation of high humidity is mainly caused by the large amount of water vapor generated during the production process or the high relative humidity required in the production, such as printing and dyeing, silk gathering, papermaking and other industries; wet deep mines; hot and humid environment formed by poor ventilation.

(3) Open-air Operation in Summer

Including the open-air operation of farmland labor, construction, transportation, etc., in addition, to the direct radiation of the sun, people are also heated by the surrounding secondary heat sources (such as high-temperature ground and objects). Although the thermal radiation intensity in open-air operation is relatively lower than the strong heat radiation workshop operation, but the duration is longer. The temperature is higher around noon, and the combined exposure of high temperature and heat radiation is often formed.

Furthermore, in laundries, restaurant kitchens, and canneries, high humidity adds to the heat burden. Occupations that require workers to wear semipermeable or impermeable protective clothing increase the risk of succumbing to heat stress.

4.4.1.2　Effect Factors of Sensitivity to High Temperature

(1) Individual Factors

The sensitivity to heat varies from individual to individual, and is affected by age, weight, physical condition, metabolism, degree of acclimatization, levels of hydration, medical conditions, and use of alcohol or medicine.

Individuals who are 45 years of age or older, overweight, and in poor physical condition are more susceptible to heat stress. Also at much increased risk are those who are not acclimatized to heat stress, with previous heat illness, and performing strenuous physical work. Medical conditions can also increase the susceptibility to heat exposure. People with respiratory disease, hypertension, cardiovascular or circulatory disorders, disease of gastrointestinal tract or renal system, and diabetes may need to take special precautions. In addition, people with skin diseases and rashes may be more susceptible to heat. Consumption of alcohol interferes with acclimatization, which means individuals who consume alcohol or are recovering from recent use are more vulnerable to the adverse effects of heat. Certain medications impair cooling mechanisms of the body. For example, hypotensives, diuretics, antipsychotics, certain types of sleeping pills, sedatives, tranquilizers, antispasmodics, antidepressants, amphetamines, medicine for Parkinson's disease decrease the capacity of the body to cope with heat.

(2) Heat Adaption and Heat Acclimatization

Heat adaption is that the body's heat tolerance increases under the stimulation of long-term thermal environment. Heat acclimatization refers to the physiological adaptation in response to heat exposure. Within a few days of the first exposure, acclimatized individuals perspire more abundantly and more uniformly over their body surface and have a faster onset of sweating than unacclimatized individuals, resulting in lower skin temperature, lower cardiovascular demand, lower heart rate, and lower core body temperature. After 2 to 3 weeks of exposure, acclimatized individuals lose less salt through sweating and can therefore withstand greater water loss.

Heat acclimatization at a certain temperature is effective only at that or lower temperature. The developed heat acclimatization can be lost quickly if the exposure is discontinued. The loss of heat acclimatization begins upon the discontinuousness of the exposure and will be noticeable after 4 days.

4. 4. 1. 3   Adverse Health Effects

(1) Health Effects of Acute Heat Exposure

In the face of heat gain from the environment or workload, the body maintains a constant core body temperature by increasing the blood flow to the skin surface and by increasing sweat production. As blood flow increases, heat is carried from the body to the surface, which allows the heat loss by radiation and convection from the surface of the body. Sweating allows the heat loss by evaporation. In this way, the body increases the rate of heat loss to balance the heat burden. Once these coping mechanisms of the body are overwhelmed, and the rate of heat gain exceeds the rate of heat loss, then the body stores heat. As it does so, the core body temperature begins to rise. Substantial deviations from normal core body temperatures cause adverse effects ranging from minor annoyance to life threatening conditions.

① Heat stroke and hyperpyrexia: Adverse health effects of exposure to heat stress may occur alone or be combined with the other. The most serious types of effects of exposure to heat are heat stroke and hyperpyrexia. According to the pathogenesis, it can be divided into three categories.

• Heat stroke: Heat stroke is generally characterized by a core body temperature of 40℃ to 41℃ or greater, a partial or complete loss of consciousness, and a hot dry skin. When heat stroke occurs, the core body temperature can rise to 41℃ or higher within 10 to 15 minutes, core body temperatures of 43℃ or higher are not uncommon. Mental status is altered, initial lethargy proceeds to irritability, confusion, stupor, and eventual loss of consciousness. Classically, sweating is said to be absent or diminished, but many individuals perspire profusely. The thermal regulatory failure in heat stroke is a life threatening emergency. In absence of immediate medical attention at an early stage, heat stroke could be fatal. Death can result from damage to the brain, heart, liver, or kidneys. Maximal recovery may occur quickly or may not occur for a period of days or weeks, and there may be permanent neurological residual. Heat stroke occurs when temperature regulation system of the body fails and the core body temperature rises to critical levels. This condition is caused by a combination of work load, environmental heat load, and dehydration overload, factors are highly variable and its occurrence is difficult to predict. The signs of heat hyperpyrexia are similar to heat stroke except that the skin remains moist.

• Heat cramps: Heat cramps are sharp pains in the muscles, typically in the muscles employed in strenuous work, which occur usually during or shortly after hard physical labor in high temperature environment. Heat cramps have been attributed to transient fluid and electrolyte imbalance caused by sweating. The fluid and electrolyte imbalance can be either insufficient or excessive salt. Heat cramps most often occur when people drink large amounts of water without sufficient electrolyte replacement. Since sweat is a hypotonic solution, excess salt can build up in the body if the water lost through sweating is not replaced, in these cases heat cramps may also occur.

● Heat exhaustion: Heat exhaustion is the response of the body to an excessive loss of the water and salts, usually through excessive sweating. It typically occurs after several days of heat stress. The signs and symptoms of heat exhaustion include heavy sweating, weakness, intense thirst, nausea, vomiting, diarrhea, headache, vertigo, visual disturbances, pale or flushed complexion, tingling and numbness of the hands and feet, fast and shallow breathing, palpitations, and muscle cramps. Body temperature is normal to moderately elevated but rarely exceeds 38.9℃. The condition may develop into heat stroke if not treated by rest, cooling, and fluids.

② Extensive adverse effects: Besides heat stroke, there are other adverse health effects of exposure to heat stress, such as heat fatigue, heat syncope, the increasing order of severity, irritability, lack of judgment and loss of critical thinking skills, and skin disorders.

● Heat fatigue: Heat fatigue is manifested with impaired performance of skilled sensorimotor, mental, or vigilance jobs. A factor that predisposes an individual to heat fatigue is lack of acclimatization.

● Heat rashes: Heat rashes are the most common disorders in high temperature occupational environments. Prickly heat is manifested as red papules with a prickling sensation that usually appear on the face, neck, back, chest, and thighs. Prickly heat occurs in skin that is persistently wetted by unevaporated sweat, and heat rash papules may become infected if they are not treated. In most cases, heat rashes will disappear when the affected individual returns to cool environments.

● Heat edema: Heat edema is swelling which generally occurs among people who are not acclimatized to working in hot conditions. Swelling is often most noticeable in the ankles. Recovery occurs after one or two days in cool environments.

● Heat syncope: Heat syncope is a transient fall in blood pressure with an associated loss of consciousness. Heat syncope is considered to arise from temporarily insufficient flow of blood to the brain due to cutaneous vasodilation in response to heat stress. Heat syncope occurs mostly among unacclimatized people who stand in place for extended periods in high temperature environments. Consciousness typically returns promptly in the recumbent posture. Recovery is normally rapid and without any long term adverse effects after rest in cool areas.

③ Increased occupational injuries: Excessive heat can also cause sweaty palms, fogged glasses, and dizziness, which in turn can result in slips, trips, and falls. It can also cause normally cool surfaces to become scorching hot, which can make accidental contact quite dangerous, resulting in serious burns.

(2) Health Effects of Chronic Heat Exposure

Prolonged exposure to heat and increase in core body temperature are associated with disorders such as fatigue, irritability, sleep disorders, increased heart rate, kidney stones, and serious gastrointestinal disease.

The lens of the eye is particularly vulnerable to infrared radiation. The lens has no heat sensors and lacks blood vessels to carry heat away. After many years of exposure to radiation from hot objects, cataracts can be developed.

A possible link between heat exposure and reproductive problems has been suggested. Among men, frequent or prolonged exposure to heat can result in elevated testicular temperature, the increase of testicular temperature of 3℃ to 5℃ may cause a substantial decrease in sperm count. Accumulated data suggest that heat stress during pregnancy may cause neural tube defects, however, currently there have been no sufficient data to prove cause and effect. To date, there is no conclusive evidence of the teratogenic effects of heat exposure in humans. The NIOSH criteria document (1986) recommends that a pregnant worker's core body temperature should not exceed 39℃ to 39.5℃ during the first trimester of pregnancy.

4.4.1.4   Prevention and Control

(1) Hygienic Standards for High Temperature Operation

During high temperature operation, the heat exchange and balance between the human body and the environment is affected by meteorological factors and labor metabolism. The development of health standards should ensure that the body's heat stress will not exceed the physiological range (for example, rectal body temperature≤38℃), formulating the standards of meteorological factors and labor intensity in order to ensure the health of workers.

The development of hygienic standards for high temperature operation refers to the WBGT. For example, the high-temperature work hygiene standards (Table 4.1) established by the International Organization for Standardization (ISO), meteorological factors are represented by WBGT. Working under the WBGT environmental conditions, the central body temperature will not exceed 38℃.

Table 4.1   Hygiene Standard of High Temperature Production Environment (ISO7243, 1989)

Metabolic Rate Level	Metabolic Rate (W/m²)	WBGT(℃)	
		Heat Adaptor	Non-heat Adaptor
0	M≤65	33	32
1	65<M≤130	30	29
2	130<M≤200	28	26
3	200<M≤260	25−26	22−23
4	M>260	23−25	18−20

At present, China has also implemented comprehensive hygienic standards for high-temperature operation, such as "Occupational Exposure Limits for Harmful Factors in Workplaces (GBZ 2.2−2007)", which uses WBGT to reflect the thermal load caused by various factors of high temperature operation environment and considers labor strength

(Table 4.2).

Table 4. 2 Different Physical Labor Intensity WBGT Limits (℃) in the Workplace

Contact Time Rate	Physical Labor Intensity(Strength Index)			
	I (≤15)	II (—20)	III (—25)	IV (>25)
100%	30	28	26	25
75%	31	29	28	26
50%	32	30	29	28
25%	33	32	31	30

Note: contact time rate is the ratio of the cumulative time that the worker contacts the high temperature operation within one working day actually to the 8-hour.

(2) Measures of Heat Control

① Engineering controls: Applications of engineering controls to reduce the metabolisms and provide cooler workplaces are the most effective means of reducing excessive heat exposure.

② Reducing metabolic heat production: Automation and mechanization of tasks reduce the physical demands and the resulting buildup of the heat in the body.

③ Reducing the radiation from hot surfaces and objects: Low emissivity materials can be used for covering hot surfaces and hot objects to reduce the heat release to work stations.

④ Insulating hot surfaces and objects: Insulation reduces the heat exchange between the source of heat and the work environment.

⑤ Shielding: Instead of reducing radiation from the source, shielding can be used to interrupt the radiation from reaching work stations. Two types of shields can be used. Stainless steel, aluminum or other bright metal surfaces reflect heat back towards the source. Absorbent shields can absorb and carry away the heat.

⑥ Ventilation and air conditioning: General ventilation is used to dilute hot air with cooler air. A permanently installed ventilation system usually works for large areas or entire buildings. Portable or local exhaust systems may be practical in small areas. When the air temperature is less than the worker's skin temperature, the increase in the air flow or convection using fans in the work area can help workers stay cooler by increasing both the convective heat exchange and the rate of evaporation. Air conditioning is the most effective method of air cooling because it reduces the temperature of the air by removing heat from the air. An alternative to air conditioning is the chillers which circulate cool water. Local air cooling can be effective in reducing air temperature in specific areas. Cool rooms can be used to enclose a specific workplace or to offer a recovery area near hot jobs. Air conditioner, dehumidification, and elimination of open hot water baths, drains, and leaky steam valves can be used for reducing humidity.

⑦ Administrative controls and work practices.

• Training programs: Training is the key to good work practices. Provide training for employees, especially the new and the young employees. The training program should include information about knowledge of the hazards of heat stress, the dangers of using drugs and alcohol in high temperature work environments, and the importance of monitoring themselves and coworkers for symptoms. The trainees should be able to recognize the predisposing factors, danger signs, and symptoms, be aware of first aid procedures for heat stroke, and use personal protective equipment.

● Acclimatization: A properly designed and applied acclimatization program decreases the risk of heat related adverse effects. Allow sufficient acclimatization period before full workload. New employees should acclimatize before assuming a full workload. It is advisable to assign a portion of the normal workload to a new employee on the first day of work and gradually increase on subsequent days. Loss of acclimatization occurs gradually when a person is moved away from a high temperature environment. A decrease in heat tolerance occurs even after a long weekend, therefore, it is often not advisable for anyone to work under very high temperature on the first day of the week.

● Pace of work: If practical, allow flexibility to permit less physically demanding activities during peak temperature periods. Hot jobs should be scheduled for the cooler part of the day, and routine maintenance and repair work in hot areas should be scheduled for the cooler seasons of the year. Reduce the physical demands of work, shorten heat exposure time, and use frequent rest breaks.

● Rest area: Provide cool rest areas.

● Fluid and salt supplements: Working in a high temperature environment causes sweating which means losing vital water and salt that must be replaced. Plenty of cool caffeine free and alcohol free drinking water should be available in the workplace and workers should be encouraged to drink frequently in small amounts even if they do not feel thirsty. An acclimatized worker loses relatively little salt in their sweat and, therefore, the salt in the normal diet is usually sufficient to maintain the electrolyte balance in the body fluids. For unacclimatized workers who may sweat continuously and repeatedly, additional salt in the food may be used. Too much salt can cause higher body temperatures, increased thirst, and nausea. Drinks with alcohol or caffeine should never be taken, as they dehydrate the body.

● Emergency action plan: In extreme environments, an emergency plan is needed. The plan should include procedures for providing affected workers with first aid and medical care. People are generally unable to notice their own heat stress related symptoms. Their survival depends on the ability of their coworkers to recognize the symptoms and seek timely first aid and medical help. Assign one person trained in first aid to each work shift.

● Identify susceptible employees: Individuals should be screened for medical conditions, and advice may be needed from an occupational health professional or medical practitioner.

● Individual protection: Provide personal protective equipment. In high temperature and humid workplaces, light, loose clothing allows maximum skin exposure and efficient body cooling by sweat evaporation. Specially designed heat protective clothing, such as ice vests and wetted clothing, is available for working in extremely high temperature conditions. Eye protection which absorbs radiation is needed when the work involves very hot objects, such as molten metals and hot ovens.

● Medical treatments: Heat stroke and heat hyperpyrexia require immediate first aid and medical attention. If signs of possible heat stroke are shown, professional medical treatment should be obtained immediately. The worker should be placed in a shady area and the outer clothing should be removed. The body temperature should be lowered by sponging the body with tepid water or fanning with cool air. Fluid should be given orally or intravenously as soon as possible. The medical outcome of heat stroke depends on the physical fitness and the timing and effectiveness of first aid treatment. Delayed treatment may result in damage to the brain, kidneys, and heart.

4.4.2　Noise

The word noise is cognate with the Latin word "nauseas", which means disgust or discomfort. Noise is sound people feel unwanted and unpleasant; WHO defines noise as sound "disagreeable or undesired sound" or other disturbance. In the hygienic sense, any sound that is annoying, unexpected, or detrimental to health is called noise, that is, besides the annoying sound which is caused by the disorderly combination of frequency and intensity is noise, other kinds of sounds, such as the sound of a conversation or music, are also noise for those who don't need it. The source of most outdoor noise referred as environmental noise is mainly caused by transportation systems, motor vehicles, aircrafts, or trains. Indoor noise caused by machines and building activities in the workplaces is called occupational noise or industrial noise. There is no great difference whether noise-induced hearing loss or other noise related health disorders are brought about by outdoor or indoor noise.

Occupational noise or industrial noise is the amount of acoustic energy received by an employee's auditory system when they are working, which is considered an occupational hazard traditionally linked to loud industries such as ship-building, mining, railroad work, welding, and construction, but can be present in any workplace where hazardous noise is present.

4.4.2.1　Characteristics, Classification and Exposure Opportunities

(1) Characteristics

Sound is a mechanical wave that is an oscillation of pressure transmitted through some medium (like air or water), composed of frequencies within the range of hearing. The characteristics of a particular sound depend on the rate at which the sound source vibrates, the amplitude of the vibration, and the properties of the conducting medium. Frequency is an objective description of the rate at which complete cycles of high-and low-pressure regions are produced by a sound source, and it is measured in Hertz (Hz). Normal human ears respond to a very wide frequency range, approximately from 20 to 20,000 Hz. Sound lower in frequency than 20 Hz, the "normal" limit of human hearing, is referred to low-frequency sound or infrasound. Sound higher in frequency more than 20,000 Hz is referred to ultrasound, which is an oscillating sound pressure wave with a frequency greater than the upper limit of the human hearing range. The sensitivity of the human ear to sound depends on the frequency or pitch of the sound. People hear some frequencies better than others.

For occupational hygiene purposes, the sound is measured to determine noise exposures. The most common instruments used for measuring noise include the sound level meter (SLM), the integrating sound level meter (ISLM), and the noise dosimeter. A basic sound level meter consists of a microphone that converts air pressure variations into an electrical signal, an amplifier/filter, an exponential time-averaging circuit, a device to determine the logarithm of the signal, and some types of output display. Decibels (dB) are a measurement of sound intensity over the standard threshold of hearing. Measurements in dBA or dB(A) are decibel scale readings that have been adjusted to attempt to take into account the varying sensitivity of the human ear to different frequencies of sound with an "A" frequency-weighting networks. Other frequency-weighting networks, such as C, B and D, have been developed, but they are not used frequently for occupational noise measurements. The main effect of the adjustment is that low and very high frequencies are given less weight than on the standard decibel scale. Many regulatory noise limits are specified in terms of dB(A) because dB(A) is better correlated with the relative risk of noise-induced hearing loss.

Industrial noise usually has the following characteristics, making it more harmful than environmental noise: ① High intensity: the intensity is more than 80 dB (A), even up to 100 dB (A) or more, and its harm is far from disturbing the work. Long-term exposure can cause damage to both the human auditory system and the non-auditory system. ② The high frequency sound has a large proportion: the industrial noise is more common with high frequency sound, and its harm is greater than the medium and low frequency sound. ③ Continuous exposure time: during the production process, the continuous contact time can last for several hours each working day. ④ Other harmful factors: production environment is often accompanied by other harmful factors such as vibration, high temperature and poison. These harmful factors can be combined with noise to produce a joint effect.

(2) Classification and Exposure Opportunities

There are many ways to classify the occupational noise. According to the generation mode of sound source it can be divided into three kinds: ① Aerodynamic noise is produced by gas vibration. Gas disturbance when there is a vortex in the gas, or when a sudden change of pressure occurs, such as ventilator, blower, air compressor, or high pressure gas release noise. ② Mechanical noise is produced by mechanical impact, friction and rotation, such as crusher, ball mill, chainsaw, machine tool. ③ Electromagnetic noise is caused by the vibration of the electrical components caused by the pulsation of the magnetic field and the frequency of the power supply, such as noise generated by generators, transformers or relays.

According to its properties, noise can be divided into two kinds-continuous steady state noise and intermittent noise (or impulse noise). If sound or noise remains constant for a long time, it is called continuous steady-state noise. If the noise varies with time, it is called impulse noise. Impulse noise is more harmful to the human health than steady-state noise.

4.4.2.2 Health Effects

With industrialization noise has become a very common problem at the workplace which can lead to auditory disorders, especially noise induced hearing loss (NIHL), and non-auditory disorders. Noise can be a nuisance and cause speech interference at 30—80 dB(A). In occupational medical practice, noise presents three fundamental risks to health: ① acutely, through blasts, explosion, or other impulse noise that lead to hearing deficits; ② chronically, through continued exposure to unsafe levels of noise that lead to sensorineural hearing loss; ③ extra-auditory effects, including mental disorders (sleep problems, anxiety, etc.), hypertension and adverse influences on existing illness such as hyperlipoproteinemia and hypertension.

(1) Hearing Mechanism

The ear comprises of outer, middle and inner ear (Figure 4.7). The outer ear provides protection to the middle and inner ear by maintaining a stable environment. The middle ear is a cavity connected to the outer ear by the tympanic membrane and the inner ear by the oval and round windows. It has three bones (ossicular chain) that can conduct sound waves from the outer ear to the cochlea. The cochlea and the semi-circular canals in the inner ear are responsible for hearing and balance, respectively. There are about 24000 hear cells in Corti's organ which are the sensory cells responsible for hearing. These cells have no ability to regenerate after birth.

The ear can be divided into two parts according to physiological functions. One is conducting apparatus including outer ear, the tympanic membrane, the ossicular chain and labyrinthine fluids. The other is the sensorineural apparatus that comprise the Corti's organ, acoustic nerve and its central connections.

Sound can be transmitted to the inner ear in three models. ① The most common way is when sound energy is transmitted to the oval window from the vibrating tympanic membrane by ossicular chain. ② Sound can be transmitted directly across the middle ear when waves fall on the round window (there is a large perforation in the ear drum). ③ Sound is transmitted by bone conduction when sound energy is transmitted to the inner ear through the bones of skull.

In the inner ear, the cochlea hair cells of Corti's organ sense the sound energy and the cochlea nerve carries sensory information from the hair cells to the brain.

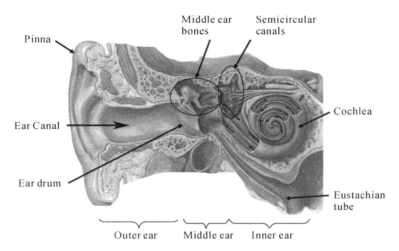

Figure 4. 7   Schematic Drawing of the Ear

(2) Noise-induced Hearing Loss (NIHL)

• Temporary threshold shift (TTS): The effects of noise on hearing may be temporary or permanent. Temporary threshold shift (TTS) is transitory hearing loss with normal hearing being restored after cessation of noise exposure. Time to recovery from TTS varies. TTS occurs as early as after two minutes of exposure and recovery begins immediately after cessation of exposure with most of the recovery occurring within 16 hours. If loss of hearing is less than 30dB, recovery usually within 16 hours. Based on recovery speed, TTS can be divided into two types, namely the auditory adaptation and auditory fatigue.

Auditory adaptation: When exposed to strong noise environment for a short time, the body's auditory organ sensitivity decreases and the auditory threshold increases by 10 to 15 dB. After getting out of the noise environment, one may have a feeling of "small" or "far" to the external sound, which can be recovered within one minute. This phenomenon is called auditory adaptation, which is a physiological protection phenomenon of the body.

Auditory fatigue: Being in a loud noise environment for a long time causes an obvious hearing loss and the increase of auditory threshold to be more than 15−30 dB. After leaving the noise environment, hearing recovery takes several hours or even tens of hours, which is called auditory fatigue. It is usually limited to the time interval (16 hours) between the time when leaving the noise and the next day before work. If the hearing cannot recover in such a period of time, and workers continue to expose to the noises, the auditory fatigue may develop into a permanent threshold shift(PTS).

• Permanent threshold shift (PTS): It refers to an increase in hearing threshold caused by noise or other factors that cannot be restored to the normal hearing threshold level. Permanent threshold shift has the basis of pathological changes, and it is an irreversible change. The size of permanent threshold shift is the basis for judging the degree of noise damaged to the auditory system, and it is also the basis for the diagnosis of occupational noise-induced deafness.

NIHL is the irreversible permanent hearing loss with no recovery on cessation of exposure which usually develops gradually and is symmetric. The hearing loss commences at 4 kHz frequency and extends to other frequencies with continued exposure. In the audiogram, the dip usually seen is bilateral and symmetrical, with a maximum at 4kHz (Figure 4. 8).

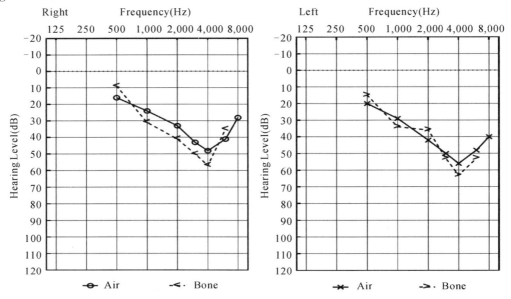

Figure 4. 8   Audiogram of a Quarry Worker with Bilateral NIHL

A combination of mechanical, metabolic, and vascular factors are involved in the destructive changes that lead to NIHL. Prolonged noise exposure is associated with disruption of the hair cells of the Corti's organ and degeneration of nerve fibers and ganglion cells. The hair cells are highly susceptible to the mechanical trauma of loud noise. The cell bodies swell with repeated exposure to loud noise, and ultimately, the hair cells are destroyed. In addition, high noise levels disrupt the vascular supply of the basilar membrane. Capillary vasoconstriction in response to loud noise may result in reduced oxygen tension and local hypoxia within the cochlea. Eventually, the Corti's organ breaks down, with separation of segments of sensory cells from the basilar membrane, leading to elimination of sensory structures and replacement by a single flat cell layer. Hair cells of the basal turn of the cochlea, which conduct sound at higher frequencies (4000 to 6000 Hz), appear to be preferentially affected, most probably due to their location in areas of high shear stress along the Corti's organ. That is why the preferential loss of hearing in this range in early NIHL. Eventually, disruption of the adjacent medial and apical areas occurs as well, leading to heating loss at a wider range of frequencies. Cochlear blood vessels and nerve endings associated with the hair cells can also be damaged.

(3) Acute Hearing Loss

Acute hearing loss, also known as acute acoustic trauma, is a kind of conductive hearing loss which may occur in any setting where loud impulsive noise is present. Exposure to such sudden intense levels of noise can cause abrupt acute and subsequent permanent damage to the middle and inner ear, in which the tympanic membrane is ruptured or/and the ossicular bones are dislocated and so on.

(4) Other Noise-related Health Effects

In addition to hearing loss, exposure to noise in the workplace can cause a variety of other health problems, including exposure to noise over a long period of time decreases coordination and concentration. This increases the chances of accidents. Noise increases stress, which can lead to a number of health problems, including heart, stomach, and nervous disorders. Noise is suspected of being one of the causes of heart disease and stomach ulcers. Workers exposed to noise may complain of nervousness, sleep disorders, and fatigue (feeling tired all the time).

4.4.2.3 Prevention and Control

Noise is the most common occupational hazard in industrial production. It is neither economical nor possible to complete elimination of noise at this stage. Therefore, enterprises should take comprehensive measures in strict accordance with relevant national laws and regulations to control the noise intensity of workplaces by controlling sound sources and blocking the spread of noise; wearing ear protectors for noise workers to reduce the exposure level of individual noise; helps to detect noise susceptible and noise sickness early; health education helps improve workers' health protection awareness and healthy behavior.

(1) Limits of Noise Exposure

According the National Institute for Occupational Safety and Health (NIOSH), noise exposure should be controlled so that the exposure is less than the combination of exposure level and duration. Recommended exposure limit (REL) for 8 hours a workday and 40 hours a workweek is 85 dB(A). Combinations of noise exposure levels and maximum exposure duration in a workday by NIOSH are expressed below Table 4.3.

Table 4.3   NIOSH Standard for REL of Noise

Sound Level [dB(A)]	Duration (Hours: Minutes: Seconds)
82	16 : 00 : 00
85	08 : 00 : 00
88	04 : 00 : 00
91	02 : 00 : 00
94	01 : 00 : 00
97	00 : 30 : 00
100	00 : 15 : 00

(to be continued)

continued

Sound Level [dB(A)]	Duration (Hours: Minutes: Seconds)
103	00 : 07 : 30
106	00 : 03 : 45
109	00 : 01 : 53
112	00 : 00 : 56
115	00 : 00 : 28
118	00 : 00 : 14
121	00 : 00 : 07
124	00 : 00 : 03
127	00 : 00 : 01

In China, RELs for stationary noise and non-stationary noise are both 85 dB(A). REL for non-stationary noise is expressed as below Table 4.4.

Table 4.4   REL for Non-stationary Noise in the Workplace of China

Exposure Time	Exposure Limit [dB(A)]	Remark
5 d/w, =8 h/d	85	Calculation of 8 h equivalent continuous sound level
5 d/w, ≠8 h/d	85	Calculation of 8 h equivalent continuous sound level
≠5 d/w	85	Calculation of 40 h equivalent continuous sound level

REL for impulse noise in China is expressed as table 4.5.

Table 4.5   REL for Impulse Noise in the Workplace of China

Impulse Noise Exposure Times (n)	Peak Sound Level [dB(A)]	Limit for Impulse Noise Exposure Times (n)
$n \leqslant 100$	140	$n \leqslant 100$
$100 < n \leqslant 1000$	130	$100 < n \leqslant 1000$
$1000 < n \leqslant 10000$	120	$1000 < n \leqslant 10000$

(2) Control the Source

As with other types of exposures, the best method of prevention is to eliminate the hazard. Therefore controlling noise at its source is the best method of noise control. It may also often be cheaper than other methods of noise control. This method of control may require that some noisy machinery be replaced. Noise can be controlled at the source by the manufacturer, so that noisy devices never reach your workplace. Many machines are now required to conform to noise standards. Therefore before new machines (such as presses, drills) are purchased, checks should be made to see that they conform to noise standards. Unfortunately, many used machines producing high noise levels (which have been replaced with quieter models) are often exported to developing countries, causing workers to pay the price with hearing loss, stress, etc.

(3) Barriers

If it is not possible to control the noise at the source, then it may be necessary to enclose the machine, place sound-reducing barriers between the source and the worker, or increase the distance between the worker and the source.

(4) Individual Protection

Controlling noise at the worker, by using ear protection (sometimes called hearing protection) is, unfortunately, the most common yet least effective form of noise control. Forcing the worker to adapt to the workplace is always the least desirable form of protection from any hazard. Generally, there are two types of ear protection: earplugs and earmuffs. Both are designed to prevent excessive noise from reaching the inner ear.

Earplugs are worn inside the ear and come in a variety of materials, including rubber, plastic, or any material that fit tightly in the ear. Earplugs are the least desirable type of hearing protection because they do not provide very effective protection against noise and they can cause ear infection if pieces of the plug are left in the ear or if a dirty plug is used. Cotton wool should not be used as ear protection.

(5) Health Supervision

Health examination should be carried out on workers exposed to noise regularly, especially hearing examination. The purpose is to detect the hearing damage at an early stage and take effective protective measures in time.

(6) Administrative Control

Administrative control is very important for not only mastering but also eliminating noise hazards. Reasonable arrangements of labor and rest are needed to avoid the continuously long-lasting noise. It is easy to aggravate auditory fatigue during the noise work. So leaving the noise environment during the break and restore the auditory fatigue is really necessary.

4.4.3　Vibration

Vibration is a mechanical phenomenon whereby oscillations occur about an equilibrium point. The oscillations may be periodic such as the motion of a pendulum or random such as the movement of a tire on a gravel road. Vibration is a physical factor, which allows electrophysical measurements and expressions in precise units.

Vibration is a very common form of motion in nature. It widely exists in people's production and life. Human body is also in a state of vibration. The vibration generated by the production or working equipment is called productive vibration. Vibration is a common occupational hazard factor, which can endanger the physical and mental health of workers and cause occupational diseases under certain conditions.

4. 4. 3. 1　Characteristics, Classification and Exposure Opportunities

(1) Characteristics

The terms used to describe the characteristics of vibration include frequency, amplitude, and acceleration. A vibrating object moves back and forth from its normal stationary position. A complete cycle of vibration occurs when the object moves from one extreme position to the other and then return.

① The number of cycles that a vibrating object completes per unit of time is called frequency. The unit of frequency is hertz (Hz).

② Amplitude is the distance from the stationary position to the extreme position on either side and is measured in meter (m). The intensity of vibration depends on amplitude.

③ The speed of a vibrating object varies from zero to a maximum during each cycle of vibration. Speed of vibration is expressed in units of meters per second (m/s).

④ Acceleration is a measure of time rate of change in speed. The measure of acceleration is expressed in units of meters per second squared (m/s^2). Measurement of acceleration can provide information about velocity and amplitude of vibration. In addition, the magnitude of acceleration is related to the degree of harm. Therefore, most regulating jurisdictions and standard agencies use acceleration as a measure of vibration exposure.

(2) Classification and Exposure Opportunities

Vibration enters the body from the organs in contact with vibrating equipment. Occupations requiring regular and frequent use of vibrating tools and equipment and handling of vibrating materials are found in a wide range of industries, for example, construction and maintenance of railways, roads, grounds, and parks; forestry; foundries; mines and quarries; manufacturing concrete products; motor vehicle manufacture and repair; and ship building and repair. On the basis of transmission pathways and adverse health effects, vibration is traditionally divided into whole body vibration (WBV) and segmental vibration.

①Whole body vibration: Whole body vibration (WBV) refers to the transmission of vibration energy to the human body through a broad contact area, such as from a machine platform through the feet, from a seat through the buttocks and back, or from the vibrating surface through the reclining body. In these cases, the entire body or a number of organs in the body can be affected. Whole body vibration exposures can be found in many occupational settings. Exposure is most likely to occur in vehicle use that includes road, off road, rail, air, and maritime use. Exposed groups also include operators who work on vibrating floors. A major emphasis for risk evaluation and remediation has been put employees who drive construction vehicles and off road vehicles over rough and uneven surfaces as a main part of their job.

② Segmental vibration: The most widely studied and most common type of segmental vibration exposure is hand arm vibration (HAV) exposure which affects the hands and arms. Hand arm vibration refers to the transmission of vibration energy to the hands and arms by the use of hand held power tools, hand guided machinery, or by holding materials being processed by machines. Exposed occupational groups include operators of sanders, grinders, cutting wheels; drills, chain saws, brush cutters, concrete breakers, polishers, chipping hammers, hedge trimmers, powered mowers, and high frequency oscillatory devices in orthopedics and dentistry.

4.4.3.2   Health Effects

The vibration caused by long-term contact can have adverse effects on the health of the body. In severe cases, it may lead to occupational diseases.

Suitable vibration can result in positive effects. One immediate effect of vibration is that muscles can be used quickly and efficiently. Another immediate effect of vibration is the improvement of circulation. Vibration can also have a positive effect on bone mineral density. Vibrations can cause compression and remodeling of the bone tissue, activating the osteoblasts while reducing the activity of the osteoclasts. However, these positive processes will only be effective if the intensity of vibration is not too high and the exposure duration of vibration is not too long. In occupational settings, the high intensity and prolonged exposure duration result in adverse health effects in human.

Vibration exposure causes vasoconstriction of the blood vessels supplying the fingers. Prolonged exposure may damage the endothelium and stimulate smooth muscle proliferation so that the lumen of the vessels gradually narrows. The resulting reduced blood flow can produce white fingers in cold environments, and the return of blood circulation to the finger is signaled by red flush. Once the circulation is permanently impaired, the fingers become cyanosed.

Damage also occurs to the peripheral nerves. Demyelinating neuropathies may reduce both the sensory and motor nerve conduction velocities. Mechanoreceptor dysfunction may impair both sensation and muscular responses. Consequently, dysfunctions in sensation and movements occur.

(1) Whole Body Vibration

Acute physical and psychological effects of whole body vibration can cause fatigue and loss of proficiency. Chronic exposure of whole body vibration can affect the entire body and result in a number of health disorders. Whole body vibration can result in increased incidence of the disorders of the neurological, circulatory, respiratory, digestive, urinary, reproductive, and musculoskeletal systems. Signs and symptoms include fatigue, headache, insomnia, psychological effects, vision problems, increased heart rate, increased oxygen uptake, increased respiratory rate, gastric problems, menstrual disturbance, and low back pain. However, the main problem associated with whole body vibration is low back pain.

(2) Hand Arm Vibration

Excessive exposure to hand arm vibrations can result in various patterns of diseases casually known as hand arm vibration syndrome(HAVS). HAVS is a disorder that affects the nerves, blood vessels, muscles, connective tissues, joints, and bones, of the fingers, hands, wrists, and arms. The development of HAVS is gradual HAVS increases in severity over time. It may take a few months to several years for the symptoms of HAVS to become clinically noticeable. Early signs and symptoms include nervous disorders such as headaches, irritability, depression, forgetfulness, and sleeping disorders. Muscular fatigue, weakness, stiffness, and pain in the hand are common. The most common and typical condition is vibration induced white finger.

Vibration induced white finger (VWF), also known as dead finger or Reynolds phenomenon of occupational origin, occurs at sites most exposed usually following exposure of the hands or the whole body to a cold environment. VWF is the result of impaired circulation and nervous system. VWF is manifested as tingling, numbness, loss of sensation, and blanching of the fingers. Initially the tips of one or more fingers rapidly become pale, which is followed by a dusky bluish phase and an intense red flush sequentially, and usually uncomfortable throbbing is accompanied. In mild cases only the tips of the fingers are affected and the symptoms may disappear after a short time. As the condition progresses, the whole finger can be affected and the occurrence is more frequent especially in the cold and wet. The thumbs are rarely affected.

In more severe forms, there is considerable pain in hands, arms and shoulders, particularly in the joints of the fingers and hands. Loss of manual dexterity and loss of grip strength in the hands, wrists, and forearms may occur. In severe cases, attacks may occur even in warm surroundings, and the numbness and loss of sensation could become permanent. Rarely the condition can progress to the extent that circulation is permanently impaired and the fingers become cyanosed.

Premature osteoarthrosis of the wrist and elbow and bone cysts in fingers and wrists can occur as well. Carpal tunnel syndrome (CTS) is a median entrapment neuropathy that causes paresthesia, pain, numbness, and other symptoms in the distribution of the median nerve in people using small hand tools. The early symptom is tingling; later symptoms can progress to intermittent numbness, usually in the thumb, index, middle, and ring fingers. Pain in the fingers, hands, and the wrist may also develop. The symptoms of CTS are frequently worse at night and a person may be awakened from sleep by pain. Long standing CTS leads to permanent nerve damage with constant numbness, atrophy and weakness of the muscles.

(3) Factors Affecting the Sensitivity to Vibration

The formation of vibration related adverse effects depends on various factors as noted in the following.

① Frequency of vibration: The frequency of vibration is generally considered the determinant of the affected organs.

② Intensity and exposure duration of vibration: The prevalence and the severity of vibration related adverse effects depend on the intensity and exposure duration of vibration. With the increase in the intensity and exposure duration of vibration, the occurrence of vibration related disorders increases while the latent period shortens.

③ Work practice: The operating posture and grip force affect the absorption and transmission of vibration energy. Vehicle age and maintenance, seat and cab design, and the presence of other vibrating equipment on the vehicle determine the magnitude of disorders in field settings.

④ Environmental factors: Low temperature and high humidity facilitate the occurrence and development of hand arm vibration syndrome.

⑤ Personal conditions and habits: Disease or prior injury in the fingers or hands, use of drugs, and smoking are susceptible factors. People with Raynauds syndrome can develop the most severe complications of vibration induced white finger very quickly.

4. 4. 3. 3　Prevention and Control

Prevention programs aim to eliminate or substitute the hazardous process where possible. Protecting workers from the effects of vibration usually requires a combination of appropriate working methods, good work practices, the use of appropriate vibration absorbing materials, and education programs.

(1) Selection of Working Methods and Equipment

Introducing working methods and equipment which eliminate or reduce exposure is the most efficient and effective way of controlling exposure to vibration. In industrial settings, anti-shock mounting of machinery, remote manipulation, and vibration isolated platform provide reduced exposure. Work equipment and tools of appropriate ergonomic design can reduce the vibration level and exposure magnitude transferred to individuals.

(2) Good Work Practices

The layout of workplace sites should be properly designed to reduce the transportation, and therefore, reduce the vibration exposure. Regular maintenance of vehicles and ground conditions throughout sites may greatly reduce shocks and jolts. Sharpened cutting tools should be properly maintained and repaired to avoid increased vibration caused by faults or general wear. The tool should be operated only when necessary and at the minimum speed and impact force to reduce vibration exposure. The duration and magnitude of exposure should be determined and reduced to as low a level as is reasonably practicable.

(3) Personal Protection

Wear anti-vibration gloves whenever possible. Anti-vibration gloves provide protection from typical industrial hazards and cold temperature. In turn, anti-vibration gloves may reduce may reduce the onset or the severity of sensation disorders and pain. Keeping the hands and body warm helps to maintain blood supply to the fingers and thereby reduces the risk of injury. Giving up or cutting down on smoking is necessary because smoking is a susceptible factor, due to it effects on blood flow.

(4) Employee Education

Training should include sufficient information on hazards of vibration, techniques of avoiding unnecessary exposure, and means of minimizing the adverse effects of vibration.

(5) Health Surveillance

Health surveillance is vital to detect and respond to early signs of damage. Health surveillance aims to identify those who develop early symptoms so that progression can be avoided.

4. 4. 4　Non-ionizing Radiation

Non-ionizing radiation is relatively low-energy ($<12\text{eV}$) radiation that does not have enough energy to ionize atoms or molecules. It includes ultraviolet (UV), visible light, infrared, radiofrequency radiation and laser.

4. 4. 4. 1　Radiofrequency Radiation

Radiofrequency radiation is a rate of oscillation in the range of 100 kHz to 300 GHz, which include high-frequency electromagnetic field and microwave.

(1) Exposure Opportunity

①High-frequency induction heating: It is a non-contact heating process. It uses high frequency electricity to heat materials that are electrically conductive. Induction heating is often used in high frequency treatment, welding, smelting and semiconductor processing. The frequency range is 300 Hz—3 MHz.

②High-frequency dielectric heating: It is the process in which radiowave or microwave electromagnetic radiation heats a dielectric material. The heating is used in plastic hot-bonding, high frequency gluing, grain drying and seed treatment, drying of paper, cloth, leather, cotton and wood. The frequency range is 1—100 MHz.

③Microwave: Microwave is a form of electromagnetic radiation with wavelengths ranging from as long as one meter to as short as one millimeter, or equivalently, with frequencies between 300 MHz and 300 GHz. The microwaves with frequency range of 3—300 GHz are used in radar navigation, exploring, communication and scientific research. The microwaves with frequencies of 2450 MHz and 915 MHz are used in food processing, material drying, killing insects, physical therapy, and cooking.

(2) Health Effects

The biological effects caused by high-frequency electromagnetic field and microwave include thermal effects and non-thermal effects. Thermal effects result from heating of tissue by radiofrequency radiation energy. High levels of radiation have the ability to heat biological tissue rapidly. Tissue damage in humans could occur during exposure to high radiation levels radiofrequency radiation because of the body's inability to cope with or dissipate the excessive heat that could be generated. Non-thermal effects occur when the emitted energy of the radiofrequency radiation does not significantly increase the temperature of biological tissue, but does bring some physical or biochemical changes. A number of authors have claimed that they could be demonstrated, but this is still an open debate in the scientific community.

① Nervous system: Radiofrequency radiation can induce changes in the nervous system and its activities. The main symptoms are nervous breakdown syndromes and autonomic nervous dysfunction syndromes. The neurological disorders such as headaches, dizziness, tremors, decreased memory and attention, decreased reaction times, sleep disturbances and visual disruption have been reported.

② Cardiovascular system: Autonomic nervous dysfunction syndromes are characteristic changes. The most common one is an increase of the excitability of the parasympathetic nervous system. The symptoms include low blood pressure, bradycardia, chest tightness, palpitation, precordial discomfort or pain. Electrocardiograms show sinus arrhythmia, bradycardia, prolongation of conduction time of atrium and ventricle.

③ Eye: The punctate and flake opacities of the lens are readily visible in the workers with long-term hard intensity microwave exposure. The range of hazardous frequency is from 1,000 MHz to 3,000 MHz. Occupational low intensity microwave exposure can accelerate lens aging.

(3) Prevention and Control

① High-frequency electromagnetic field: Field source shielding is the most effective and fundamental protective measure. The thin metal sheet or metal mesh and cover with ground connection are used to shield the field source of high-frequency electromagnetic field. Distance protection is also important in the protections of high-frequency electromagnetic field. Adopt automatic and semi-automatic techniques to keep the workers far away from the field source of high-frequency electromagnetic field. Implement hygienic standard is needed. Hygienic Standard for the Design of Industrial Enterprises (GBZ1—2002) provides the electromagnetic radiation intensity in workplace shall not exceed the limit. The threshold limits of 8h daily exposure time are 0.05 mW/cm² (14 V/m) for continuous wave, and 0.025 mW/cm² (10 V/m) for impulse wave.

② Microwave: The first protective measure is to absorb the radiation energy of microwave. The equivalent antenna must be applied in debugging microwave equipment. Use the materials having the ability to absorb and reflect microwave to shield microwave. The microwave operation point should be set up the place with the lowest levels of radiation intensity. The personal protection equipment are essential in the protections of microwave. Wear protective clothing, protective caps and protective glasses in the workplace. Implement hygienic standard is needed. Hygienic Standard for the Design of Industrial Enterprises (GBZ1—2002) provides the electromagnetic radiation intensity in workplace shall not exceed the limit. Average power density is 50 μW/cm², and daily total amount is 400 W/cm² for continuous wave. Average power density is 25 μW/cm², and daily total amount is 200 W/cm² for impulse wave.

4.4.4.2   Infrared Radiation

Infrared radiation also called infrared light is electromagnetic radiation with longer wavelengths than those of visible light, extending from the nominal red edge of the visible spectrum at 700 nm to 1 mm. Infrared is broken into three categories including near, mid and far-infrared. Near-infrared refers to the part of the infrared spectrum that is closest to visible light and far-infrared refers to the part that is closer to the microwave region. Mid-infrared is the region between the two categories. The primary source of infrared radiation is heat or thermal radiation. Sunlight is composed of nearly thermal-spectrum radiation that is slightly more than half infrared. Sources of infrared radiation include furnaces, melting metals and glasses, strong infrared light source, and baking and heating equipment.

The primary targets of an infrared radiation exposure are the skin and the eye. Infrared radiation will not penetrate the skin very deeply. Therefore, exposure of the skin to very strong infrared radiation may lead to local thermal effects of different severity, and even serious burns. Especially at longer wavelengths, an extensive exposure may cause a high local temperature rise and burns. The threshold values for these effects are time dependent, because of the physical properties of the thermal transport processes in the skin. Short wave infrared radiation can be effectively absorbed by the cornea. The absorption may lead to increased temperatures in the eye due to thermal conduction. Because of a quick turnover rate of the surface corneal cells, any damage limited to the outer corneal layer can be expected to be temporary. The exposure can cause a burn on the cornea similar to that on the skin. Corneal burns are not very likely to occur, however, because of the aversion reaction triggered by the painful sensation caused by strong exposure. The infrared radiation can also affect the retina, because of the transparency of the ocular media.

The most effective standard protection from exposure to infrared radiation is the total enclosure of the source and all of the radiation pathways that may exit from the source. Personal protection is applicable. Available eye protection in the form of suitable goggles or visors or protective clothing should be used. If the work conditions will not allow for such measures to be applied, administrative control and restricted access to very intense sources may be necessary. In some cases a reduction of either the power of the source or the working time (work pauses to recover from heat stress), or both, might be a possible measure to protect the workers.

4.4.4.3 Ultraviolet Radiation

Ultraviolet (UV) radiation is defined as the portion of the electromagnetic spectrum between x rays and visible light, with the wavelength range between 100 and 400 nm. The UV spectrum is divided into UV-C (100—290 nm), UV-B (290—320 nm) and UV-A (320—400 nm). They differ in their biological activity and the depth to which they penetrate into the skin. The sun is the greatest natural source of UV radiation. Artificial UV sources include tanning booths, black lights, curing lamps, germicidal lamps, mercury vapor lamps, halogen lights, high-intensity discharge lamps, fluorescent and incandescent sources. Unique hazards apply to the different sources depending on the wavelength range of the emitted UV radiation.

UVC rays do not have any effect on the body because they are completely absorbed by atmospheric ozone and hence do not reach the body. UV-A and UV-B rays on the other hand do reach the earth and can penetrate the skin quite rapidly. Some UV exposure is essential for good health. It stimulates vitamin D production in the body. However, excessive exposure to UV radiation is associated with acute and chronic health effects on the skin and eye. Too much UV radiation exposure can cause sunburn, premature ageing and skin damage leading to skin cancer. Sunburn is an acute injury following excessive exposure to UV radiation. Sunburn is not immediate. Skin redness reaches a maximum at about $8-12$ hours after exposure and fades within a few days. The red appearance of the skin (erythema) results from an increased blood content near the skin's surface. The exposure to ultraviolet radiation of wavelength shorter than 320 nm can cause erythema, in which wavelength with 297 nm is the most effective. Chronic UV-A and UV-B exposure can cause a number of degenerative changes in the cells, fibrous tissue and blood vessels of the skin. Long-term exposure can cause prematurely aged skin, wrinkles, loss of skin elasticity, dark patches (lentigos, sometimes called age spots or liver spots), and pre-cancerous skin changes (such as dry, scaly, rough patches called actinic keratoses). If exposure to sunlight continues for several years, the damaged skin has an increased chance of developing certain skin cancer. Exposure to ultraviolet radiation increases the risk of developing these cancers. Three different types of skin cancer are linked to sunlight exposure basal cell cancer, squamous cell cancer and malignant melanoma. An unprotected eye exposed to UV radiation may accumulate a sufficient dose to cause an adverse effect in the cornea of the eye. This condition is popularly referred to as snowblindness or welders flash. Within six hours such an exposure gives rise to a gradual transition symptoms forming a feeling of itchiness, increased tearing, severe pain and photophobia (light sensitivity). This is caused by an inflammatory reaction in the cornea and conjunctiva known as photokeratoconjunctivitis, which leads to a swelling and loss of the superficial cells in the cornea and the conjunctiva.

Protection against UV radiation emitted from artificial sources is generally straightforward where sources are used in a controlled work environment. The basic principles of control by engineering measures, administration, and the provision of protective clothing, can be applied. A notable exception is arc welding, where the process may be carried out in a place, to which others not directly involved in the welding process, may have access. When the nature of the work requires accomplishment of a task close to a source where neither engineering controls nor administrative controls are practical, personal protective clothing should be provided and worn.

4.4.4.4   Laser

The term originated as an acronym for Light Amplification by Stimulated Emission of Radiation (Laser). It is a kind of non-ionizing radiation through a process of optical amplification based on the stimulated emission of electromagnetic radiation. In industry, laser is used to drill, weld, cut, and mark all sorts of material. In the military field and aerospace industry, laser is used in laser radar, laser communication, laser distance measuring, laser guidance and laser aiming. Laser in medicine is used to treat many diseases in ophthalmology, surgery, dermatology and oncology. Laser is also widely used in life science research and nuclear physics.

The effects of laser on organic tissues including thermal effects, mechanical effects, photochemical reactions and electromagnetic effects. The radiation from a laser source constitutes of light rays, which can be considered as quasi-parallels. The unprotected human eye is extremely sensitive to laser radiation and can be permanently damaged from direct or reflected beams. When a high-power laser-beam travels through the eye, its power gets focused on a smaller spot, and localized on the retina. This power concentrated on a small diameter spot creates irreversible damages to the eye. However, the power itself is not the only danger for the eye. Indeed, some factors are as relevant as the power concerning the potential damages including wavelength, exposure duration and continuous/pulsed nature of the exposition. The retina, cornea, and lens are the areas most commonly damaged. Visible and near infrared laser light pose a critical hazard on the retina. Infrared A is transmitted by the cornea to the lens of the eye which narrowly focuses it on the retina, concentrating the radiant exposure of the laser by up to 100,000 times. Since the tissue structures of the retina are unable to undergo any repair, lesions caused by the focusing of visible or near-infrared light on the retina may be permanent. Laser light in the ultraviolet or far infrared spectrum can cause damage to the cornea or the lens. The effects of laser radiation are less important on skin than on the eye. Thermal (burn) injury is the most common cause of laser induced skin damage, which can cause pigmentation and erythema.

Hazard control measures of laser can be grouped into three general categories including engineering, administrative and personnel protective equipment. Maximum emphasis should be placed on engineering control measures. However, if engineering controls are impractical or inadequate, warning devices, personnel protective equipment or administrative controls must be used. For all uses of lasers and laser systems, it is recommended that the minimum laser beam energy or power be used for the application and the beam location maintained at a height other than eye level for a sitting or standing position. If it is not feasible to locate the beam at a height other than eye level, the beam should be enclosed.

4.4.5　Ionizing Radiation

Ionizing radiation is radiation with enough energy ($> 12\text{eV}$) so that during an interaction with an atom, it can remove tightly bound electrons from the orbit of an atom, causing the atom to become charged or ionized. The main forms of ionizing radiation include gamma (γ) rays, X rays, alpha (α) particles, beta (β) particles and neutrons. Ionizing radiation is widely used in industry and medicine and can present a significant health hazard.

4.4.5.1　Exposure Opportunity

Along with natural radioactive sources present in the Earth's crust and cosmic radiation, man-made sources also contribute to our continuous exposure to ionizing radiation. The radiation sources can pose a considerable health risk to affected workers if not properly controlled.

(1) Nuclear Power Industry

The workers are always exposed to radiation from mining, smelting and processing radioactive materials. Nuclear reactors, nuclear power station building and running are also sources of ionizing radiation exposure.

(2) Production and Use of Ray Generator

The exposure can come from accelerator, X- and γ-radiation source used in medicine, industrial and agricultural production.

(3) Production and Use of Radionuclide

The compounds mixed with radionuclide such as radioactive luminescent paint and radioactive reagent contribute to human exposures. The materials are used in a variety of industries for testing, inspection, manufacturing, and other applications. Medical procedures include diagnosing and treating a health problem accounted for the radiation exposures.

(4) Mineral Associated with Radionuclide

Radionuclide contains in raw minerals and soil samples and the associated radiological risk from some mining sites. Phosphate fertilizer, rare earth ore, tungsten ore mining and processing can produce radiation.

4.4.5.2   Radiation Quantities and Units

For applying ionizing radiation, the following basic radiation quantities need to be understood, including exposure (X), absorbed dose (D), equivalent dose (H) and effective dose (E). In summary, exposure may be described as the amount of ionizing radiation that may strike an object such as the human body when in the vicinity of a radiation source. Absorbed dose is the deposition of energy per unit mass by ionizing radiation in the patient's body tissue. Equivalent dose also attempts to take into radiation the variation in biologic harm that is produced by different types of radiation. Effective dose is radiation quantity used for radiation protection purpose. It begins with E and, by applying modifying factors, attempts to take into account the part of the body that is being irradiated to arrive at an index of overall harm to a human. E is the quantity that attempts to summarize the overall exposure to ionizing radiation. Each radiation quantity has its own special unit of measure. These units are discussed in detail in the following section.

(1) Exposure

When a volume of air is irradiated with X-rays or gamma-rays, the interaction that occurs between the radiation and neutral atoms in the air results in some electrons being liberated from those air atoms as they are ionized. Consequently the ionized air can function as a conductor and carry electricity because of the negatively charged free electrons and positively charged ions that have been created. As the intensity of X-ray exposure of the air volume increases, the number of electron-ion pairs produced also increases. Thus, the amount of radiation responsible for the ionization of a well-defined volume of air may be determined by measuring the number of electron-ion pairs or charged particles in that volume of air. This radiation ionization in the air is termed exposure.

Exposure (X) is defined as the total electrical charge of one sign, either all pluses or all minuses, per unit mass that X-ray and γ-ray photons with energies up to 3 MeV generate in dry (i. e. non-humid) air at standard temperature and pressure (760 mmHg or 1 atmosphere at sea level and 22℃).

The coulomb (C) is the basic unit of electrical charge. The ampere is the SI unit of electrical current. In the International System, the exposure unit is measured in coulombs per kilogram (C)/kg. This exposure unit is equal to an electrical charge of 1 C produced in a kilogram of dry air by ionizing radiation. The roentgen (R) is precisely defined as the photon (either X-ray or γ-ray) exposure that under standard conditions of pressure and temperature produces a total positive or negative ion charge of 2.58×10^{-4} C/kg of dry air. An exposure of 1C/kg equals $1/2.58 \times 10^{-4}$ R (or 3.88×10^{3} R). Therefore conversion from R (the traditional unit of exposure) to C/kg (the SI unit) may be accomplished by multiplying the number of roentgens by 2.58×10^{-4}. On the other hand, conversion of coulombs C/kg to R may be accomplished by dividing by 2.58×10^{-4}.

(2) Absorbed Dose

As ionizing radiation passes through an object such as a human body, some of the energy of that radiation is transferred to that biologic material. It is actually absorbed by the body and stays within it. The quantity absorbed dose (D) is defined as the amount of energy per unit mass absorbed by an irradiated object. This absorbed energy is responsible for any biologic damage resulting from the tissues being exposed to radiation.

The SI unit of absorbed dose is the gray (Gy), which is defined as energy absorption of 1 joule (J) per kilogram of matter in the irradiated object. One gray is therefore determined by the following simple equation:

$$1 \text{ Gy} = 1 \text{ J/kg}$$

A joule (a unit of energy) may be defined as the work done or energy expended when a force of 1 newton (N) acts on an object along a distance of 1 meter (m). Traditionally the rad has been used as the unit of absorbed dose. Rad stands for radiation absorbed dose. This unit has been used to indicate the amount of radiant energy transferred to an irradiated object by any type of ionizing radiation. The rad is equivalent to an energy transfer of 100 erg (another unit of energy and work) per gram of irradiated object. One rad may be expressed mathematically as follows:

$$1 \text{ rad} = 100 \text{ erg/g or, } 1 \text{ rad} = 1/100 \text{ J/kg} = 1/100 \text{ Gy}$$

Thus, gray and rad units are easily translated to compare absorbed dose values. If the absorbed dose is stated in rad, the equivalent number of gray may be determined by dividing by 100. On the other hand, if the absorbed dose is stated in gray, the number of rad may be determined by multiplying by 100.

(3) Equivalent Dose

Equivalent dose (H) is the product of the average absorbed dose in a tissue or organ in the human body and its associated radiation weighting factor (W_R) chosen for the type and energy of the radiation in question. The radiation weighting factor (W_R) takes this into account. W_Rs places risks associated with biologic effects on a common scale. Each type and energy of radiation has a specific radiation weighting factor, the numeric value of which may be found in Table 4.6.

H is used for radiation protection purposes when a person receives exposure from various types of ionizing radiation. H for measuring biologic effects may be determined and expressed in sieverts (SI units) or in rem (traditional units). It is obtained by multiplying the absorbed dose (D) by the radiation weighting factor (W_R) as follows:

$$H = D \times W_R$$
$$Sv = Gy \times W_R$$

Table 4.6   Radiation Weighting Factors for Different Types and Energies of Ionizing Radiation

Radiation Type and Energy Range	Radiation Weighting Factor (W_R)
X-ray and gamma-ray photons and electrons (every energy)	1
Neutrons, energy <10 keV	5
10 keV—100 keV	10
>100 keV—2 MeV	20
>2 MeV—20 MeV	10
>20 MeV	5
Protons	2
Alpha particles	20

Source: International Commission on Radiological Protection (ICRP): Recommendations, ICRP Publication No. 60[M]. New York, Pergamon Press, 1991.

(4) Effective Dose

Effective Dose (E) provides a measure of the overall risk of exposure to ionizing radiation, it is defines as "the sum of the weighted equivalent doses for all irradiated tissues or organs". E incorporates both the effect of the type of radiation used (e. g., X-ray radiation, gamma, neutron) and the variability in radiosensitivity of the organ or body part irradiated through the use of appropriate weighting factors. These factors determine the overall harm to those biologic components for risk of developing a radiation-induced cancer or, for the reproductive organs, the risk of genetic damage. The weighting factor that takes into account the relative detriment to each organ and tissue is called the tissue weighting factor (W_T). The tissue weighting factor is a conceptual measure for the relative risk associated with irradiation of different body tissues.

The tissue weighting factor (Table 4.7) is a value that denotes the percentage of the summed stochastic (cancer plus genetic) risk stemming from irradiation of tissue (T) to the all-inclusive risk, when the entire body is irradiated in a uniform fashion. W_T accounts for the risk to the entire organism brought on by irradiation of individual tissues and organs.

To determine E, an absorbed dose (D) is multiplied by a radiation weighting factor (W_R) to obtain E and by a tissue weighting factor (W_T). E may be expressed in sieverts (SI unit) or in rem (traditional unit).

$$E = D \times W_R \times W_T$$

E can be used to compare the average amount of radiation received by the entire body from a specific radiologic examination with that from natural background radiation. It is possible to describe the examination radiation dose in terms of the length of time it would take to acquire a comparable E from environmental sources.

Table 4.7　Organ or Tissue Weighting Factors

Organ or Tissue	Weighting Factor (W_T)
Gonads	0.20
Red bone marrow	0.12
Colon	0.12
Lung	0.12
Stomach	0.12
Bladder	0.05
Breast	0.05
Liver	0.05
Esophagus	0.05
Thyroid	0.05
Skin	0.01
Bone surface	0.01

Source: National Council on Radiation Protection and Measurements (NCRP): Limitation of Exposure to Ionizing Radiation, Report No. 116, Bethesda, NCRP, 1993.

4.4.5.3　Health Effects

(1) Influencing Factors

If the persons are exposed to ionizing radiation, many factors including ionizing radiation and human factors determine whether it will cause health effects. These factors include the dose (how much), the duration (how long), and the type of radiation, and also include the age, sex, diet, family traits, lifestyle, and state of health.

① Physical characteristics of ionizing radiation: The amount of biological damage depends on how many particles of ionizing radiation passes through the living tissue and how densely the ionizing is: high ionization density causes more damage than low ionization density. Therefore penetrating power and ionization density are important factors to affect the biological damage caused by ionizing radiation. For example, inhaling or ingesting an alpha-emitting isotope can do lots of damage, because the densely-ionizing alphas are already inside the body and are not stopped by the skin.

②Rate of absorption: The rate at which the radiation is administered or absorbed is most important in the determination of what effects will occur. Since a considerable degree of recovery occurs from the radiation damage, a given dose will produce less effect if divided (thus allowing time for recovery between dose increments) than if it is given in a single exposure. Thus, the same amount of radiation is more dangerous if delivered in a short time.

③Area exposed: The portion of the body irradiated is an important exposure parameter because the larger the area exposed, other factors being equal, the greater the overall damage to the organism. This is because more cells have been impacted and there is a greater probability of affecting large portions of tissues or organs. Even partial shielding of the highly radiosensitive blood-forming organs such as the spleen and bone marrow can mitigate the total effect considerably. An example of this phenomenon is in radiation therapy, in which lethal doses if delivered to the whole body are commonly delivered to very limited areas, e. g. to tumor sites. Generally when expressing external radiation exposure without qualifying the area of the body involved, whole-body irradiation is assumed.

④Variation in species and individual sensitivity: There is a wide variation in the radiosensitivity of various species. Lethal doses for plants and microorganisms are usually hundreds of times larger than those for mammals. Even among different species of rodents, it is not unusual for one to demonstrate three or four times the sensitivity of another. Within the same species, individuals vary in sensitivity. Within the same individual, a wide variation in susceptibility to radiation damage exists among different types of cells and tissues. In general, those cells which are rapidly dividing or have a potential for rapid division are more sensitive than those which do not divide.

(2) Biological Effects of Ionizing Radiation

From the biological effects of radiation on human body, radiation effects are generally divided into two categories namely deterministic effects and stochastic effects. It has been discovered that severity of certain deterministic effects on human beings will increase with increasing doses. There exists a certain level, the threshold, below which the effect will be absent. The examples of deterministic effects include cataract, erythema, infertility, etc. The severity of stochastic effects is independent of the absorbed dose. Under certain exposure conditions, the effects may or may not occur. There is no threshold and the probability of having the effects is proportional to the dose absorbed. The examples of stochastic effects include radiation inducing cancer and genetic effect.

If radiation interacts with the atoms of the DNA molecule, or some other cellular components of the cell, it is referred to a direct effect. Such an interaction may affect the ability of the cell to reproduce and survive. If enough atoms are affected such that the chromosomes do not replicate properly, or if there is significant alteration in the information carried by the DNA molecule, the cell may be destroyed by direct interference with its life-sustaining system. If a cell is exposed to radiation, the probability of the radiation interacting with the DNA molecule is very small since these critical components make up such a small part of the cell. However, each cell, just as the case for the human body, is mostly water. Therefore, there is a much higher probability of radiation interacting with the water that makes up most of the cell's volume. When radiation interacts with water, it may break the bonds that hold the water molecule together, producing fragments such as hydrogen and hydroxyls. These fragments may recombine or interact with other fragments or ions to form compounds, such as water, which would not harm the cell. However, they could combine to form toxic substances, such as hydrogen peroxide, which can contribute to the destruction of the cell. The effect is called indirect effect.

Not all radiation effects are irreversible because cells have a tremendous ability to repair damage. In many instances, the cells are able to completely repair any damage and function normally. If the damage is severe enough, the affected cell dies. In some instances, the cell is damaged but is still able to reproduce. However, the daughter cells may be lacking in some critical life-sustaining components, and they may die. The other possible result of radiation exposure is that the cell is affected in such a way that it does not die but is simply mutated. The mutated cell reproduces and thus perpetuates the mutation. This could be the beginning of a malignant tumor.

4. 4. 5. 4   Radiation Sickness

Radiation sickness or radiation poisoning is defined as the damage to the organ tissues due to the excessive exposure to ionizing radiation. The exposure to radiation interferes with the process of cell division. There are two types of radiation poisoning, including acute radiation syndrome and chronic radiation syndrome. Radiation may be external radiation and internal radiation. External radiation happens when the source of radiation is outside the exposed body, while internal radiation occurs when the source of radiation is present inside the exposed body. An example of external radiation is when a space traveler gets exposed to cosmic rays. An example of internal radiation is when a human consumes radioactive cow's milk.

(1) Acute Radiation Syndrome

When the radiation is delivered to the whole body in large doses, generally over 100 rad, the whole body signs and symptoms occur. This type of injury occurs only when the dose is received over a short period of time, and the total effect may vary from mild to death. Acute radiation syndrome progresses including the following stages prodrome, latent stage, manifest illness stage, recovery or death. Acute radiation syndrome is classically divided into three main presentations including hematopoietic, gastrointestinal and neurological. Hematopoietic type is marked by a drop in the number of blood cells, called aplastic anemia. This may result in infections due to low white blood cells, bleeding due to low platelets, and anemia due to low red blood cells. In gastrointestinal type, nausea, vomiting, loss of appetite and abdominal pain are usually seen within two hours. Vomiting in this time-frame is a marker for whole body exposures that are in the fatal range above 4 Gy. Without exotic treatment such as bone marrow transplant, death with this dose is common. The death is often due to infection than gastrointestinal dysfunction. Neurological type presents with neurological symptoms such as dizziness, headache, or decreased level of consciousness, occurring within minutes to a few hours, and with an absence of vomiting. It is invariably fatal.

(2) Chronic Radiation Syndrome

Chronic radiation syndrome is a constellation of health effects that occur after months or years of chronic exposure to low level exposure of ionizing radiation. The main effects are related to hematopoietic system. The symptoms include recurrent infections, low grade fever, loss of appetite, weakness and fatigue, fainting, dehydration, anemia, unhealed open wounds, hair loss, bruises, and skin burns. Large amounts of or long term exposure can cause birth defects and cancer.

4. 4. 5. 5   Prevention and Control

The only way to prevent radiation is to reduce the dose of the radiation that is suffered by the human being.

(1) Protection and Control of External Radiation

①Reducing the time of radiation: The longer a person is exposed to radiation, greater the risk of radiation sickness . Thus, it is in the best interest to reduce the time frame of radiation exposure of the human being.

②Increasing the distance from the radioactive substance: The more distant a person is from the radioactive substance, the risk of exposure is reduced. If the distance is doubled, the rate of exposure is quartered. Hence, workers in highly radioactive areas are advised to pick up radioactive materials with a pair of tongs.

③Shields: People working with radioactive materials wear protective clothing. Apart from that, it is also believed that the amount of radiation exposure can be reduced by placing a layer of material between the source of radiation and the person. The material, however, must be such that it absorbs the radiation. This is why nuclear fallout shelters are made of thick stone blocks.

(2) Protection and Control of Internal Radiation

However, all radiation is not bad. Its use in cancer prevention has been found. Radiation therapy is used for the treatment of cancer patients because radiation is known to prevent cell division. Cancer cells are the fastest dividing cells in the body and therefore cancer radiation therapy is helpful in preventing the growth and spread of cancer cells in the human body.

4. 5　Occupational Cancer

It has been known for more than 300 years that exposures to certain agents at the workplace may cause cancers. In 1775, Sir Percivall Pott, one of the leading British surgeons of the day, described some cases of cancer of the scrotum among English chimney sweeps. He ascribed this condition, which was known in the trade as "soot wart", to the chimney sweeps' pitifully dirty working conditions and to the "lodgment of soot in the rugae of scrotum". In the ensuing century, the syndrome became widely known, but it remained the only recognized occupationally caused cancer until the latter part of the nineteenth century. In 1875, Volkmann described a syndrome identical to "chimney sweeps cancer" of the scrotum among a group of coal tar and paraffin workers. Apparent clusters of scrotal cancer were thereafter reported among shale oil workers and mule spinners in the cotton textile industry. By 1907 the belief in the carcinogenicity of "pitch, tar, and tarry substances" was widespread enough that skin cancers among exposed workers were officially recognized as compensable in the UK. Other types of cancer were also implicated as occupationally induced. In the late nineteenth century, following several centuries of informal observations of unusually high incidence of lung tumors in residents of Joachimsthal, Czechoslovakia, and Schneeberg, Germany, it was shown that these risks were related to work in local metal mines. At about the same time, Rehn reported a striking cluster of bladder cancer cases among workers from a German plant which produced dyestuffs from coal tar. The era of initial identification of occupational cancer by the clinicians has extended into the 20th century. Following the accumulation of several of these clinical case reports of high-risk occupations, the scientific investigation of cancer etiology began in earnest at the beginning of the twentieth century with experimental animal research. A major breakthrough came with the experiments of Yamagiwa and Ichikawa, in which they succeeded in inducing skin tumors in rabbit ears by applying coal tar. Several important experimental discoveries were made in the next 20 years, particularly by an English group led by Kennaway. In a series of experiments, they managed to isolate dibenz anthracene and benzo pyrene, both polycyclic aromatic hydrocarbons (PAHs) and active ingredients in coal tar. The period of formal epidemiological assessment of the occurrence of cancer in relation to occupational exposures started after World War II. The era of modern cancer epidemiology began around 1950 with several studies of smoking and lung cancer. In the field of occupational cancer epidemiology, this era saw the conduct of some important studies of gas workers, asbestos workers, and workers producing dyestuffs in the chemical industry. The findings of these early studies were important in highlighting significant workplace hazards, and the methods that these pioneering investigators developed for studying occupational cohorts have strongly influenced the conduct of occupational cancer research. Knowledge of the occupational carcinogen and cancer grew rapidly during 1950 to

1975. However, relatively few occupational carcinogens have been identified in the last 25 years of the twentieth century.

Occupational cancer is likely to be a more important problem in the medium-and low-resource countries than in high-resource countries because of the importance of the informal sector, the lack of stringent implementation of existing regulations, the low level of attention paid by management and the workforce to industrial hygiene, and the presence of child labour. However, detailed information on prevalence of exposure and of cancer risk is currently lacking.

4.5.1   Common Carcinogens and Characteristics of Occupational Cancer

4.5.1.1   Common Carcinogens

In general, the occupational tumor has a clear etiology and has a history of exposure to occupational carcinogens. Occupational carcinogens are divided into chemical, physical and biological carcinogens, the most common of which are chemical carcinogens. Notably, the incidence of occupational cancer could be reduced when the associated carcinogen is controlled.

The IARC Monographs on the Evaluation of Carcinogenic Risks to Humans evaluate data relevant to the carcinogenic hazard to humans as a consequence of exposure to the carcinogen. Accordingly, evidence of carcinogenicity for most known or suspected occupational carcinogens has been evaluated in the IARC Monographs programme. At present, there are 47 chemicals, groups of chemicals and mixtures for which exposures are mostly occupational, that are human carcinogens (Table 4.8). An additional 42 occupational agents are classified as probably carcinogenic to humans (Group 2A) such as diesel engine exhaust and trichloroethylene (Table 4.9). A large number of important occupational agents are classified as possible human carcinogens (Group 2B).

Table 4.8   Occupational Agents Classified as Established Human Carcinogens (Group 1),

by the IARC Monographs, Volumes 1-123

Exposure	Target Organ	Use
Chemical Agents		
Acid mists, strong inorganic	Larynx	Chemical
4-Aminobiphenyl	Bladder	Rubber
Arsenic and inorganic arsenic compounds	Lung, skin, bladder	Glass, metals, pesticides
Asbestos	Larynx, lung, mesothelium, ovary	Insulation, construction, renovation

(to be continued)

continued

Exposure	Target Organ	Use
Benzene	Leukemia	Starter and intermediate in chemical production, Solvent
Benzidine	Bladder	Pigments
Benzo[α]pyrene	Lung, skin(suspected)	Coal liquefaction and gasification, coke production, coke ovens, coal tar distillation, roofing, paving, aluminum production
Beryllium and beryllium compounds	Lung	Aerospace, metals
Bis (chloromethyl) ether, chloromethyl methyl ether	Lung	Chemical
1,3-Butadiene	Leukemia and/or lymphoma	Plastic, rubber
Cadmium and cadmium compounds	Lung	Pigment, battery
Chromium[VI] compounds	lung	Metal plating, pigments
Coal-tar pitch	Skin, lung	Construction, electrodes
Engine exhaust, diesel	Lung	Transport, mining
Ethylene oxide	—	Chemical, sterilizing agent
Formaldehyde	Nasopharynx, leukemia	Plastic, textile
Ionizing radiation (including radon-222 progeny)	Thyroid leukemia, salivary gland, lung, bone, esophagus, stomach, colon, rectum, skin, breast, kidney, bladder, brain	Radiology, nuclear industry, underground mining
Leather dust	Nasal cavity	Shoe manufacture and repair
Lindane	Lymphoma	pesticides
4,4'-Methylenebis (2-chloroaniline) (MOCA)	—	Rubber
Mineral oils, untreated or mildly treated	Skin	Lubricant
2-Naththylamine	Bladder	Pigment
Nickel compounds	Nasal cavity, lung	Metal, alloy
Polychlorinated biphenyls	Skin, lymphoma, breast	Waste incineration, fires, and waste recycling
Shale-oils	Skin	Lubricant, fuel

(to be continued)

continued

Exposure	Target Organ	Use
Silica dust, crystalline, in the form of quartz or cristobalite	Lung	Construction, mining
Solar radiation	Skin	Outdoor work
Soot	Skin, lung	Chimney sweeps, masons, firefighters
2, 3, 7, 8-Tetrachlorodibenzo-p-dioxin	—	Chemical
Tobacco smoke, secondhand	Lung	Bars, restaurants, offices
ortho-Toluidine	Bladder	Pigments
Trichloroethylene	Kidney	Solvent, dry cleaning
Vinyl chloride	Liver	Plastics
Wood dust	Nasal cavity	Furniture
Occupation or industry without specification of the responsible agent		
Acheson process	Lung	Synthesize graphite and silicon carbide
Aluminum production	Lung, bladder	—
Auramine production	Bladder	—
Coal gasification	Lung	—
Coal tar distillation	Skin	—
Coke production	Lung	—
Hematite mining (underground)	Lung	—
Iron and steel founding	Lung	—
Isopropyl alcohol manufacture using strong acids	Nasal cavity	—
Magenta production	Bladder	—
Painter	Bladder, lung, mesothelium	—
Rubber manufacture	Stomach, lung, bladder, leukemia	—
Fumes and ultraviolet radiation from welding	Lung, kidney, ocular melanoma	Welding

**Table 4. 9 Occupational Agents Classified as Probable Human Carcinogens (Group 2A),
by the IARC Monographs, Volumes 1-123**

Exposure	Target Organ	Use
Chemical Agents		
Acrylamide	—	Plastics
Bitumens (combustion products during roofing)	Lung	Roofing
Captafol	—	Pesticide
α-Chlorinated toluenes (benzal chloride, benzotrichloride, benzyl chloride) and benzoyl chloride (combined exposures)	—	Pigments, chemicals
4-Chloro-o-toluidine	Bladder	Pigments, textiles
Cobalt metal with tungsten carbide	Lung	Hard metal production
Creosotes	Skin	Wood
Diazinon	Lymphoma or leukemia, lung	Organophosphate insecticide
Dichloromethane	Biliary tract, lymphoma	paint stripping, spray painting, and metal and printing-press cleaning
Diethyl sulfate	—	Chemical
Dimethylcarbamoyl chloride	—	Chemical
1,2-Dimethylhydrazine	—	Research
Dimethyl sulfate	—	Chemical
Epichlorohydrin	—	Plastics
Ethylene dibromide	—	Fumigant
Glycidol	—	Pharmaceutical industry
Hydrazine	Lung	Chemical
Indium phosphide	—	Semiconductors
Lead compounds, inorganic	Lung, stomach	Metals, pigments
Malathion	Lymphoma, prostate	Organophosphate insecticide
Methyl methanesulfonate	—	Chemical
N,N-dimethylformamide	Testes	Acrylic-fiber and synthetic-leather
2-Nitrotoluene	—	Production of dyes
Non-arsenical insecticides	—	Agriculture

(**to be continued**)

continued

Exposure	Target Organ	Use
PAHs (several apart from BaP)	Lung, skin	Coal liquefaction and gasification, coke production, coke ovens, coal tar distillation, roofing, paving, aluminum production
1,3-Propane sultone	—	Manufacture of lithium batteries
Polybrominated biphenyls	—	Plastics
Silicon carbide whiskers	Lung	Silicon carbide production
Styrene	—	Reinforced plastics and rubber industries
Styrene-7,8-oxide	—	Plastics
Tetrabromobisphenol A	—	electronic products, recycling facilities
Tetrachloroethylene (perchloroethylene)	—	Solvent
1,2,3-Trichloropropane	—	Solvent
Tris(2,3-dibromopropyl)phosphate	—	Plastics, textiles
Vinyl bromide	—	Plastics, textiles
Vinyl fluoride	—	Chemical
Occupation or Industry Without Specification of the Responsible Agent		
Art glass, glass containers, and pressed ware (manufacture of)	Lung, stomach	—
Carbon electrode manufacture	Lung	—
Food frying at high temperature	—	—
Hairdressers or barbers	Bladder, lung	—
Petroleum refining	—	—
Occupation Circumstance Without Specification of the Responsible Agent		
Shift work involving circadian disruption	Breast	Nursing, several others

4.5.1.2 Characteristics of Occupational Cancer

It is instructive to estimate the number of cancers that might be caused by occupational exposure to carcinogens. Estimating the total proportion of cancers attributable to workplace carcinogens involves two approaches. One method draws on studies of specific occupational groups (usually "cohort studies") in which the numbers of attributable cases can be estimated. Along with some estimate of the total number of exposed workers, the total burden can thus be estimated. This approach is somewhat uncertain as there is usually very limited quantitative information on the extent and level of exposure across occupational groups collected in a comparable way to the specific epidemiological studies from which risk estimates derive. A more satisfactory method is to estimate the attributable fraction directly from case-control studies in communities. This fraction is specific to the place where the study was conducted, but if there are a number of similar studies which can be synthesized, a global estimate may be possible. There are now many occupational case-control studies and the proportions summarized here derive from these types of studies.

Comparing with non-occupational cancers, the common cause of occupational cancers is considered to have exposed with occupational carcinogens. The incubation periods of occupational cancers are varied among occupational carcinogens. For example, benzene could result in leukemia with exposure period of 4 to 6 months, while the longest incubation period of asbestos-induced mesothelioma could be forty years. Although whether there exists a threshold doses of carcinogens for occupational cancers contains an open question, current evidence demonstrates a considerable dose-reaction relationship between carcinogens and occupational cancers. Additionally, occupational cancer generally occurred several organs that directly exposed by carcinogens. Further, several cancers exhibit special pathological type after exposed with varied intensity of carcinogens.

4.5.2　Common Types of Occupational Cancer

The sites of cancer which contribute most numbers to the estimated burden of occupational cancer include lung, mesothelioma, bladder, sinonasal and laryngeal cancers. Estimated burdens in terms of the proportions of cases attributable to occupation are summarized here.

4.5.2.1　Lung Cancer

Lung cancer almost exclusively involves carcinomas, these tumors arising from epithelia of the trachea, bronchi or lungs. There are several histological types, the most common being squamous cell carcinoma, adenocarcinoma, and small (oat) cell carcinoma.

Lung cancer was a rare disease until the beginning of the twentieth century. Since then, its occurrence has increased rapidly. This neoplasm has become the most frequent malignant neoplasm among men in most countries and represents the most important cause of cancer death worldwide, particularly among men. Survival from lung cancer is poor (5%—10% at five years). The most important occupational lung carcinogens are reported to be asbestos, silica, radon, heavy metals, and polycyclic aromatic hydrocarbons.

Many case-control studies in different countries have shown that some lung cancers are attributable to known occupational carcinogens. Two recent studies have been carried out in very large populations to overcome the small numbers inherent in individual studies. One is a four-country analysis of the entire Nordic population followed prospectively for cancer incidence from the 1970 censuses, and using exposures inferred from the occupation reported at the census. In this study, about 18% of male lung cancers and less than 1% of female lung cancers are attributed to occupational exposures. This compares with an estimate derived from a reanalysis of eight case-control studies in five European countries of 13% for male cancers and 3% for females. Both results are close to the earlier estimate for the USA of 15% for males and 5% for females. Overall, an estimate of 15% for males and 2%—3% for females would seem appropriate.

4.5.2.2　Mesothelioma

Mesothelioma is the most important primary tumor of the pleura. It can also originate from the peritoneum and the pericardium. Mesotheliomas were considered very rare tumors until large series of cases were reported in the 1960s among workers employed in asbestos mining and manufacturing. In most high-resource countries, the incidence of pleural mesothelioma is of the order of 1—1.5/100,000 in men and around 0.5/100,000 in women. Lower rates are reported from low-resource countries. In areas with a high prevalence of occupational exposure to asbestos such as shipbuilding and mining centers, the rates might be as high as 5/100,000 in men and 4/100,000 in women.

Pleural mesothelioma death rates are rising in several European countries where surveillance is most effective, particularly in Finland, UK and Netherlands. Extrapolation of current trends suggests that death rates will continue to rise, reaching a peak around 2018, before falling again. Asbestos is the main cause of mesothelioma and the proportion attributable to asbestos may be considered to be over 80%. Some of these are not directly occupational (e.g. family members exposed while living near asbestos factories or exposed to dust brought home by asbestos workers), but most of cases are due to occupational exposures. As a proportion of cancers, the approximately 1,200 per year in the UK amount to about 0.5% of all cancers per annum and this is expected to rise to 2% of cancers at the mortality peak in 20—30 years' time. In terms of absolute numbers it has been estimated that asbestos-related mesothelioma deaths will amount to 250,000 in total in Western Europe alone in the first 35 years of 21st century. The number of occupational mesotheliomas is hard to estimate in the developing countries like India and China due to lacking of strict occupational diseases reporting system and well-designed epidemiology studies. It is similar for other occupational cancers in developing countries, but definitely, the absolute number and proportion are much higher than European countries.

4.5.2.3　Bladder Cancer

Bladder cancer is the ninth most common cancer worldwide, with 330,000 new cases and more than 130,000 deaths per year. More than 90% of bladder cancers are transitional cell carcinomas. Much less common are adenocarcinoma (6%), squamous cell carcinoma (2%) and small cell carcinoma (less than 1%).

A high risk of bladder cancer has been reported among workers in industries that involve exposure to aromatic amines, in particular 2-naphthylamine, 4-aminobiphenyl and benzidine, including the rubber and dyestuff industries. Working in aluminum production, auramine manufacture, coal gasification and magenta manufacture also significantly increases the susceptibility to bladder cancer. Other occupations that might increase the risk of bladder cancer include leather workers, painters, hairdressers and barbers, coke production workers, and petroleum refining workers, possibly because of exposure to a variety of chemicals including polycyclic aromatic hydrocarbons, polychlorinated biphenyls, formaldehyde and solvents. The uncertainty surrounding these occupations is partly due to the difficulty of measuring past exposure to specific chemical agents.

For bladder cancer, a pooled reanalysis of 11 case-control studies of occupational risks for males found an overall attributable fraction for known occupational risks of 4%. While in the Nordic study, it was estimated 2%. These are both somewhat lower than the 10% estimated by Doll and Peto (1981) for the USA. For females, both studies estimated the attributable fractions are very low.

4.5.2.4　Sinonasal Cancer

Sinonasal cancer is relatively uncommon in the general population, accounting for less than 1% of all neoplasms and less than 4% of those arising in the head and neck region. The incidence of sinonasal cancer is from $0.5 \times 100,000$ to $1.5 \times 100,000$ person per year in men and from $0.1 \times 100,000$ to $0.6 \times 100,000$ in women. A strong relationship between sinonasal cancer and exposure to wood, leather dust, and nickel compounds has been established long time ago. Other suspected causative factors include hexavalent chromium compounds, welding fumes, arsenic, mineral oils, organic solvents, and textile dust. Sinonasal cancer, particularly adenocarcinomas, are characterized by a high occupational etiologic fraction, the attributable fraction for all sinonasal cancers together is estimated as 30%—41% for males by the Nordic and European pooled reanalysis of eight case-control studies, respectively. For females the results are less consistent, with the equivalent estimates being 2% and 7% of all sinonasal cancers.

4.5.2.5　Laryngeal Cancer

Most laryngeal cancers are squamous cell carcinomas, reflecting their origin from the squamous cells which form the majority of the laryngeal epithelium. Cancer can develop in any part of the larynx, but the cure rate is affected by the location of the tumor. For the purposes of tumor staging, the larynx is divided into three anatomical regions: the glottis (true vocal cords, anterior and posterior commissures); the supraglottis (epiglottis, arytenoids and aryepiglottic folds, and false cords); and the subglottis. Most laryngeal cancers originate in the glottis. Supraglottic cancers are less common, and subglottic tumors are least frequent.

Smoking is the most important risk factor for laryngeal cancer. Death from laryngeal cancer is 20 times more likely for heavy smokers than for nonsmokers. Heavy chronic consumption of alcohol, particularly alcoholic spirits, is also significant. When combined, these two factors appear to have a synergistic effect. The attributable fraction of occupational risks for laryngeal cancers together is estimated as 6%—8% for males by the Nordic and European pooled reanalysis of six case-control studies. For females, the attributable fraction was close to zero in these studies.

Evidence on occupational cancer has been obtained mainly in developed countries. To a large extent, the critical data concern the effects of high exposure levels as a consequence of industrial practice during the first half of the 20th century. Few studies have been conducted in developing countries, other than some in China. Since forty years ago, there have been major changes in the geographical distribution of industrial production. These have involved extensive transfer of technology, sometimes obsolete, from highly-industrialized countries to developing countries in Asia and in South America. For example, the manufacture of asbestos-based products is moving to countries such as Brazil, China, India, Pakistan and the Republic of Korea, where health and safety standards and requirements may not be so stringent. Occupational exposures to carcinogenic environments are increasing in these developing countries as a result of transfers of hazardous industries and the establishment of new local industries as part of a rapid global process of industrialization.

A particular problem in developing countries is that much industrial activity takes place in multiple small-scale operations. These small industries are often characterized by old machinery, unsafe buildings, employees with minimal training and education. Protective clothing, respirators, gloves and other safety equipment are rarely available or used. The small operations tend to be geographically scattered and inaccessible to inspections by health and safety enforcement agencies. Although precise data are lacking, the greatest impact of occupational carcinogens in developing countries is likely to be in the less organized sectors of the relevant industries. Examples include the use of asbestos in building construction, exposure to crystalline silica in mining, and the occurrence of polycyclic aromatic hydrocarbons and heavy metals in small-scale metal industries and in mechanical repair shops.

The most generally accepted estimates of the proportion of cancers attributable to occupational exposures in developed countries are in the range of 4%—5%. Lung cancer is probably the most frequent of these cancers. However, the estimates do not apply uniformly to both sexes or to the different social classes. Among those actually exposed to occupational carcinogens (e. g. those doing manual work in mining, agriculture and industry), the proportion of cancer attributable to such exposure is estimated to be about 20%.

4. 5. 3　Strategies for Prevention of Occupational Cancer

Virtually, occupational tumor has a clear etiology and has a history of exposure to occupational carcinogens. In theory, therefore, occupational cancer is largely preventable by promoting healthier workplaces and substantially reducing cancers associated with exposure to occupational carcinogens. Several avenues exist for the primary prevention of occupational cancer.

4.5.3.1 Risk Identification

A most effective approach to the prevention of occupational cancer is premarket testing of all new chemical compounds and industrial processes. Systematic cancer risk identification is performed by a number of national and international organizations. For example, IARC is a WHO organization producing evaluations of carcinogenicity to humans from both environmental and occupational exposure and naturally occurring substances. Since 1971, more than 1,000 agents have been evaluated, of which more than 400 have been identified as carcinogenic, probably carcinogenic, or possibly carcinogenic to humans. However, considering the very large number of chemical substances and exposure circumstances worldwide, this is a small fraction, and many substances are unevaluated.

4.5.3.2 Legal Initiatives

Restriction of the use of human carcinogens in the workplaces, after they have been identified by IARC, is the simplest but bluntest way available for risk reduction. Banning the use of a substance has been successfully used with occupational carcinogens, while regulation is quite different from restriction. Regulation requires that anyone who deals with the substance should keep to certain minimum standards to minimize the exposure and consequently the toxic effects. Known human carcinogens are strictly regulated in the workplaces, through standards, at least in industrialized countries. In China, for example, the permissible concentration-time weighted average (PC-TWA) of carcinogen benzene in the workplace is no higher than 6 mg · cm^{-3}.

4.5.3.3 Risk Elimination/Reduction

Industrial hygiene, workplace technology and general knowledge on the safety issues have been continuously improving in industrialized countries over the last 50 years. As a consequence, exposures in the workplace are now less intense than in the past. However, the possibility of low-level exposures still exists, sometimes to a multitude of chemicals or mixtures of chemicals with possibilities for various types of interactions.

Elimination of carcinogens in the workplace, by removing a process or a substance completely, is the definitive way of reducing occupational cancer risk. However, the drastic step of eliminating a process central to a workplace may result in the closing down of an industry. Elimination is often rejected in favor of more practicable control alternatives. Substitution of a new, less hazardous material for a material of known carcinogenicity is a more efficient way for the prevention of occupational cancers. It is important to ensure that the new material is less hazardous. Other approaches include process enclosure or isolation, or use of ventilation are also effective for controlling the carcinogenic exposures.

4.5.3.4 Surveillance and Monitoring in the Workplace

Biological monitoring and medical screening of workers usually uses information from health records and results from periodical physical and laboratory examinations to estimate the exposure levels and to assess the early health effects. Surveillance of workers is very useful for identifying unforeseen hazards and to protect workers working in the risk workplaces, with the idea of detecting the cancer in its presymptomatic stages when it still can be controlled or cured. Screening for occupational cancer in highly exposed populations for purposes of early diagnosis or treatment is not usually applied, but has been applied in the certain situations. Medical surveillance of populations at risk of getting cancer is only effective in the following situations: first, if the screening test is easy to perform and sensitive enough; second, if it can detect premalignant abnormalities or tumors at an early stage; finally, if there is an effective intervention that can greatly reduce morbidity and mortality when applied to early tumors.

4.5.3.5　Publicity, Education and Training

The publicity, education and training of the union's occupational health services propagate to the workers can help them receive occupational healthy knowledge and improve the awareness of the risk of carcinogens. The content of training usually includes the identification of hazard factors, the prevention and treatment measures of occupational-cancer-inductive factors, the reasonable use of personal labor protection articles, the operation rules of the post, etc.

4.5.3.6　Use of Personal Protective Equipment

Personal protective equipment is essential to reduce employee exposure to hazards when engineering controls and administrative controls are not feasible or effective to reduce carcinogens to acceptable levels. Respirators, gloves and other forms of protective clothing are all common forms of protective equipment in use throughout industry. These equipments are important in reducing carcinogenic exposures provided that specifically designed equipment is in use and that equipment is properly used and maintained.

(Li Huangyuan, Ma Junxiang, Zhang Liping, Zhou Fang, Li Jing, Wu Qiuyun, Zhao Ran, Ni Chunhui, Zhao Jinshun, Feng Zhihui, Xu Jin, Li Zhen, Yu Guangxia)

Exercises

Chapter 5   Food Nutrition and Health

5.1   Introduction

Food is essential for human survival. The relationship between food and human health includes two aspects: one is that we obtain nutrients through food to meet the physiological needs of the body; the other is that harmful pollutants in food may be harmful to the human body when they enter the body.

Nutrition is the science that interprets the interaction of nutrients and other substances in food in relation to maintenance, growth, reproduction, health and disease of any organism. It includes food intake, absorption, assimilation, biosynthesis, catabolism, and excretion. Nutrition has developed rapidly in recent years. With the application of molecular biology technology, some new functions of nutrients have been discovered, especially the relationship between phytochemicals and human health becomes the research hotspot. The integration of nutrition, genomics, and molecular biology has opened a whole new world of study called nutritional genomics—the science of how nutrients affect the activities of genes and how genes affect the interactions between diet and disease.

Nutrition has always played a significant role in your life. Every day, you select foods that influence your body's health, for several times a day. Each day's food choices may benefit or pose a certain degree of damage to health, but over time, the consequences of these choices become significant. That being the case, paying close attention to current good eating habits supports health benefits in the future. Conversely, carelessness about food choices can contribute to chronic diseases. Although most people realize food habits affect health, they often choose foods for other reasons. After all, foods bring pleasures, traditions, and connect people as well as nourishment. In recent years, with the improvement of living standards, the incidence of nutrient deficiency is getting lower and lower, but the incidence of nutrition-related chronic diseases caused by excess energy is rising.

While people pay more attention to health, they pay more attention to food hygiene and food safety than ever before. Food-borne diseases caused by food contamination continue to occur, while new food processing technology, new food raw materials and health food development, nano-food, genetically modified food safety problems also emerging health threats.

The relationship between food and health will be described from both nutrition and food hygiene and safety. The nutrition part includes basic of nutrients, life cycle nutrition, public nutrition, nutrition and disease, and clinical nutrition therapy. And the food borne illness is also discussed.

5.2   Basic of Nutrients

5.2.1   Definition of Nutrients

Nutrients are chemical substances obtained from food and used in the body to provide energy, structural materials, and regulating agents to support growth, maintenance, and repair of the body's tissues. Nutrients may also reduce the risks of some diseases. There are six major classes of nutrients: carbohydrates, lipids, proteins, vitamins, minerals and water. Carbohydrates, lipids, and proteins are sometimes called macronutrients because the body requires them in relatively large amounts (many grams daily), they can be used to provide energy, so they are also called energy-yielding nutrients. In contrast, vitamins and minerals are called micronutrients, required only in small amounts (milligrams or micrograms daily).

5.2.2   Introduction of Dietary Reference Intake (DRI)

Using the results of research, nutrition experts have produced a set of recommended values that define the amounts of energy, nutrients, other dietary components, and physical activity that best support health. These recommendations are called Dietary Reference Intakes (DRIs). They include Estimated Average Requirements (EAR), Recommended Nutrient Intake [RNI, it equals Recommended Dietary Allowances (RDA)], Adequate Intakes (AI), Tolerable Upper Intake Levels (UL), Acceptable Macronutrient Distribution Ranges (AMDR), Proposed Intakes for Preventing Non-communicable Chronic Diseases (PI-NCD, PI), and Specific Proposed Levels (SPL).

The DRIs system is used by the United States, Canada, Japan, China and many other countries in the world and is intended for the general public and health professionals. In China, The Chinese Nutrition Society implemented the current Dietary Reference Intakes in 2013. This DRIs are composed of several items:

① EAR: Expected to satisfy the needs of 50% of the people in that age group based on a review of the scientific literature.

② RNI or RDA: The daily dietary intake level of a nutrient considered sufficient by the Food and Nutrition Board to meet the requirements of 97%—98% of healthy individuals in each life-stage and sex group. It is calculated based on the EAR and is usually approximately 20% higher than the EAR.

③ AI: A recommended average daily nutrient intake level, based on experimentally derived intake levels or approximations of observed mean nutrientintake by a group (or groups) of apparently healthy people that are assumed to beadequate.

④ UL: To caution against excessive intake of nutrients (like vitamin A) that can be harmful in large amounts. This is the highest level of daily consumption that current data have shown to cause no side effects in humans when used indefinitely without medical supervision.

⑤ AMDR: A range of intake specified as a percentage of total energy intake. Used for sources of energy, such as fats, proteins and carbohydrates. Different country proposed different percentages for fats, proteins and carbohydrates, the Chinese current criterion for fats, proteins and carbohydrates is 20%—30%, 10%—15% and 50%—65%, respectively. This item was proposed on the basis of meeting the requirements of most healthy individuals and reducing the risks of non-communicable chronic diseases.

⑥ PI: Chinese Nutrition Society (CNS) proposed this item in 2013 aimed at reducing the risks of non-communicable chronic diseases.

⑦ SPL: The amount specific to non-nutrient substances proposed by CNS, such as lycopene 18 g/d, lutein 10 g/d, soybean isoflavones 55 g/d.

In most countries, the DRIs include EAR, RNI or RDA, UL, and AMDR.

The relationship among EAR, RDA and UL are showed in Figure 5.1.

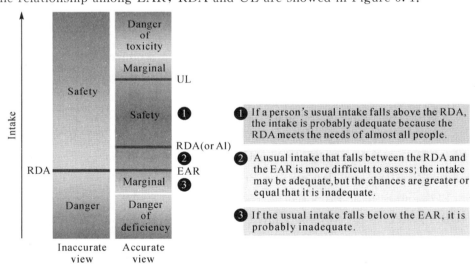

Figure 5.1　Inaccurate *versus* Accurate View of Nutrient Intakes

Source: WHITNEY E, ROLFES. Understanding Nutrition[M]. 14th ed. Canada: Cengage Learning, 2016.

5.2.3　Nutrients

There are more than 40 essential nutrients for human. The table 5.1 is the essential nutrients in the human diet and their classes.

Table 5. 1　Essential Nutrients in the Human Diet and Their Classes*

Carbohydrate	Energy-Yielding Nutrients Lipids (Fats and Oils)	Protein (Amino Acids)
Glucose (or a carbohydrate that yields glucose)	Linoleic acid (omega-6) a-Linolenic acid (omega-3)	Histidine Isoleucine Leucine Lysine Methionine Phenylalanine Threonine Tryptophan Valine

Non-Energy Yielding Nutrients					
Vitamins		Minerals			
Water-Soluble	Fat-Soluble	Major	Trace	Some Questionable Minerals	Water
Thiamin	A	Calcium	Chromium	Arsenic	Water
Riboflavin	D	Chloride	Copper	Boron	
Niacin	E	Magnesium	Fluoride	Nickel	
Pantothenic acid	K	Phosphorus	Iodide	Silicon	
Biotin		Potassium	Iron	Vanadium	
B-6		Sodium	Manganese		
B-12		Sulfur	Molybdenum		
Folate			Selenium		
C			Zinc		

This table includes nutrients that the current *Dictary Reference Intakes* and related publications list for humans. Some disagreement exists over the questionable minerals and certain other minerals not listed. Fiber could be added to the list of essential substances, but it is not a nutrient. The vitamin-like compound choline plays essential roles in the body but is not listed under the vitamin category at this time. Alcohol is a source of energy but is not an essential nutrient.

5. 2. 3. 1　Proteins

Proteins, like fats and carbohydrates, are composed of carbon, hydrogen, and oxygen; in addition, they must contain nitrogen. Most proteins contain about 16% nitrogen; for this reason, nitrogen determination is used to study protein metabolism and protein content of foods. Nitrogen content is multiplied by 6.25 to calculate the protein content.

(1) Functions of Protein

① As the fundamental structural element of the body; ② maintenance and repair of body tissues; ③ contribute to the energy pool of the body (4 kcal/g); ④ essential Amino Acids.

Essential amino acids that the body cannot synthesize in adequate amounts are called essential or indispensable because they must be supplied by the diet in proper proportions and amounts to meet the requirements for maintenance and growth of tissue. Nonessential or dispensable amino acids are those that the body can synthesize in sufficient amounts to meet its needs if the total amount of nitrogen supplied by protein is adequate.

Nitrogen balance studies involve the evaluation of dietary nitrogen intake and the measurement and summation of nitrogen losses from the body. They can be conducted when subjects consume a diet with a protein (nitrogen) intake that is at or near a predicted adequate amount, less than (including protein-free nitrogen) a predicted adequate amount, or greater than a predicted adequate amount. To determine nitrogen balance or status, nitrogen intake and output must be assessed. Assessment of nitrogen intake is based upon protein intake. To calculate grams of nitrogen consumed from grams of protein, the following calculation can be used: 0.16 $\times$ protein ingested (measured in g) = nitrogen (measured in g). Expressed alternately, ingested protein (g)/6.25 = ingested nitrogen (g). So, for example, 80 g of protein intake provides 12.8 g of nitrogen. To reverse the calculations and convert grams nitrogen into grams of protein: protein (g) = nitrogen (g) $\times$ 100/16, or protein (g) = nitrogen (g) $\times$ 6.25. Nitrogen losses are measured in the urine (U), feces (F), and skin (S). To calculate nitrogen balance/status, nitrogen losses are summed and then subtracted from nitrogen intake (In). Thus, nitrogen balance/status = In$-[(U-U_e)+(F-F_e)+S]$. The subscript e (in Ue and Fe) in the equation stands for endogenous (also called obligatory) and refers to losses of nitrogen that occur when the subject is on a nitrogen-free diet. Positive nitrogen balance, that is, nitrogen intake from protein greater than nitrogen loss in urine and feces, occurs only when new tissues are synthesized, as in growth and pregnancy, or in replacement of tissue loss due to injury or disease.

Nine amino acids are essential for maintenance of nitrogen equilibrium in humans. Infants and children have proportionally greater demands for essential amino acids than adults. The nonessential amino acids in protein also affect the quality of the protein. For example, the amount required of the sulfur-containing essential amino acid, methionine, may be somewhat reduced if cysteine, a sulfur-containing non-essential amino acid, is supplied in the diet. Similarly, the presence in the diet of tyrosine, a nonessential amino acid similar in structure to phenylalanine, may reduce the requirement for phenylalanine. These amino acids are listed in Table 5.2.

Table 5.2   The Amino Acids Contribute to Human Body

Essential Amino Acids	Conditionally Essential Amino Acids	Nonessential Amino Acids
Histidine	Arginine	Alanine
Isoleucine	Cysteine	Aspartic acid
Leucine	Glutamine	Asparagine

(**to be continued**)

continued

Essential Amino Acids	Conditionally Essential Amino Acids	Nonessential Amino Acids
Lysine	Glycine	Glutamic acid
Methionine	Proline	Serine
Phenylalanine	Tyrosine	Selenocysteine
Threonine		Pyrrolysine
Tryptophan		
Valine		

（3）Quality of Protein

Proteins are normally classified as complete, partially incomplete, and incomplete. A complete protein contains all the indispensable amino acids in the approximate amounts needed by humans. Sources of complete proteins are mostly foods of animal origin such as milk, yogurt, cheese, eggs, meat, fish, and poultry. The exceptions are gelatin, which is of animal origin but lacks the indispensable amino acid tryptophan, and soy protein, which is of plant origin but is a complete protein. Incomplete proteins, or low-quality proteins, are derived from plant foods such as legumes, vegetables, cereals, and grain products. Proteins from plant sources are usually not of as good quality as those from animal sources because one or more of the following essential amino acids are in short supply: lysine, methionine, threonine, and tryptophan. They are therefore incomplete or partially incomplete. The best quality plant proteins are found in legumes, such as beans, peas, lentils, and peanuts, and in nuts. The proteins in bread, cereals and vegetables other than those mentioned, and fruit are incomplete. These proteins, nevertheless, are an important part of the food intake because their amino acids contribute to the total nitrogen of the body that must be available for nonessential amino acids and other nitrogen-containing compounds in the tissues.

Protein quality is a measure of the efficiency with which a protein is used for growth or maintenance and depends primarily on the essential amino acid composition of the protein. When the diet is adequate in energy and total nitrogen (protein), protein quality can be calculated by comparing the essential amino acids in an unknown protein with those in a reference protein. The amino acid score (chemical score) can be calculated as follows: [(1 mg of limiting amino acid in 1 g of test protein) ÷ (1 mg of same amino acid in 1 g of reference protein) ×100].

The amino acid score for the protein would be the score for the most limiting essential amino acid. If the most limiting essential amino acid is 80% of the reference pattern, then the amino acid score is considered to be 80. The proteins in egg and human milk have been used as the protein reference patterns.

The protein digestibility corrected amino acid score (PDCAAS) is a commonly used indicator of protein quality. In fact, foods intended for individuals over 1 year of age or with health claims must use the protein digestibility corrected amino acid score method to provide information on the product's food label. This method involves comparing the amount of the limiting amino acid for a test protein to the amount of the same amino acid in 1 g of a reference protein (usually egg or milk). The value is then multiplied by the test protein's digestibility, as shown in the following formula.

$$PDCAAS(\%) = \frac{\text{Amount(mg) of limiting amino acid in 1 g test protein}}{\text{Amount(mg) of same amino acid in 1 g reference protein}} \times \text{True digestibility}(\%)$$

Biologic value (BV) is another term used to describe protein quality and is defined as the percentage of absorbed nitrogen retained by the body. It can be calculated as follows: {[nitrogen retained (g)] ÷ [(nitrogen absorbed (g)]} × 100%. This is determined by a carefully standardized assay in which the nitrogen intake and losses of rats are measured to determine the efficiency of utilization. Animal proteins in eggs, milk, cheese, meat, poultry, and fish have high biologic values compared with lower values for most of the vegetable proteins. The amino acid score should correspond with the biologic value for proteins that are completely digested.

Another method of evaluating protein quality is the protein efficiency ratio (PER). The PER is a measure of the weight gain per amount of protein consumed by a growing animal. It can be calculated as follows: {[gain in bodyweight (g)] ÷ [amount of protein consumed (g)]}. It is the method used to determine protein quality for food labeling.

Fortunately, most of our foods contain a mixture of proteins, one of which often supplements another. More to the point, however, is the fact that we combine several different foods in a meal in which the proteins tend to supplement one another because of their varying amino acid content. This complementary action is the complementary action of different foods that complement each other with their essential amino acid deficiencies. For instance, cereals. which are low in lysine, are usually eaten with milk, which provides a generous amount of this substance. For this reason, cereal and milk or bread and cheese are good combinations. It is obvious that this type of complementary value among foods makes a varied diet more desirable than a restricted one.

(4) Protein Allowances

Any quantitative estimate of protein requirement must take into account the quality of the proteins involved. The Chinese Nutrition Society (CNS) recommends a daily intake of 1. 16 g protein per kg of body weight for Chinese adults consuming the mixed protein diet. The DRIs of protein for the Chinese residents are listed in table 5. 3. The acceptable macronutrient distribution ranges (AMDR) of protein for Chinese adults is 10%—15% of total energy intake. The recommended dietary allowance of protein for infants is based upon the amount of milk protein that is known to produce a satisfactory growth rate. It is highly desirable that at least one-third of the daily protein intake to be derived from animal sources.

Table 5. 3   The DRIs of Protein for the Chinese

Age/Year	Gender	
	Male	Female
0—	9（AI）	9（AI）
0.5—	20	20
1—	25	25
2—	25	25
3—	30	30
4—	30	30
5—	30	30
6—	35	35
7—	40	40
8—	40	40
9—	45	45
10—	50	50
11—	60	55
14—	75	60
18—	65	55
50—	65	55
65—	65	55
80—	65	55
Pregnant women early stage	—	+0
Middle stage	—	+15
Later stage	—	+30
Lactating women		+25

"+": The extra amount of protein for the pregnant women based on the RNI of protein for the non-pregnant women with same age.

(5) Food Sources of Protein

The proteins of milk are casein and lactoalbumin, they are both complete proteins and contain a good balance of amino acids. Meat, poultry, and fish are forms of animal tissue protein synthesized by each species to meet its specific needs for growth and maintenance. Such proteins are remarkably similar in amino acid content to the amino acid requirements of humans. Meat, poultry, and seafood vary in protein content in inverse ratio to the moisture content: beef 25 g, lamb 24 g, poultry 20 g, and fish 15 g to 20 g of protein per 100g of fresh product. Vegetables are poor sources of protein, which only provide 1% or 2%

protein. Soybeans, which have the highest protein content among the legumes, are now available in a variety of forms suitable for use in the fabrication of foods. Roasted peanuts and peanut butter contain about 26% protein. The protein of uncooked grains ranges from 7% to 14%. The grain proteins are low in one or more essential amino acids; for example, wheat is low in lysine, corn in tryptophan, rice in tryptophan and the sulfur-containing amino acids, cystine and methionine. Plant proteins, however, may supplement each other in such a way that a combination may provide a better balance of amino acids than any one food alone.

5. 2. 3. 2　Carbohydrates

Carbohydrates, mainly in the form of cereal grains and root vegetables, are the major sources of energy for most peoples of the world. They are the cheapest and the most easily digested form of human and animal energy. Carbohydrates are a primary fuel source for cells, especially the cells of the central nervous system and red blood cells.

（1）Classifications of Carbohydrates

According to the Food and Agriculture Organization/World Health Organization Expert Consultation in 1997, carbohydrates are divided into three groups: sugars, oligosaccharides and polysaccharides.

① Sugars: the degree of polymerization (DP) of sugars is 1—2 and the term "sugar" is conventionally used to describe the mono-and disaccharides.

• Monosaccharides are the simplest carbohydrate units and are classified according to whether they are aldehyde or ketone derivatives and the number of carbon atoms in the molecule. Hexoses, sugars containing six carbon atoms, are the nutritionally significant sugars found in foods, whereas others, particularly the pentoses, ribose, and deoxyribose, which each contain five carbon atoms, are produced in the metabolism of foodstuffs. The single hexoses-glucose, fructose, and galactose-require no digestion and are readily absorbed from the intestine directly into the blood stream.

• Disaccharides, containing two hexose units—that are commonly encountered in foods include: sucrose, maltose, arid lactose. Disaccharides are hydrolyzed by specific enzymes in the digestive tract into monosaccharides or, commercially, by acid hydrolysis. Each of the three disaccharides has distinct characteristics that are of interest in human nutrition.

② Oligosaccharides contain 3 to 9 single sugar units (DP is 3—9). Several oligosaccharides are known as the prebiotics that are very important to maintain the probiotics in the colon, providing certain health benefits. For instance, two oligosaccharides of nutritional importance are raffinose and stachyose, which are found in onions, cabbage, broccoli, whole wheat, and legumes, such as kidney beans and soybeans. Oligosaccharides cannot be broken down by our digestive enzymes. Thus, when we eat foods with raffinose and stachyose, these oligosaccharides pass undigested into the large intestine, where bacterial metabolism takes place, producing gas and other by-products. Although many people have no symptoms after eating legumes, others experience unpleasant side effects from intestinal gas.

③ Polysaccharides or complex carbohydrates (DP is more than 10), the molecules of which may contain several hundred times as many glucose units as those of the sugars, such as sugars-dextrin, starch, cellulose, and glycogen. Consequently, they are much less soluble and more stable but differ markedly among themselves in digestibility and resistance to spoilage. To be suitable for human food, however, carbohydrate must be subjected to digestion by the enzymes in the digestive tract. Starches and dextrins fall into this category, but celluloses and hemicelluloses, which also found in food, cannot be digested by humans.

Starch, the chief form of carbohydrate in the diet, occurs in two forms:

• Amylose, a straight chain polysaccharide of glucose units linked together the same as maltose (1,4 glucosidic bonds);

• Amylopectin, a branched structure of glucose units with a linkage different from maltose at the branchings (1,6 glucosidic bonds) but similar throughout the rest of the chain. Starch is found in cereal grains, vegetables, and other plants.

Cellulose, found in the framework of plants, is also a polysaccharide of glucose units but with linkages different from those of maltose and starch. It is the chief constituent of wood, stalks and leaves of all plants, and the outer coverings of seeds and cereals. No cellulose-splitting enzyme is secreted by the mucosa of the human gastrointestinal tract, but bacterial fermentation or disintegration may play a role in dissolving the substances that bind the cellulose fibers or particles together.

The indigestibility of cellulose is its major asset, as the undigested fiber furnishes the bulk necessary for efficient and normal peristaltic action of the intestines. Research has demonstrated that the normal colon performs better when a reasonable amount of bulk or residue is present.

(2) Glycemic Index and Glycemic Load

Our bodies react uniquely to different sources of carbohydrates. For example, a serving of high-fiber brown rice results in lower blood glucose levels, compared with the same-size serving of mashed potatoes. As researchers investigated the glucose response to various foods, they noted that it was not always as predicted. Thus, 2 tools were developed: the glycemic index and the glycemic load, to indicate how blood glucose responds to various foods.

① The glycemic index (GI) is a ratio of the blood glucose response of a given food, compared with a standard (typically, glucose or white bread). Glycemic index is influenced by a food's starch structure (amylose vs. amylopectin), fiber content, food processing, physical structure (small vs. large surface area), and temperature, as well as the amount of protein and fat in a meal. Generally, foods that elicit glycemic responses similar to that of pure glucose are considered high-GI foods (GI>70), whereas those that cause a lower or more gradual rise in blood glucose are considered low-GI foods (GI ≤55). Foods with particularly high glycemic index values are potatoes, breads, short-grain white rice, honey, and jelly beans. A major shortcoming of the glycemic index is that it is based on a serving of food that would provide 50 grams of carbohydrate. However, this amount of food may not reflect the amount typically consumed.

② Glycemic load (GL) takes into account the glycemic index and the amount of carbohydrate consumed, so it better reflects a foods effect on blood glucose than does the glycemic index alone. To calculate the glycemic load of a food, the number of grams of carbohydrate in a serving is multiplied by the foods glycemic index, then divided by 100 (because the glycemic index is a percentage). For example, vanilla wafers have a glycemic index of 77, and a serving of 5 cookies contains 15 g of carbohydrate. This yields a glycemic load of approximately 12. Even though the glycemic index of vanilla wafers is considered high, the glycemic load calculation shows that the impact of this food on blood glucose levels is fairly low. Generally, Low-GL foods: GL <10; Medium GL foods: $10 \leqslant GL \leqslant 20$; High GL foods: GL$>20$.

(3) Probiotics and Prebiotics

Driven by the increasing burden of gastrointestinal disease, the functional foods market has moved heavily toward gut-derived events. Specifically, these foods target the human gut to stimulate beneficial microbial genera either directly, by providing growth substrates to promote the growth of an individual's autochthonous " healthy flora " selectively (prebiotics), or by using live microbial additions (probiotics). *Bifidobacteria* and *lactobacilli* are the most common targets for *in vivo* within the large intestine for such fortification. The use of probiotics and prebiotics carries little to no risk for consumers, but it holds much promise for improved health and well-being.

① A more recent formal definition of probiotics was proposed by the World Health Organization (WHO): " Live microorganisms which, when administered in adequate amounts, confer a health benefit to the host. " This definition relies on viability of the strains during ingestion and within the product. This requirement is key for probiotic efficacy. Probiotics are usually strains of lactic acid—producing bacteria, in particular members of the *Lactobacillus* and *Bifidobacterium* genera. Other microorganisms have also been developed as potential probiotics, namely *Bacilluscoagulans*, *Escherichia coli*, and *Saccharomyces*.

② A prebiotic is defined as "a non-digestible food ingredient that beneficially affects the host by selectively stimulating the growth and/or activity of one or limited number of bacteria in the colon that confer benefits upon host well-being and health". Most of the interest in the development of new prebiotics aims at non-digestible oligosaccharides—short-chain polysaccharides that consist of 2 to 20 saccharide units. Examples of these include inulin-type fructans, galactooligosaccharides (GOSs), isomaltooligosaccharides (IMOs), xylooligosaccharides (XOSs), soy oligosaccharides (SOSs), glucooligosaccharides, and lactosucrose. Prebiotics owe their derivation to the probiotic concept and were first developed to influence gut microbiota but without survival issues in the intervention used.

Prebiotics alter the indigenous flora components in a selective manner. The health outcomes are more or less similar to those of probiotics.

(4) Functions of Carbohydrates

① Digestible carbohydrates:

● Providing energy (4 kcal/g).

● Sparing protein from use as an energy source. When dietary carbohydrate intake is adequate to maintain blood glucose levels, protein is "spared" from use as energy.

● Preventing ketosis. When carbohydrate intake falls below this level (50 to 100 g/day), the release of the hormone insulin decreases, resulting in the release of a large amount of fatty acids from adipose tissue to provide energy for body cells. The subsequent incomplete breakdown of these fatty acids in the liver results in the formation of acidic compounds called ketone bodies, or keto-acids, and a condition called ketosis, or ketoacidosis.

● Detoxification, glucuronic acid, an oxidation product of glucose metabolism, is important in the detoxification of a number of intermediary products of normal metabolism and of certain drugs.

② Indigestible carbohydrates: Although the carbohydrates indigestible (e. g. Dietary fiber), they play the important role in maintaining the integrity of the gastrointestinal tract and overall health.

● Fiber helps prevent constipation and diverticular disease and enhances the management of body weight, blood glucose levels, and blood cholesterol levels.

● Prebiotics promote the growth of beneficial bacteria in the large intestine. Probiotic bacteria are thought to colonize in the large intestine and provide certain health benefits. For instance, probiotics may help prevent and treat diarrhea, prevent food allergies and colon cancer, and treat irritable bowel syndrome and inflammatory bowel disease.

(5) Carbohydrates Allowances

According to the latest version of DRIs for Chinese (DRIs 2013), the EAR of carbohydrate for Chinese adults is 120 g per day and the AMDR of carbohydrate is 50%—65% of total energy intake. The AI of dietary fiber for Chinese adults is 25—30 g per day.

(6) Sources of Food

Carbohydrates are found in a wide variety of foods. Foods such as table sugar, jam, jelly, fruit, fruit juices, soft drinks, baked potatoes, rice, pasta, cereals, and breads are predominantly carbohydrates. Other foods, such as dried beans, lentils, corn, peas, and dairy products (milk and yogurt), also are good sources of carbohydrate, although they contribute protein, and in some cases fat, to our diets as well.

5. 2. 3. 3　Lipids

Lipids include fat and lipoid. They serve multiple purposes in the diet. In addition to their high energy value, they contain essential fatty acids and act as carriers for the fat-soluble vitamins. That fat makes a meal more satisfying is due partially to its slow gastric emptying time and therefore its satiety value, and partially to the flavor it gives to other foods.

(1) Structure, Classification and Function of Lipids

Fats are a form of stored energy in animals as important as carbohydrates are in plants. Fat is also called triglyceride (TG) and is composed of 1 molecule glycerol and 3 molecule fatty acids through ester bond.

Triglycerides are esters of glycerol with three fatty acids. Triglycerides usually contain a mixture of two or three different fatty acids rather than three identical ones. The number 2 position on the triglyceride molecule is the central position and is occupied by different types of fatty acids depending on the origin of the fat. Seed fats, such as cottonseed oil, usually have unsaturated fatty acids (oleic or linoleic acids) in this position. Fats made up of different fatty acids have different properties and physiological functions.

Fatty acids, the type and configuration of the fatty acids in fats, are responsible for differences in flavor, texture, melting point, absorption, essential fatty acid activity, and other characteristics. Fatty acids vary in length from four to about 24 carbon atoms including, with few exceptions, only the even-numbered members of the series. They are referred to as short chain (less than 6 carbons), medium chain (8 to 12 carbons) and long chain (more than 12 carbons). Reference may also be made to extra long chain fatty acids, or those over 20 carbons.

Fatty acids are also classified as saturated or unsaturated, depending on the presence or absence of double bonds. A double bond occurs when two adjoining carbons each have one less hydrogen atom than they normally hold. Then a double bond between the two carbons satisfies the carbon valence of 4. Fatty acids, such as oleic, are called monounsaturated fatty acids (MUFA) because they contain one double bond, whereas linoleic, linolenic, and arachidonic acids, which contain two, three, and four double bonds respectively, are called polyunsaturated fatty acids (PUFA). The polyunsaturated fatty acids have been shown in certain instances to lower blood cholesterol level, whereas saturated fatty acids(SFA) tend to raise the serum cholesterol level. Saturated fatty acids, particularly the long chain fatty acids and their glycerides, have higher melting points and accordingly tend to be solid in form at room temperature. These fats are found in greater amounts in animal sources. Oils, for the most part, contain large amounts of unsaturated fatty acids, have lower melting points, and are mainly of vegetable origin. Coconut oil, however, is a notable exception because it is almost 90% saturated; short and medium chain acids account for its being oil. The fat of fish is always fluid at cold temperatures and is therefore called an oil fish fats can contain a higher proportion of polyunsaturated extra long chain fatty acids than do the meat or poultry fats. Animals, including humans, are metabolically able to increase or decrease the chain length of fatty acids by the addition or removal of two carbon fragments and can convert the saturated fatty acid stearic to the monounsaturated fatty acid oleic by removal of two hydrogens (Figure 5. 2).

Humans, however, cannot synthesize the polyunsaturated fatty acid, such as linoleic

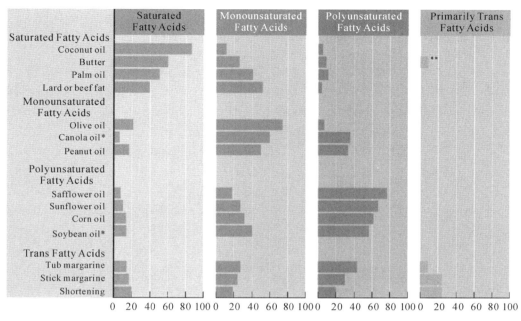

Figure 5. 2   Fatty Acid Composition of Common Fats and Oils (Expressed as % of All Fatty
Acids in the Product)

acid and a-linolenic acid; for this reason, linoleic acid and a-linolenic acid are considered to
be essential fatty acid (EFA). An EFA is one that is essential for normal nutrition and that
cannot be synthesized by the body from other substances. Derivatives of EFA,
eicosapentaenoic acid (EPA), docosahexaenoic acid (DHA) and arachidonic acid (AA),
play important roles in the development of brain and visual function, participate in the
regulation of immunity, inflammation, heart rate, blood coagulation and vasomotor in vivo,
and regulate blood lipids. Deficiency of EFA can cause skin eczema-like lesions, alopecia,
growth retardation of infants, and etc.

Trans-fatty acids: In nature, most double bonds are *cis*—meaning that the hydrogens
next to the double bonds are on the same side of the carbon chain. Only a few fatty acids
(notably a small percentage of those found in milk and meat products) naturally occur as
trans-fatty acids—meaning that the hydrogens next to the double bonds are on opposite sides
of the carbon chain (Figure 5.3). In the process of making margarine from vegetable oil by
hydrogenation, double bonds are formed from cis to trans. It comes from artificial butter,
cakes, biscuits, fried foods, cheese products, peanut butter and other foods. In the body,
trans-fatty acids behave more like saturated fats, increasing blood cholesterol and the risk of
heart disease.

Lipoid includes phospholipids (PL) and cholesterol, which are the important
components of biomembrane. Phospholipids, structural compounds found in cell
membranes, are essential components of certain enzyme systems and are involved in the
transport of lipids in the plasma and are a source of energy. Lecithins, phosphatidylcholine,

are the most abundant of the phospholipids in both tissues and foods where, because of their emulsifying properties, they serve as solubilizers and stabilizers.

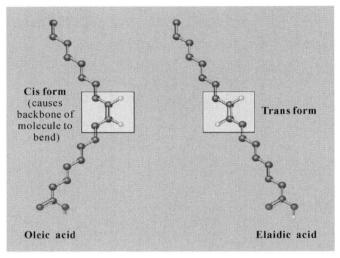

Figure 5. 3   *Cis*-and *Trans*-fatty Acids Compared

Cholesterol, an essential constituent of many animal cells, especially the myelin sheath around nerve fibers and in glandular tissues, is found in high concentration in the liver, where it is synthesized and stored. Egg yolks and brains are particularly rich sources of cholesterol in the diet. Other important food sources include butter, cream, cheese, heart, kidneys, liver, sweetbreads, lobster, shrimp, crab, and fish roe. The maintenance of a normal level of blood cholesterol is of great physiological importance. It is a precursor of vitamin D and closely related to the steroid hormones in the body, the corticoids, androgens, and estrogens. It should not therefore be considered an abnormal substance in the body but one that has vital functions to perform.

(2) Sources and Reference Intake of lipids

① Main food sources of lipids: Human dietary fat mainly comes from animal adipose tissue and meat as well as seeds of nuts and plants (Table 5. 4). Most animal fats contain 40%—60% SFA, 30%—50% MUFA and a small amount of PUFA. Most vegetable oils contain 10%—20% SFA and 80%—90% MUFA and PUFA.

Table 5. 4   **Fat Content in Common Foods (g/100g, edible part)**

Food	Fat Content	Food	Fat Content	Food	Fat Content
Pork (fat)	88. 6	Sesame paste	52. 7	Beijing Roast Duck	38. 4
Pine nut	70. 6	Braised Soy Sauce Pork	50. 4	Pork (fat and lean)	37. 0
Pork neck	60. 5	Bacon (raw)	48. 8	Eggpowder (whole egg)	36. 2

(**to be continued**)

continued

Food	Fat Content	Food	Fat Content	Food	Fat Content
Pork rib	59. 0	Potato chips (Fried)	48. 4	Bacon	36. 0
Walnut	58. 8	Sausage	40. 7	Broiler(fat)	35. 4
Egg yolk powder	55. 1	Chocolate	40. 1	Duck egg yolk	33. 8
Peanut butter	53. 0	Beef jerky	40. 0	Spring roll	33. 7

② Recommended intake of dietary fat: Due to the lack of research on average fat requirement, RNI can not be calculated. Therefore, the recommended intake of dietary fat and fatty acids is AI or AMDR, which is the ideal range of nutrients intake. The upper limit is U-AMDR (Table 5. 5).

Table 5. 5 Reference Intakes of Dietary Fats and Fatty Acids for Chinese Residents

Population(year)	Total fat	SFA	n-6 PUFA	(LA)	n-3 PUFA	(ALA)	EPA+DHA	
	AMDR /%E	U-AMDR /%E	AI /%E	AMDR /%E	AI /%E	AMDR /%E	AI/mg	AMDR/g
0—	48(AI)	—	7. 3(ARA 150 mg)	—	0. 87	—	100(DHA)	—
0. 5—	40(AI)	—	6. 0	—	0. 66	—	100(DHA)	—
1—	35(AI)	—	4. 0	—	0. 60	—	100(DHA)	—
4—	20~30	<8	4. 0	—	0. 60	—	—	—
7—	20~30	<8	4. 0	—	0. 60	—	—	—
18—	20~30	<10	4. 0	2. 5—9. 0	0. 60	0. 5—2. 0	—	0. 25~3. 0
≥60	20~30	<10	4. 0	2. 5—9. 0	0. 60	0. 5—2. 0	—	0. 25~3. 0
Pregnant and lactating women	20~30	<10	4. 0	2. 5—9. 0	0. 60	0. 5—2. 0	250 (DHA 200)	—

5. 2. 3. 4 Energy

Proteins, fats and carbohydrates can produce energy after oxidation *in vivo* to meet the energy required for life activities. One g carbohydrate can produce 16. 8 kJ (4 kal) energy, 1 g fat can produce 37. 8 kJ (9 kal) energy, and 1 g protein can produce 16. 8 kJ (4 kal) energy. The three substances mentioned above are also called energy-yielding nutrients, and the energy value produced is also called heat production coefficient.

Proteins, fats and carbohydrates are also called energy-yielding nutrients, and the energy value produced is also called heat production coefficient. Table 5. 5 gives the DRIs of dietary fats and fatty acids for Chinese residents.

(1) Energy Requirement of the Human Body

The body's need for energy is consistent with its consumption. Energy consumption includes three aspects: basic metabolism, labor and activity needs, and specific dynamic action (Figure 5. 4). There is also energy required for growth and development during the growth period.

① Basic metabolism: It is the energy consumption necessary to maintain the basic life activities of human body. Fasting 12—14 hours, awakening and sleeping, room temperature kept 20—25℃, no physical activity and nervous thinking activity, systemic muscle relaxation and digestive system in a static state were measured. In fact, the body is in the state of maintaining the most basic life activities, that is, energy consumption for maintaining the most basic life activities such as body temperature, heartbeat, breathing, basic functions of organs, tissues and cells. The level of basal metabolism is expressed by basal metabolic rate (BMR), which refers to the energy consumed by human basal metabolism per unit time. BMR can be expressed in kJ/(m^2 • h), kJ/(kg • h), and MJ/d.

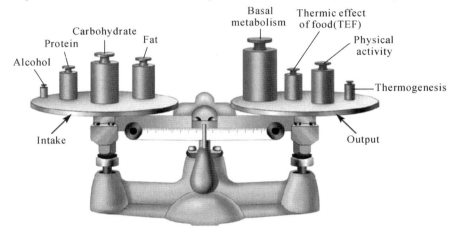

Figure 5. 4　　Major Components of Energy Intake and Expenditure

Factors affecting basal metabolic rate:

• Body shape and constitution, body shape affect body surface area. The larger the body surface area, the greater the body heat dissipation to the external environment, and the higher the basic metabolism. The lean constitution of the body or lean body mass is an active metabolic tissue, and its energy consumption is significantly higher than that of adipose tissue. Slender people have higher basal metabolic rate than shorter people.

• Age, with the increase of age, the basal metabolic rate decreases gradually.

• Gender, the proportion of lean body mass in women is lower than that in men, and the proportion of fat is higher than that in men, so the basal metabolic rate is lower than that in men. During pregnancy or lactation, women need to synthesize new tissues and increase their basal metabolic rate.

• Endocrine, many hormones play a regulatory role in cell metabolism, when the glands (such as thyroid, adrenal) secrete abnormally, it can affect the basic metabolic rate.

• Stress state, all stress states, such as fever, trauma, psychological stress, can increase the basic metabolism. In addition, climate, race, sleep, mood and other factors may also affect basal metabolism.

② Energy consumption of physical activities: In addition to basic metabolism, the energy expended by physical activity is an important part of the total energy expenditure of the human body. The energy consumed by daily activities depends mainly on the intensity and duration of physical activities. Physical activities are generally divided into occupational activities, social activities and leisure activities, ect. Among them, occupational activities have the largest difference in energy consumption. The difference of human energy requirement is mainly due to the difference of physical activity. Approximate energy costs of various activities are showed as follow (Table 5. 6).

Table 5. 6　Approximate Energy Costs of Various Activities

Activity	Kcal/kg per Hour	Activity	Kcal/kg per Hour	Activity	Kcal/kg per Hour
Aerobics-heavy	8. 0	Dressing/showering	1. 6	Running or jogging (10 mph)	13. 2
Aerobics-medium	5. 0	Driving	1. 7	Downhill skiing (10 mph)	8. 8
Aerobics-light	3. 0	Eating(sitting)	1. 4	Sleeping	1. 2
Backpacking	9. 0	Food shopping	3. 6	Swimming (0. 25 mph)	4. 4
Basketball-vigorous	10. 0	Football-touch	7. 0	Tennis	6. 1
Cycling(5. 5 mph)	3. 0	Golf	3. 6	Volleyball	5. 1
Bowling	3. 9	Horseback riding	5. 1	Walking (2. 5 mph)	3. 0
Calisthenics-heavy	8. 0	Jogging-medium	9. 0	Walking (3. 75 mph)	4. 4
Calisthenics-light	4. 0	Ice skating(10 mph)	5. 8	Water skiing	7. 0
Canoeing (2. 5 mph)	3. 3	Jogging-slow	7. 0	Weight lifting-heavy	9. 0
Cleaning (female)	3. 7	Lying-at ease	1. 3	Weight lifting-light	4. 0
Cleaning (male)	3. 5	Racquetball-social	8. 0	Window cleaning	3. 5
Cooking	2. 8	Roller skating	5. 1	Writing (sitting)	1. 7
Cycling (13 mph)	9. 7				

③ Specific dynamic action (SDA): SDA is also known as thermic effect of food, refers to the additional energy consumption caused by the human body in the process of ingestion. This is the energy consumed in a series of digestion, absorption, synthesis activities and the mutual transformation between nutrients and nutrient metabolites after ingestion. Eating different foods increases energy expenditure differently, protein has the greatest special dynamic effect, equivalent to 30% of its own production capacity, carbohydrate 5%—6%, fat 4%—5%. In general, adults consume a mixed diet, with additional energy expenditure due to the special dynamic effect of food, which is equivalent to 10% of their basal metabolism.

④ Growth and development: The growth and development of infants, children and adolescents need energy, mainly including the energy needed to form new tissues for the growth and development of the body, and the energy needed for metabolism of newly generated tissues. Infant needs about 20.9 kJ (5 kcal) energy for every 1 g weight gain. The growth and development of uterus, breast, placenta, fetus and body fat reserve of pregnant women need energy. The synthesis and secretion of milk by lactating mothers also need additional energy.

(2) Energy Sources and Reference Intake

The energy supply of the three major energy-yielding nutrients mentioned above should be appropriately proportioned. The reasonable energy ratio is suggested by CNS as follows: carbohydrate accounts for 50%—65%, fat accounts for 20%—30%, protein accounts for 10%—15%.

(3) Energy Balance

Healthy adults should always keep a balance energy intake and energy expenditure. Too little energy intake leads to weight loss; excessive intake leads to overweight or obesity. Body mass index, waist circumference, waist-to-hip ratio and body fat content are commonly indicators used to determine whether energy intake meets the needs of the body.

5.2.3.5　Vitamins

Vitamins are organic compounds that are essential micronutrients that the body needs in small quantities for the proper functioning of its metabolism. Vitamins do not provide energy. They cannot be synthesized in the body, either at all or not in sufficient quantities, and therefore must be obtained through the diet.

Vitamins are classified as fat-soluble vitamins and water-soluble vitamins. In humans there are 13 vitamins: 4 fat-soluble vitamins (A, D, E, and K) and 9 water-soluble vitamins (8 B vitamins and vitamin C). Water-soluble vitamins dissolve easily in water and, in general, are readily excreted from the body, to the degree that urinary output is a strong predictor of vitamin status. Because they are not as readily stored, more consistent intake is important. Fat-soluble vitamins can be dissolved in organic solvent and fat. They are absorbed through the intestinal tract with the help of lipids (fats). Over consumption of vitamins A and D can accumulate in the body, which can result in hypervitaminosis.

(1) Vitamin A

Vitamin A was the first fat-soluble vitamin to be recognized. Three different forms of vitamin A are active in the body: retinol, retinal, and retinoic acid. Collectively known as retinoids, these compounds are commonly found in foods derived from animals, also called preformed vitamin A. Foods derived from plants provide carotenoids. There are more than 700 carotenoids in plant foods, some of which (about 10%) can be converted into vitamin A. They are called provitamin A carotenoids, such as α-carotene, β-carotene, γ-carotene. The most studied provitamin A carotenoids is β-carotene, which can be converted into retinol in the intestine and liver.

① Functions of vitamin A.

• Components of visual pigments: Vitamin A plays a crucial role in vision as part of the compound rhodopsin in the rod cell of the retina. When light hits the retina, rhodopsin separates, changes shape, and sends a nerve impulse to the brain. When vitamin A is inadequate, the lack of rhodopsin makes it difficult to see in dim light;

• Regulation of gene expression: Retinoic acid (RA) and its isomers (all-trans-RA and 9-cis-RA) act as hormones to affect gene expression and thereby influence numerous physiological processes. All-trans-RA and 9-cis-RA are transported to the nucleus of the cell bound to cytoplasmic retinoic acid-binding proteins (CRABP). Within the nucleus, RA binds to retinoic acid receptor proteins. Specifically, all-trans-RA binds to retinoic acid receptors (RAR) and 9-cis-RA binds to retinoid X receptors (RXR), retinoic acid plays a major role in cellular differentiation;

• Maintenance of healthy epithelial tissue: It is the protective tissue that body surfaces, i. e. the skin and the inner mucous membranes in the respiratory tract, gastrointestinal tract, and genitourinary tract. These tissues are the primary barrier to infections. Retinoic acid maintains skin health by activating genes that cause immature skin cells to develop into mature epidermal cells;

• Maintenance of normal immune function: Vitamin A influences the immune system in important ways. It helps maintain the health of epithelial tissues. Vitamin A also supports the generation of T-lymphocytes;

• Growth and development: Both vitamin A excess and deficiency are known to cause birth defects. Retinol and RA are essential for embryonic development. During fetal development, RA functions in limb development and formation of the heart, eyes, and ears. Additionally, RA has been found to regulate expression of the gene for growth hormone.

② Vitamin A deficiency.

Vitamin A status depends mostly on the adequacy of vitamin A stores, 90% of which are in the liver. Vitamin A status also depends on a person's protein status because retinol-binding protein serves as the vitamin's transport carrier inside the body. If a person were to stop taking vitamin A-containing foods, deficiency symptoms would not begin to appear until after stores were depleted—one to two years for a healthy adult but much sooner for a growing child. Then the consequences would be profound and severe.

Vitamin A deficiency is a major nutrition problem in many developing countries. An estimated 250 million children worldwide have some degree of vitamin A deficiency and thus are vulnerable to infectious diseases and blindness. With an estimated 250,000 to 500,000 children becoming blind annually worldwide, vitamin A deficiency constitutes the leading preventable cause of blindness in low-and middle-income nations. About half of them dying within a year of losing their sight. Routine vitamin A supplementation and food fortification can be a life-saving intervention.

• Vitamin A deficiency and vision: The earliest symptom of vitamin A deficiency is impaired dark adaptation known as night blindness. The next clinical stage is the occurrence of abnormal changes in the conjunctiva, manifested by the presence of Bitot's spots. Severe or prolonged vitamin A deficiency eventually results in a condition called xerophthalmia, characterized by changes in the cells of the cornea that ultimately result in corneal ulcers, scarring, and blindness.

● Vitamin A deficiency and infectious disease: Vitamin A deficiency can be considered a nutritionally acquired immunodeficiency disease. Even children who are only mildly deficient in vitamin A have a higher incidence of respiratory disease and diarrhea as well as a higher rate of mortality from infectious disease compared to children who consume sufficient vitamin A.

● Vitamin A deficiency and keratinization: Elsewhere in the body, vitamin A deficiency affects other surfaces. On the body's outer surface, the epithelial cells change shape and begin to secrete the protein keratin. The skin becomes dry, rough, and scaly as lumps of keratin accumulate (keratinization). Without vitamin A, the goblet cells in the GI tract diminish in number and activity, limiting the secretion of mucus. With less mucus, normal digestion and absorption of nutrients falter, and this worsens malnutrition by limiting the absorption of nutrients in the diet. Similar changes in the cells of other epithelial tissues weaken defenses, making infections of the respiratory tract, the GI tract, the urinary tract, and inner ear likely.

● Vitamin A deficiency and growth retardation: Vitamin A deficiency is associated with reduced appetite, weight loss and failure to grow adequately.

③ Hypervitaminosis A: The condition caused by vitamin A toxicity is called hypervitaminosis A. It is caused by overconsumption of preformed vitamin A, not carotenoids. Preformed vitamin A is rapidly absorbed and slowly cleared from the body. Therefore, toxicity from preformed vitamin A may result acutely from high-dose exposure over a short period of time or chronically from a much lower intake. Acute vitamin A toxicity is relatively rare, and symptoms include nausea, headache, fatigue, loss of appetite, dizziness, dry skin, desquamation, and cerebral edema. Signs of chronic toxicity include dry itchy skin, desquamation, loss of appetite, headache, cerebral edema, and bone and joint pain. Symptoms of vitamin A toxicity in infants include bulging fontanels. Severe cases of hypervitaminosis A may result in liver damage, hemorrhage, and coma. Generally, signs of toxicity are associated with long-term consumption of vitamin A in excess of ten times the RDA (8,000 to 10,000 mcg/day or 25,000 to 33,000 IU/day).

④ Dietary reference intakes: The RDA of the United States for men and women is 900 and 700 μg retinol activity equivalents (RAE)/day, respectively. In China, the RNI of CNS about vitamin A for men and women is 800 and 700 μg RAE/day, respectively. The UL for both Chinese and American adults is 3,000 μg/day of preformed vitamin A.

⑤ Food Sources: There are two main dietary sources of vitamin A.

Retinoids: Preformed vitamin A found in foods of animal origin, such as liver, cod liver oil, fish roe, whole milk, butter, egg.

Carotenoids: Found in foods of plant origin in the form of common plant pigments, such as green leafy, red, yellow-orange pigment. Some of them can be converted into vitamin A in the body, they are called provitamin A carotenoids, Such as α-carotene, β-carotene, γ-carotene and β-cryptoxanthin.

(2) Vitamin D

There are two major compounds with vitamin D activity: vitamin D_3 (cholecalciferol) and vitamin D_2 (ergocalciferol). Vitamin D_3 can be synthesized by humans in the skin upon exposure to ultraviolet-B (UV-B) radiation from sunlight, or it can be obtained from the diet. Plants synthesize ergosterol, which is converted to vitamin D_2 (ergocalciferol) by ultraviolet light. When exposure to UVB radiation is insufficient for the synthesis of adequate amounts of vitamin D_3 in the skin, adequate intake of vitamin D from the diet is essential for health.

Vitamin D itself is biologically inactive, and it must be metabolized to its biologically active form. After it is consumed in the diet or synthesized in the epidermis of skin, vitamin D enters the circulation and is transported to the liver. In the liver, vitamin D is hydroxylated to form 25-hydroxyvitamin D [25(OH)D], the major circulating form of vitamin D. Increased exposure to sunlight or increased dietary intake of vitamin D increases serum levels of 25(OH)D, making the serum 25(OH)D concentration a useful indicator of vitamin D nutritional status. In the kidney, the 25(OH)D_3-1-hydroxylase enzyme catalyzes a second hydroxylation of 25 (OH) D, resulting in the formation of 1alpha, 25-dihydroxyvitamin D [1, 25 (OH)$_2$D]—the most potent form of vitamin D. Most of the physiological effects of vitamin D in the body are related to the activity of 1,25(OH)2D.

① Functions of vitamin D.

• Maintenance of calcium balance via vitamin D endocrine system: Maintenance of serum calcium levels is vital for normal functioning of the nervous system, bone growth and maintenance of bone density. Vitamin D is essential for the efficient utilization of calcium by the body. The parathyroid glands sense serum calcium levels and secrete parathyroid hormone (PTH) if calcium levels drop too low. Elevations in PTH increase the activity of the 25 (OH) D_3-1-hydroxylase enzyme in the kidney, resulting in increased production of 1,25(OH)$_2$D. Increasing 1,25(OH)$_2$D production results in changes in gene expression that normalize serum calcium by: a. increasing the intestinal absorption of dietary calcium; b. increasing the reabsorption of calcium filtered by the kidneys; c. mobilizing calcium from bone when there is insufficient dietary calcium to maintain normal serum calcium levels. Parathyroid hormone and 1,25(OH)$_2$D are required for these latter two effects.

• Regulation of cell differentiation: The active form of vitamin D, 1, 25 (OH)$_2$D, inhibits proliferation and stimulates the differentiation of cells. Laboratory studies also show that vitamin D keeps cancer cells from growing and dividing.

● Vitamin D and immunity: Vitamin D in the form of $1,25(OH)_2D$ is a potent immune system modulator. There is considerable scientific evidence that $1,25(OH)_2D$ has a variety of effects on immune system function, which may enhance innate immunity and inhibit the development of autoimmunity.

② Vitamin D deficiency: Vitamin D deficiency may lead to decreased calcium absorption, secondary hyperparathyroidism, rickets in children, osteomalacia and osteoporosis in adults and elderly, muscle weakness and pain. Vitamin D deficiency may also increase the risk of a host of chronic diseases, such as osteoporosis, heart disease, some cancers, and multiple sclerosis, as well as infectious diseases, such as tuberculosisand even the seasonal flu.

③ Hypervitaminosis D: Excessive intake of vitamin D is toxic. Usually, toxicity is not manifest except after huge doses, which result in calcification of soft tissues due to persistent hypercalcemia. In adults, hypercalcemia has been accompanied by such symptoms as anorexia, nausea, weight loss, polyuria, constipation, and azotemia. Similar symptoms are seen in infants, and in certain rare severe forms, mental retardation also occurs.

④ Dietary reference intakes and the sources.

DRIs: The CNS recommends AI of vitamin D to 10 μg (400 IU) for everyone ages 0—65, and 15 μg (600 IU) for elderly older than age 65. The UL is 50 μg (2,000 IU) for everyone ages 11 years old and above; the National Institute of Medicine of the United States increased the RDA of vitamin D to 600 international units (IU) for everyone ages 1—70, and raised it to 800 IU for adults older than age 70 to optimize bone health. The safe upper limit was also raised to 4,000 IU.

Sources of vitamin D: Vitamin D activity could be produced by irradiation. It is obvious that an adequate natural source of ultraviolet light is impossible in northern climates during the winter months. For this reason, some other source of vitamin D is needed. The natural distribution of vitamin D in common foods is limited, but only in significant amounts in fatty fish, cream, butter, eggs, and liver. Consequently, we have come to depend on fortified foods, fish-liver oil, other vitamin D supplements, or concentrates for preventive and therapeutic use.

(3)Vitamin E

Vitamin E is a family of 8 naturally occurring compounds 4 tocopherols (alpha, beta, gamma, delta) and 4 tocotrienols (alpha, beta, gamma, delta)—with widely varying degrees of biological activity. Vitamin E has a long carbon chain tail attached to a ringed structure. This tail exists in many possible isomer forms. The most active form of the vitamin E is alpha tocopherol (Figure 5.5). This is the form found in some foods and in varying amounts in vitamin supplements.

① Functions of vitamin E: Vitamin E is a fat-soluble antioxidant and one of the body's primary defenders against the adverse effects of free radicals. Its main action is to stop the chain reaction of free radicals from producing more free radicals. In doing so, vitamin E

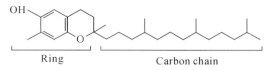

Vitamin E (alpha tocopherol)

Figure 5. 5   Structure of Alpha Tocopherol

protects the vulnerable components of the cells and their membranes from destruction. Most notably, vitamin E prevents the oxidation of the polyunsaturated fatty acids, but it protects other lipids and related compounds (for example, vitamin A) as well.

② Human requirement: The RDA for vitamin E is 15 mg/day of alpha-tocopherol for both men and women. The recommendation is based on the amount of vitamin E needed to prevent the breakdown of red blood cell membrane, a process called hemolysis.

Adults consume, on average, only two-thirds of the RDA for vitamin E each day. In addition to an increased intake of vitamin Erich foods, the daily consumption of a ready-to-eat breakfast cereal containing vitamin E or the use of a supplement can close the gap between typical vitamin E intakes and needs.

Food and supplement labels often report vitamin E activity in IUs. When converting IUs of vitamin E in synthetic form (as in most supplements) to milligrams, 1 IU equals about 0. 45 mg. If the vitamin E is from a natural source, 1 IU equals 0. 67 mg because the natural form of vitamin E is more potent than the synthetic form.

③ Food sources: Vitamin E is widespread in foods. Much of the vitamin E in the diet comes from vegetable oils and products made from them, such as margarine and salad dressings. Wheat germ oil is especially rich in vitamin E. Because vitamin E is readily destroyed by heat and oxidation, fresh foods are preferable sources. Most processed and convenience foods do not contribute enough vitamin E to ensure an adequate intake.

④ Vitamin E deficiency: As a fat-soluble vitamin, absorption of vitamin E relies on normal digestion and absorption of dietary fat. Deficiency can occur in children or adults who are unable to absorb or utilize vitamin E adequately. Without vitamin E, the red blood cells break and spill their contents, probably because of oxidation of the polyunsaturated fatty acids in their membranes. This classic sign of vitamin E deficiency, known as erythrocyte hemolysis, is seen in premature infants born before the transfer of vitamin E from the mother to the infant that takes place in the last weeks of pregnancy. Vitamin E treatment corrects hemolytic anemia. Prolonged vitamin E deficiency, as can occur with some genetic disorders, also causes neuromuscular dysfunction. Common symptoms include loss of muscle coordination and reflexes and impaired vision and speech. Vitamin E treatment helps to correct these neurological symptoms of vitamin E deficiency.

⑤ Vitamin E toxicity: Vitamin E supplement has risen in recent years as its protective actions against chronic diseases have been recognized. Fortunately, the liver carefully regulates vitamin E concentrations. Toxicity is rare, and vitamin E appears safe across a broad range of intakes. The UL for vitamin E (1,000 milligrams) is more than 65 times greater than the recommended intake for adults (15 milligrams). Extremely high doses of vitamin E may interfere with the blood-clotting action of vitamin K and enhance the effects of drugs used to oppose blood clotting, causing hemorrhage.

(4) Vitamin K

The family of compounds known as vitamin K, or the quinones, include phylloquinones (vitamin K1) from plants and menaquinones (vitamin K2) found in fish oils and meats. Menaquinones also are synthesized by bacteria in the human colon. A synthetic compound, called menadione, can be converted to menaquinone in body tissues. Phylloquinone, the main dietary form of the vitamin K, is the most biologically active form.

① Functions of vitamin K: More than a dozen different proteins and the mineral calcium are involved in making a blood clot. Vitamin K is essential for the activation of several of these proteins, among them prothrombin, made by the liver as a precursor of the protein thrombin. When any of the blood-clotting factors is lacking, it may cause hemorrhagic disease. If an artery or vein is cut or broken, bleeding goes unchecked. Of course, this is not to say that hemorrhaging is always caused by vitamin K deficiency. Another cause is the genetic disorder hemophilia, which is neither caused nor cured by vitamin K.

Vitamin K also participates in the metabolism of bone proteins, most notably osteocalcin. Without vitamin K, osteocalcin cannot bind to the minerals that normally form bones, resulting in low bone density. An adequate intake of vitamin K helps to decrease bone turnover and protect against fractures. The effectiveness of vitamin K supplements on bone health is inconclusive.

Vitamin K is historically known for its role in blood clotting, and more recently for its participation in bone building, but researchers continue to discover proteins needing vitamin K's assistance. These proteins have been identified in the plaques of atherosclerosis, the kidneys, and the nervous system.

② Human requirement: Vitamin K requirement is believed to be very small and easily met by bacterial synthesis and dietary intake. The daily requirement for man appears to be about 0.03 mg/kg for the adult. Newborn infants tend to be deficient in vitamin K due to minimal stores of prothrombin at birth and lack of an established intestinal flora. Soon after birth, all infants or those at increased risk should receive a single intramuscular dose of a vitamin K preparation (0.1—0.2 mg of menadione sodium bisulphite or 0.5 mg of vitamin K1) by way of prophylaxis.

③ Food sources: Vitamin K occurs in three chemical forms.

Phylloquinone: Most of our dietary intake comes from this form, which occurs in green leafy vegetables and to a lesser extent in a wide range of foods including fruits, cereal, meat, dairy produce and vegetable oils.

Menaquinones: These are produced by bacteria, particularly those found in the gut.

Menadione: This is synthetic water-soluble from which is rarely used because it can cause jaundice.

④ Vitamin K deficiency: A primary deficiency of vitamin K is rare, but a secondary deficiency may occur in two circumstances. First, whenever fat absorption falters, as occurs when bile production fails, vitamin K absorption diminishes. Second, some drugs disrupt vitamin K's synthesis and action in the body: antibiotics kill the vitamin K-producing bacteria in the intestine, and anticoagulant drugs interfere with vitamin K metabolism and activity. Excessive bleeding due to vitamin K deficiency can be fatal. Newborn infants present a unique case of vitamin K nutrition because they are born with a sterile intestinal tract, and the vitamin K-producing bacteria take weeks to establish themselves. Furthermore, vitamin K is minimally transported across the placenta and its concentration in breast milk is low. At the same time, plasma prothrombin concentrations are low, which reduces the likelihood of fatal blood clotting during the stress of birth.

⑤ Vitamin K toxicity: Vitamin K Toxicity is not common, and no adverse effects have been reported with high intakes of vitamin K. Therefore, a UL has not been established. High doses of vitamin K can reduce the effectiveness of anticoagulant drugs used to prevent blood clotting. People taking these drugs can continue eating their usual diets. Their blood clotting times should be monitored closely and drug dosages adjusted accordingly.

(5) Vitamin C

Vitamin C exists naturally in foods in two forms, namely the reduced form (usually designated as ascorbic acid) and the oxidized form (dehydroascorbic acid). Both forms are physiologically active and are found in body tissues. Further oxidation of dehydroascorbic acid to diketogulonic acid results in irreversible inactivation of the vitamin. Ascorbic acid in fruits and vegetables and the synthetic form are equally well utilized.

Of all the vitamins, ascorbic acid is unstable under heat, oxidation, drying, and storage. Alkalinity, even to a slight degree, is distinctly destructive to this vitamin. Acidic fruits and vegetables lose much less ascorbic acid when heated than non-acidic foods. Vitamin C is extremely soluble in water and dissolves out of some vegetables during the first few minutes of the cooking process.

① Functions of vitamin C: Vitamin C has complex functional roles in the body, including collagen synthesis, carnitine synthesis, tyrosine synthesis and catabolism, and neurotransmitter synthesis. These above-various reactions need a mineral (copper or iron) cofactor, Vitamin C acts as a reducing agent (antioxidant) to maintain the iron and copper atoms in the metalloenzyme in a reduced state. In addition, Vitamin C also has the functions of antioxidant, anti-free radicals, and inhibits the formation of tyrosinase.

② Human requirement: The RNI of Vitamin C is 100 mg per day for adults formulated by CNS. UL for Vitamin C is 2,000 mg per day for adults. High levels of vitamin C in the body help prevent coronary heart disease, stroke, cancer and other diseases. The PI-NCD value of vitamin C in adults is 200 mg. It is generally difficult to exceed the standard only through food intake.

③ Food sources: The commonly used fruits and vegetables are the richest sources of Vitamin C, with citrus fruits, strawberries, cantaloupe, and a number of raw, leafy vegetables topping the list. Many factors affect the Vitamin C content of fruits and vegetables: variety, maturity, length of storage, part of the plant, and seasonal and geographical factors.

④ Lack or excess: Vitamin C deficiency occurs when the vitamin C storage in the body is reduced with the reduced dietary intake or increased body need and no replenishment in time. If the amount of storage in the body is less than 300 mg, it will result in scurvy. The clinical manifestations are as follows:

Prodromal symptoms: Patients generally have malaise and loss of appetite. In the early stage of adulthood, it will also cause gingival swelling, sometimes infections and inflammation. Deficiency in infants and young children may cause growth retardation, irritability and indigestion.

Bleeding: Punctiform hemorrhage of whole body, initially confined around the hair follicles and gums, further may occur in subcutaneous tissue, muscles, joints and tendon sheath bleeding, and even form hematoma or ecchymosis.

Gingivitis: Hemorrhage and looseness can be seen in the gums, especially at the tip of the gums.

Osteoporosis: Collagen synthesis disorders, and poor bone mineral formation leads to osteoporosis.

Vitamin C is a water-soluble vitamin, if the excess, the unabsorbed ones in the blood will rapidly excrete in the urine, so it exhibits remarkably low acute toxicity. More than two to three grams may cause indigestion, particularly when taken on an empty stomach. Other symptoms for large doses include nausea, abdominal cramps and diarrhea. These effects are attributed to the osmotic effect of unabsorbed vitamin C passing through the intestine.

(6) Thiamin

Thiamin or vitamin B_1 is a water-soluble vitamin of the B complex. It is a colorless organosulfur compound with a chemical formula $C_{12}H_{17}N_4O_S$. Its structure consists of aminopyrimidine and a thiazole ring linked by a methylene bridge. Thiamine is soluble in water, methanol, and glycerol and practically insoluble in less polar organic solvents. It is stable at acidic pH, but is unstable in alkaline solutions.

① Functions of thiamin: Thiamin plays essential coenzyme and non-coenzyme roles in the body, including energy transformation, synthesis of pentoses and nicotinamide adenine dinucleotide phosphate (NADPH) and membrane and nerve conduction.

Thiamin is essential for energy metabolism in the human body, especially for sugar metabolism. Therefore, the amount of thiamin required by the human body is usually related to the caloric intake. When the body's energy is mainly derived from sugar, thiamin is most needed.

② Human requirement: The RNI for thiamin of the CNS is 1 4 mg per day for men and 1. 2 mg per day for women. Recommendations of thiamin for pregnant women and breastfeeding mother is 1. 5,1. 8 mg per day, respectively.

③ Food sources: Thiamin is widely distributed in a large variety of animal foods and vegetables; enrichment of bread and cereals was instigated to make it easier for the average person to meet his requirement economically. Dry yeast and wheat germ are the richest natural sources of thiamin, but they are eaten only in relatively small amounts. Except for pork, which is outstanding, muscle meats contain less than the organs, such as liver, heart, and kidney. Fruits in general are poor sources of this vitamin.

④ Lack or excess: Thiamin deficiency generally affects the neural, cardiac, and gastrointestinal functions, and the symptoms of beriberi include peripheral neuropathy and weakness, muscle pain and tenderness, enlargement of the heart, difficulty breathing, edema, anorexia, weight loss, poor memory, and confusion. Thiamine deficiency is a medical condition of low levels of thiamine (vitamin B1). A severe and chronic form is known as beriberi. Beriberi presents three types, including dry beriberi, wet beriberi and infantile beriberi. In dry beriberi, the main symptoms are muscle weakness and wasting, especially in the lower extremities, and peripheral neuropathy. In wet beriberi, the cardiovascular system is affected. The main symptoms are cardiomegaly, rapid heart beat, right-side heart failure. Infantile beriberi is associated with anorexia, vomiting, lactic acidosis, altered heart rate, and cardiomegaly.

Thiamin generally does not cause excessive poisoning. It may cause headache, convulsions and arrhythmia when taking a dose more than 100 times of RNI during a short period of time.

(7) Riboflavin

Riboflavin, also known as vitamin B2 is the central component of the cofactors riboflavin mononucleotide (FMN) and flavin adenine dinucleotide (FAD), and is therefore required by all flavoproteins. The name "riboflavin" comes from "ribose" and "flavin", the ring-moiety which imparts the yellow color to the oxidized molecule. The reduced form, which occurs in metabolism along with the oxidized form, is colorless. Riboflavin is stable to ordinary cooking processes but unstable in alkaline solutions.

① Functions of riboflavin: Riboflavin serves as a co-enzyme in oxidation-reduction reactions within the energy-producing metabolic pathways of carbohydrates and fat. Deficiency of riboflavin damages some types of tissues more than others. Fissures on the lips and at the corners of the mouth and scaly, sometimes greasy dermatitis around the nose are characteristic of riboflavin deficiency in humans. Anemia has been observed in some studies. Ocular symptoms appear on a low riboflavin diet and may precede all other manifestations. Eye strain and fatigue, itching and burning, sensitivity to light, and frontal headaches are the most frequent complaints.

② Human requirement: The RNI of riboflavin is 1. 4 mg per day for men and 1. 2 mg per day for women announced by CNS. Riboflavin intake should be increased when energy requirement is increased or accelerated.

③ Food sources: Riboflavin is widely distributed in animal and vegetable foods but only in small amounts in most of them. Meats, milk, and green leafy vegetables are the outstanding food sources. An average person is not likely to get an optimum amount of riboflavin unless he consumes a generous amount of milk.

④ Lack or excess: Riboflavin deficiency (also called ariboflavinosis) results in stomatitis including painful red tongue with sore throat, chapped and fissured lips (cheilosis), and inflammation of the corners of the mouth (angular stomatitis). Deficiency of riboflavin during pregnancy can result in birth defects including congenital heart defects and limb deformities. In humans, there is no evidence for riboflavin toxicity produced by excessive intakes.

(8) Niacin

Niacin (also known as vitamin B3, nicotinic acid, or less commonly vitamin PP) is an organic compound with the formula $C_6H_5NO_2$. This colorless, water-soluble solid is a derivative of pyridine, with a carboxyl group (COOH) at the 3-position. Other forms of vitamin B3 include the corresponding amide, nicotinamide ("niacinamide"), where the carboxyl group has been replaced by a carboxamide group, as well as more complex amides and a variety of esters. The amino acid tryptophan can be converted to niacin in the body. It has been found that approximately 60 mg of tryptophan are equivalent to 1 mg of niacin. Animal and vegetable proteins contain about 1.4% and 1% of tryptophan, respectively. Total niacin equals the preformed niacin plus the niacin available from protein. Niacin equivalent (NE) is equal to 1 mg of niacin or 60 mg of dietary tryptophan.

① Functions of niacin: One of the main functions of niacin, along with the other B vitamins, is to convert food to fuel that the body can use. The B vitamins also help metabolize fats and proteins. Niacin helps keep the skin, hair, eyes and liver healthy and is necessary to keep the nervous system functioning properly.

② Human requirement: The RNI of CNS for niacin is 15 mg niacin equivalence (NE) per day for men and 12 mg NE per day for women.

③ Food sources: In general, meat, poultry, and fish are better sources of niacin than plant products. Whole grain and enriched products also make a contribution. A bound form of niacin, that is, niacytin, in wheat, corn, and rye bran is practically unavailable to humans, unless released by the method of preparation, for example, lime-treated corn. Fruits and vegetables (other than mushrooms and legumes) are insignificant sources of niacin.

④ Lack or excess: Early signs of niacin deficiency are nonspecific and include lassitude, anorexia, weakness, mild digestive disturbances, and emotional changes such as anxiety, irritability, and depression.

Insufficient niacin in the diet can cause nausea, skin and mouth lesions, anemia, headaches, and tiredness. The lack of niacin may also be observed in pandemic deficiency diseases, which are caused by a lack of five crucial vitamins (niacin, vitamin C, thiamin, vitamin D, and vitamin A) and are usually found in areas of widespread poverty and malnutrition. Chronic Niacin deficiency leads to a disease called pellagra, which are characterized by the four "D's"—Dirarrhea, Dermatitis, Dementia and Death.

The most common adverse effects of niacin at relatively low doses (50—500 mg) are flushing (e. g. warmth, redness, itching or tingling), headache, abdominal pain, diarrhea, dyspepsia, nausea, vomiting, rhinitis, pruritus and rash. The acute adverse effects of high-dose niacin therapy (1—3 g/day)—which is commonly used in the treatment of hyperlipidemias—further include hypotension, fatigue, glucose intolerance and insulin resistance, heartburn, blurred or impaired vision, and macular edema.

(9) Vitamin B6

Vitamin B6 includes three naturally occurring forms, pyridoxine, pyridoxal and pyridoxamine, which are similar in property and all have vitamin B6 activity. The basic structure of vitamin B6 is 3-methyl-3-hydroxy-5-methylpyridine, which are soluble in water and ethanol, slightly soluble in organic solvents, stable under air and acidic conditions, and easily destroyed under alkaline conditions. Various forms are sensitive to light.

① Functions of vitamin B6: The plasma levels of pyridoxal-5-phosphate (PLP) coenzyme form of vitamin B6 is associated with a vast number (>100) of enzymes, the major functions are as follows:

- Amino acid metabolism;
- Fat metabolism;
- Promoting niacin synthesis;
- Hematopoiesis;
- Promoting antibody synthesis;
- Promoting the absorption of vitamin B12, iron and zinc.

② Human requirement: The human body's need for vitamin B6 is affected by the level of dietary protein, the synthesis of vitamin B6 by the intestinal bacteria, the degree of utilization of the human body, the physiological condition, and taking the drug. Under normal circumstances, vitamin B6 deficiency is uncommon. China proposes an AI of 1. 2 mg/d for adults and appropriate increasement during pregnancy and lactation.

③ Food sources: Vitamin B6 is widely found in a variety of foods. The highest levels of food are white meat (such as chicken and fish), followed by liver, beans, nuts, and egg yolk. There are also more vitamin B6 in fruits and vegetables, among which banana, cabbage and spinach are rich in content, but they are less in the citrus fruits and milk.

④ Lack or excess: Vitamin B6 deficiency is due to insufficient dietary intake. In addition, some certain drugs such as cycloserine can form a complex with PLP to induce its deficiency.

The lacks of vitamin B6 in the human body can cause seborrheic dermatitis around the eyes, nose and mouth, and can be extended to the face, forehead, behind the ears, scrotum and perineum. Vitamin B6 deficiency can also cause impaired humoral and cell-mediated immune function, hyperhomocysteinemia and hyperuricemia.

The toxicity of vitamin B6 is relatively low. There is no adverse reaction when a large amount of vitamin B6 is ingested by food sources. Serious adverse reactions, and neurotoxicity and photosensitivity reaction may occur when the dose of vitamin B6 reaches 500 mg/d.

(10) Vitamin B12

Vitamin B12 contains heavy metal element cobalt, which is also called cobalamin. It is the largest and most structurally complex vitamin. Vitamin B12 is a red crystal with a very high melting point (insoluble in 320 degrees Celsius), and it is soluble in water and ethanol, but insoluble in chloroform and ether. It is easily destroyed by sunlight, oxidants and reducing agents.

① Functions of vitamin B12: Vitamin B12 exerts physiological effects in the form of two coenzymes, namely methylcobalamin (methyl B12) and adenosylcobalamin (coenzyme B12), which participate in biochemical reactions *in vivo*. The reaction requiring methylcobalamin as a coenzyme is the conversion of homocysteine into methionine. The second reactions require adenosylcobalamin for methylmalonyl-CoA mutase, which converts L-methylmalonyl-CoA to succinyl-CoA.

② Human requirement: The RNI of CNS of vitamin B12 for adults, pregnant and breastfeeding women is 2.4, 2.9 and 3.2 μg per day, respectively.

③ Food sources: Vitamin B12 in the diet is derived from animal food. The main food sources are meat, animal offal, fish, poultry and eggs. And milk and dairy products contain less Vitamin B12. Plant foods are basically free of vitamin B12.

④ Lack or excess: Vitamin B12 deficiency is most commonly caused by low intakes, but can also result from malabsorption, certain intestinal disorders, low presence of binding proteins, and use of certain medications. The main manifestations of vitamin B12 deficiency include megaloblastic anemia, nervous system damage, and hyperhomocysteinemia.

Vitamin B12 is relatively low in toxicity, no obvious adverse reactions are observed when daily oral dose reaches 100 μg.

(11) Folic acid

Folic acid is one of the B vitamins, which can be taken by mouth or by injection. It is especially important during periods of frequent cell division and growth, such as infancy and pregnancy. Besides folic acid is used to treat anemia caused by its deficiency, it is also used as a supplement by women during pregnancy to reduce the risk of neural tube defects (NTDs) in the baby. Up to now, more than 80 countries use fortification of certain foods with folic acid as a measure to decrease the rate of NTDs.

① Functions of folic acid: Folic acid is essential for maintaining DNA stability through donating one-carbon-unit for cellular metabolism. Therefore, it plays an important role in

DNA synthesis and replication. Folic acid is necessary for fertility in both men and women. It contributes to spermatogenesis. Therefore, receiving sufficient folic acid through the diet or supplements is necessary to avoid low fertility. It is also found that folic acid intake from food and folate supplementation over years is associated with reduced risk of cardiovascular disease and cancers such as colorectal, breast, pancreas and prostate cancer.

② Human requirement: The RNI of CNS of folic acid for adults, pregnant and breastfeeding women is 400, 600 and 550 μg dietary folic acid equivalent (DFE) per day, respectively. UL for folic acid is 1000 μg DFE per day. The recommended adult daily intake of folic acid in the U. S. is 400 μg from foods or dietary supplements.

③ Food sources: Folic acid naturally presents in a wide variety of foods. Rich sources include yeast extract, lentils, broad beans, common bean, chickpeas, dark green leaf vegetables and red bell peppersat. Folic acid naturally found in food is susceptible to high heat and ultraviolet light.

④ Lack or excess: Folic acid deficiency can be caused by unhealthy diets that do not include enough vegetables and other folate-rich foods, which may lead to glossitis, diarrhea, depression, confusion, anemia, and fetal neural tube and brain defects. Folic acid deficiency is also associated with other symptoms include fatigue, gray hair, mouth sores, poor growth, and swollen tongue. The risk of toxicity from folic acid is low, because folic acid is a water-soluble vitamin and is regularly removed from the body through urine. One potential issue associated with high doses of folic acid is that it has a masking effect on the diagnosis of pernicious anaemia due to vitamin B12 deficiency.

5.2.3.6　Minerals

The importance of minerals is noted although they constitute only a small proportion (4%) of the total body weight. They impart hardness to bones and teeth and provide the medium essential for normal cellular activity. They also determine the osmotic properties of body fluids, and show the function as obligatory cofactors in metalloenzymes. For instance, the amount and ratio of calcium and phosphorus is important for bone formation as the ratio of potassium and calcium in the extracellular fluid is important for the normal muscular activity. Minerals such as iron in hemoglobin, iodine in thyroxine, cobalt in vitamin B_{12}, and sulfur in thiamin and biotin, may act as catalysts in enzyme systems or as integral parts of organic compounds in the body.

Minerals are frequently classed as major minerals and trace minerals, also called as macro minerals and microminerals, depending on their abundance in the body. The major minerals of the human body include calcium, phosphorus, potassium, sulfur, chlorine, sodium, and magnesium. The contents of them are higher than 0.01% in the body. Distinguished from the major minerals, the contents of trace minerals, including iron, iodine, fluorine, zinc, copper, chromium, selenium, cobalt, manganese, molybdenum, vanadium, tin, silicon, and nickel are lower than 0.01% in the body. In this part, two macro minerals (calcium, phosphorus), four microminerals (iron, iodine, zinc, and selenium will be introduced.

(1) Calcium and Phosphorus

Calcium is the most abundant divalent cation in the body, representing 1. 5%—2% of total body weight, or between 1,000 and 1,400 g in the human body. Phosphorus is the second most abundant mineral in the body, which represents about 0. 8%—1. 2% of body weight, or between 560 and 850 g in the body. Of total body calcium and phosphorus, 99% of the calcium and 85% of the phosphorus are in the bones and teeth, providing them strength and rigidity. The other 1% of calcium, existing in its ionic form Ca^{2+}, are found in intra-and extra-cellular fluids. For the rest of phosphorus, 1% is in the blood and body fluids and 14% present in the soft tissues such as muscles.

① Functions of calcium and phosphorus.

Calcium: Calcium plays several crucial roles in the body, such as: a. being a structural component of bones and teeth formation and maintenance; b. being importantin cellular processes, muscle contraction, blood clotting, and enzyme activation. The major and widely known function of calcium is developing and maintaining bones. Calcium and phosphorous along with hydroxyl groups form hydroxyapatite, a crystal latticelike substance, which binds to the collagen fibers, allowing bone to be resilient and strong.

Phosphorus: structural component of bones, teeth, cell membranes, phospholipids, nucleic acids, nucleotide coenzymes, ATP-ADP phosphate transferring systems in cells, pH regulation.

② Deficiency symptoms: Deficiency of calcium can lead to rickets, osteomalacia, osteoporosis, or tetany.

Deficiency of phosphorus can lead to neuromuscular, skeletal, hematologic, and cardiac manifestations; rickets, or osteomalacia.

③ Food sources of calcium and phosphorus: The best and most important food sources of calcium include dairy products, especially milk, cheese, and yogurt, as well as some seafood such as salmon, clams, and oysters. For instance, a cup of milk and yogurt can provide between 200 and 400 mg calcium. Selected green vegetables such as turnip, broccoli, and kale are good sources of calcium. Legumes and legume products (especially tofu), and nuts also provide some calcium. Half cup of tofu can provide 125 to 227 mg calcium.

Phosphorus is more widely distributed than calcium and is more likely to be higher than deficient in the average diet. Protein-rich foods such as poultry, fish, meats, cereals, nuts, and legumes, as well as milk and milk products are all good sources. For example, per 85 g serving of meat, fish, and poultry can provide about 150—250 mg of phosphorus. Phosphate additives used in a wide variety of food products, such as carbonated beverages, processed meats and cheeses, dressings, and refrigerated bakery products, may contribute significantly to the total phosphorus intake.

④ Factors affecting absorption and retention.

Calcium and phosphorus absorption in the small intestines involve two transport systems: a. saturable, carrier-mediated, active transport; b. diffusion. For calcium, it is present in foods and dietary supplements as relatively insoluble salts, which can be solubilized (as free Ca^{2+}) from most calcium salts at acidic pH in our stomach. However, free Ca^{2+} can bind to other dietary constituents, limiting the bioavailability. There are various factors influencing the calcium absorption. Adequate vitamin D, diets with low amount of calcium (<400 mg), dietary components including lactose, sugars, sugar alcohols (such as xylitol), and protein can enhance calcium absorption. For instance, ingesting lactose along with calcium source can improve overall calcium absorption possibly by increasing solubility. In addition, different life cycle including growth, pregnancy, and lactation also improve absorption because of the high requirement. However, several dietary components influence the calcium absorption in a negative way by diminishing absorption or promoting its secretion from blood into gastrointestinal tract. For example, large amounts of phytates (phosphorus compounds found in cereals) or oxalates, which can form insoluble compounds with calcium or increase fecal calcium excretion, inhibit calcium absorption. In addition, divalent cations such as magnesium and zinc can interact with calcium to decrease the calcium absorption. Steatorrhea due to impaired absorption of fat is associated with high loss of calcium in feces, believed to result from the formation of insoluble calcium salts with free fatty acids which are present in excessive amounts in the intestine.

The same as calcium, there are several positive and negative factors affecting phosphorus absorption. For instance, calcitriol can stimulate carrier-mediate absorption of phosphorus in both duodenum and the jejunum. However, several minerals including magnesium, aluminum, and calcium can reduce the phosphorus absorption. For instance, aluminum hydroxide can reduce phosphorus adsorption from 30% to 70%. In addition, consuming phytic acid-containing foods with Ca^{2+} food can prevent the adsorption of calcium and phosphorus due to the cation-phytic acid complexes.

⑤ Dietary requirements.

Calcium: The CNS RNI of Calcium is 800 mg per day for adults. The UL for calcium is 2,000 mg per day for adults.

Phosphorus: The CNS RNI of phosphorus is 720 mg per day for adults. UL for Phosphorus is 3,500 mg per day for adults.

A 2:1 ratio of calcium to phosphorus (as found in human milk) has been shown to result in maximum calcium absorption and retention in animals. Although evidence for humans is less definitive, a higher Ca:P ratio may be beneficial and certainly is not harmful as is evident in breast-fed infants. A 1.5:1 ratio of calcium to phosphorus is recommended for the first year of life.

(2) Iron

There is about 2 to 4 g of iron in the body of a healthy adult, but its importance to our wellbeing is strikingly out of proportion to the quantitative requirement. In the body, 60% to 70% of the iron is found in hemoglobin. Iron stores in the liver, spleen, and bone marrow (as ferritin and hemosiderin) account for the next largest concentration of iron (30% to 35%). Small but essential amounts of iron (up to 10%) are found in muscle myoglobin, in transport form (bound to protein-transferrin) in the blood serum, and in every cell as a constituent of heme enzymes (notably cytochromes, oxidase, peroxidase, and catalase) and other enzymes involved in cellular respiration (iron-containing flavoproteins and iron-sulphur proteins). The only stable states of iron in body and in food are the ferric (Fe^{3+}) and the ferrous (Fe^{2+}) forms.

① Functions of iron.

• Essential part for hemoglobin and myoglobin synthesis;

• Cofactor as an active component of cytochromes and other enzymes, especially those associated with the respiratory chain of the mitochondria;

• Important part for amino acid metabolism; antioxidant; carnitine, collagen, and thyroid hormone synthesis.

② Deficiency symptoms: Being lack of iron for heme and hemoglobin synthesis results in the development of iron deficiency anemia, which impairs oxygen transport in the blood, resulting in fatigue and a decreased ability to perform normal activities. It also compromises immune function, impairs energy metabolism, and delays cognitive development.

③ Food sources: The best food sources of iron are found in the meat, fish, poultry, and egg group. Green, leafy vegetables, potatoes, dried fruits, and enriched bread and cereal products are the best plant sources. Milk and its products are conspicuously low in iron. It is now well recognized that the availabilities of iron from heme and nonheme sources are different and that the composition of the meal consumed with iron has a major influence on the absorption of nonheme iron. On the average, about 40% of iron in meat, fish, and poultry is heme iron (hemoglobin and myoglobin). The two dietary factors that are known to increase substantially the absorption of nonheme iron are ascorbic acid and an unknown "meat factor". In contrast to an "animal protein factor", this meat factor is present in beef, lamb, pork, chicken, liver, and fish, but not in milk, cheese, and eggs.

④ Factors affect iron absorption: Physiologic control of iron balance is primarily achieved by regulating iron absorption from the gastrointestinal tract. Body iron status and iron demand determine the magnitude of iron absorption under any given set of conditions, but the actual rate of uptake is influenced by the form and level of dietary iron and by the composition of the meal in which it is consumed. In healthy people with adequate iron stores and intake, iron is absorbed at a rate that tends to maintain the body iron content at a relatively constant level. However, in people with iron deficiency, the rate of absorption may be two to three times that in healthy people.

Factors include acids such as ascorbic, citric, lactic acids, sugars especially fructose and sorbitol, amino acids, and mucin can promote ion absorption. For instance, ascorbic acid (vitamin C) acts as a reducing agent of transforming ferric to ferrous iron and forms low-molecular iron chelates, which increase the absorption of iron from neutral or slightly alkaline duodenal contents in which ferric iron would otherwise be poorly soluble. However, there are many dietary factors inhibit the absorption of iron, namely: oxalic acid (found in spinach, chocolate, etc.), phytic acid (found in maize), polyphenols such as tannin derivatives of gallic acid, and divalent cations such as calcium, zinc, and manganese. In addition, gastric acidity is essential for solubilization of food iron and its conversion to an absorbable form. Increased pH of the gastrointestinal tract will also decrease the iron absorption. In addition, although there is evidence that high fiber intake decreases the absorption of iron, the impact of diets high in foods containing fiber on the bioavailability of iron is not defined well enough to determine its practical significance.

⑤ Dietary requirements for iron: Iron requirements are determined by the demands for tissue growth and hemoglobin accretion and by the need to replace iron lost in the urine, feces, and sweat, and in the female in menstruation, pregnancy, and lactation. The three periods of greatest demand for iron are during the first 2 years of life, adolescence, especially in girls, and the childbearing period. The CNS RNI of iron is 12 mg per day for men and 20 mg per day for women. UL for iron is 42 mg per day for adults. After menopause, the sex difference in the iron requirement no longer exists.

(3) Iodine

Of the estimated 25 mg of iodine in an adult, 10 mg to 15 mg is found in the thyroid in thyroglobulin, an iodinated glycoprotein, which serves as a reserve of the thyroid hormones.

① Functions of iodine: The main function of iodine is to synthesize thyroid hormones, triiodothyronine (T3), and thyroxine (T4). Although iodine has a singular function as above, which has widespread consequences because of the pivotal role that thyroid hormones play in maintaining normal metabolism. For instance, iodine is involved in the regulation of many important metabolic and developmental functions, including the regulation of basal energy expenditure, macronutrient metabolism, growth, brain development, and organ maturation.

② Deficiency symptoms: Iodine deficiency results in iodine deficiency disease (IDD), including goiter, cretinism, decreased fertility rate, increased infant mortality, and mental retardation.

③ Food sources: The best sources of iodine are sea foods. About 90% of iodine comes from foods eaten, the remainder from drinking water.

④ Iron and vitamin A deficiencies may magnify the effects of inadequate iodine. For instance, vitamin A deficiency reduces iodine uptake by the thyroid gland and decreases the synthesis of T4.

⑤ Dietary requirements for iodine: The CSN RNI of iodine is 120 μg per day for adults. UL for iodine is 600 μg per day for adults.

(4) Zinc

The human body contains about 1. 5 to 3. 0 g of zinc, highly concentrated in the hair, skin, eyes, nails, and testes, but some is found in all human tissues and fluids and in all subcellular fractions. Muscle and bone tissues contain about 90% of the total body zinc because of their large mass.

① Functions of zinc: Zinc, is a component of numerous metalloenzymes, appears to influence many body systems and functions, including growth, bone formation, brain development, behavior, fertility and reproduction, fetal development, sensory functions (taste, smell and, perhaps, vision), immune mechanisms, membrane stability, and wound healing.

② Deficiency symptoms: Deficiency of zinc leads to skin rash, diarrhea, decreased appetite and sense of taste, hair loss, as well as poor growth and development.

③ Food sources: Zinc is found in foods complexed with nucleic acids and with amino acids. Good sources of zinc are red meats (especially organ meats) and seafood (especially oysters and mollusks). Other animal foods such as poultry, and milk are dependable sources.

④ Factors affect zinc absorption: Enhancers: ligands or chelators including organic acid and prostaglandins may bind and promote zinc absorption. Glutathione and products of protein digestions such as peptide and amino acids help to serve as ligands to enhance zinc absorption. In addition, an acidic environment can enhance the absorption of zinc.

Inhibitors: phylic acid, oxalic acid, polyphenols are thought to significantly inhibit zinc absorption. For instance, polyphenols in tea and coffee and certain fibers found in fruits and vegetables can bind zinc and inhibits its absorption. In addition, folate, iron, and calcium may inhibit zin absorption.

⑤ Dietary requirements for zinc: The CNS RNI of zinc is 12. 5 mg per day for men and 7. 5 mg per day for women. UL for zinc is 40 mg per day for adults.

(5) Selenium (Se)

The total body selenium content is about 20 mg. Selenium, which is an essential micronutrient required for animal and human health, exists in several oxidation states, including Se^{2-}, Se^{4+}, and Se^{6+}. Selenium is distributed to target tissues with the highest concentrations found in the blood, liver, muscle, kidneys and skeleton. Within tissues, selenomethionine provides a "storage pool" of selenium. Selenium deficiency is associated with changes in thyroid hormone metabolism and a possible increased risk of certain cancers.

① Functions of selenium: Selenium in the food is incorporated into a number of selenium-containing proteins, the selenoproteins. The physiological functions of selenium are thought to be brought about by these selenoproteins. In humans, over 25 selenoproteins have been identified. One of its most recognized functions is the antioxidant defense network, as a part of glutathione peroxidase (GPX) enzymes, thioredoxin reductase enzymes, and selenoprotein P. These proteins primarily function in antioxidant capacities, and thus regulate cell redox status. Selenium helps prevent lipid peroxidation and cell membrane damage. Selenium is also necessary for iodine metabolism and may regulate thyroid hormone production. Selenium also plays an important role in immune function.

② Food sources of selenium: The selenium content of food is highly dependent on the concentration of selenium in the soil on which the plants were grown or on which the fodder for animals was raised. Consequently, the selenium content of foods is extremely varied. In general, the best sources of selenium are seafood, meats, cereals, grains and nuts. Selenium presents naturally in foods primarily in the organic forms, selenomethionine and selenocysteine. Selenomethionine tends to be found primarily in plant foods, such as grains and some vegetables like mushrooms, whereas selenocysteine is found mostly in animal foods. Inorganic forms of selenium include selenide (H_2Se or HSe^-), selenite (H_2SeO_3), and selenate (H_2SeO_4). There inorganic forms present in a few vegetables (such as broccoli, cucumber, beets and cabbage) as well as in yeast.

③ Factors affect selenium absorption: Selenium, in organic and inorganic forms, is efficiently absorbed throughout the small intestine. Selenium balance is achieved primarily through urinary excretion, rather than intestinal absorption. Factors enhancing selenium absorption include vitamins C, A and E, as well as the presence of reduced glutathione in the intestinal lumen. Heavy metals (such as mercury) and phytic acid are thought to inhibit selenium absorption through chelation and precipitation.

④ Selenium deficiency: Chinese scientists firstly confirmed that selenium deficiency is associated with Keshan disease. Keshan disease is a heart disease characterized by insufficient cardiac function, and is prevalent in regions of China where the soil and foods lack selenium. It has since been diagnosed in other regions, including New Zealand and Finland. Although Keshan disease can be prevented through selenium supplementation, the related cardiac disorders are not corrected by selenium once the disease has developed. Selenium deficiency is associated with changes in thyroid hormone metabolism and a possible increased risk of certain cancers. Symptoms of selenium deficiency include impaired cognition and poor immunity.

⑤ Dietary requirements for selenium: The CNS RNI of selenium is 60 μg per day for adults. UL for selenium is 400 μg per day for adults. RNI is based on the amount of selenium needed to maximized glutathione peroxidase activity in the blood. RNI for selenium for pregnancy and lactation were set at 65 and 78 μg per day, respectively.

5.2.4 Phytochemicals and Functional Foods

5.2.4.1 Definition, Classification and Bioactivity of Phytochemicals

Nowadays, there is a global high prevalence of non-communicable chronic diseases (NCDs) such as obesity, diabetes, and cardiovascular diseases (CVDs). Plant-based foods (whole grains, vegetables, fruits, etc.) are widely recognized by nutritionists and food scientists and recommended by global dietary guidelines because of their bioactivities of preventing NCDs and maintaining good health. In addition to their nutrients, plant-derived foods contain phytochemicals which usually confer color, taste, and other characteristics to them. The "phyto" is from Greek and pronounced "FYE-toe", and means "plant". In the past few decades, there has been a considerable interest in phytochemicals in the area of nutrition and food science. Moreover, the scope of "phytochemicals" has expanded beyond their initial applications to food to include therapeutics, pharmaceuticals and cosmeceuticals.

Phytochemicals have been also referred to as phytonutrients, nutraceuticals and functional ingredients. In fact, there is no absolutely conclusive definition of phytochemicals. Currently, phytochemicals may be defined as bioactive, non-nutrient plant compounds (secondary metabolites) that are associated with reduced risks of chronic diseases. First, phytochemicals are secondary metabolites in plants. Plants produce primary and secondary metabolites during the process of energy metabolism. In comparison to primary metabolites (protein, lipids, carbohydrates, etc.), secondary metabolites usually have smaller molecular weights and are far less in the quantities. Secondly, phytochemicals are not considered as nutrients. One exception is carotenoids some of which (like β-carotene) is belonged to the precursors to vitamin A. The main characteristic of nutrients (carbohydrates, protein, lipids, vitamins, minerals and water) is essentiality. To date, there is no convincing scientific evidence to support that phytochemicals are essential to human body. No report is available that deficiency of phytochemicals cause diseases. A lot of scientific evidences have shown that phytochemicals have health-promoting bioactivities such as anti-oxidation, anti-inflammation, chemoprevention, hypoglycemia, hypolipidemia, and immunomodulation. These biological activities are usually associated with the reduced risks of chronic diseases. Human ingests various phytochemicals through eating plant foods. The daily intake of phytochemicals is about 1.5 g for people who consume a mixed diet and much higher for vegetarian. The study on how phytochemicals promote human health has been a hot area in nutrition and food sciences.

(1) Classification

Phytochemicals can be classified based on their chemical structure or functions. There are millions of phytochemicals in natural plants. However, only some of them, especially these with high daily dietary intake, have relatively been investigated in detail. In general, phytochemicals can be classified into polyphenols, carotenoids, terpenes, organosulphur compounds, saponins, phytoestrogens, phytic acids and phytosterols.

① Polyphenols: Polyphenols are a group of compounds containing at least 2 ring structures that each have at least 1 hydroxyl group (OH) attached. Many polyphenols present naturally in plants, such as tea, dark chocolate (cacao beans), and wine (grapes). The polyphenols, which include more than 8,000 compounds, can be divided into a variety of classes. One of the largest of these classes is the flavonoids, which includes several subclasses-flavonols, flavanols, flavones, flavanones, anthocyanidins, and isoflavones.

② Carotenoids: Carotenoids (often referred to as provitamin A) consist of an expanded carbon chain containing conjugated double bonds, usually, but not always, with an unsubstituted β-ionone ring at one or both ends of the chain. Three provitamin A carotenoids, which are found most often in the all-trans form but can occur as cis isomers, are β-carotene, α-carotene, and β-cryptoxanthin. Although not all carotenoids are vitamin A precursors, many carotenoids, such as lycopene (an open-chain analog of β-carotene), and many oxycarotenoids (also called oxygenated carotenoids), such as canthaxanthin, lutein, and zeaxanthin, are thought to be of physiological importance to the body. Carotenoids are synthesized by a wide variety of plants and thus are found naturally in many fruits and vegetables. One of the most abundant carotenoids is β-carotene, which exhibits the greatest amount of provitamin A activity. Other common dietary carotenoids include α-carotene and β-cryptoxanthin (both provitamin A carotenoids) along with lycopene, lutein, and zeaxanthin. In general, yellow, orange, and red (brightly colored) fruits and vegetables such as carrots, watermelon, papayas, tomatoes, tomato products (ketchup, chili sauce, spaghetti sauce), squash, pink grapefruits, and pumpkins provide significant amounts of carotenoids. Green vegetables also contain some carotenoids, but the pigment is masked by (green) chlorophyll. Carrots typically represent a major source of both α-and β-carotene in American diets; ½ carrot provides about 4, 550 μg of β-carotene. Other major dietary contributors of β-carotene include broccoli (725 μg β-carotene/½ cup cooked), cantaloupe (1,616 μg/½ cup), squash (136 μg/cup cooked), peas (600 μg/½ cup cooked), and spinach (5,660 μg/½ cup cooked). Fruits provide much of the dietary β-cryptoxanthin, and tomatoes, along with tomato sauces and watermelon, are good sources of dietary lycopene, a carotenoid that is red in color. Good sources of zeaxanthin include peppers (orange), corn, potatoes, and eggs. Broccoli, beets, kiwi fruit, and eggs provide some lutein. Canthaxanthin, a red-orange carotenoid, is found in plants as well as in fish and seafood such as sea trout and crustaceans. Meat and fish are not major sources of carotenoids, but because animals and fish feed on plants, they can accumulate some carotenoids. Carotenoids also may be added to foods. β-carotene and canthaxanthin, for example, are approved by the Food and Drug Administration for use as food color additives.

③ Terpenes: The term "terpenes" originates from turpentine (balsamum terebinthinae), the so-called "resin of pine trees". Terpenes are also designated as terpenoids or isoprenoids and the largest group of natural products comprising approximately 36,000 terpene structures. They comprise single to several hundreds of repetitive five-carbon (5C) units of isopentenyl diphosphate (IPP) and its isomer dimethylallyl diphosphate (DMAPP). Based on the number of isoprenoid units present in the structures, terpenes are classified into hemiterpene (C5), monoterpenes (C10), sesquiterpenes (C15), diterpenes (C20), sesterterpenes (C25), triterpenes (C30), tetraterpenes (C40) and polyterpenes ($>$ $C40-C5 \times 10^{3-4}$).

All living organisms manufacture terpenes for certain essential physiological functions including growth, development, reproduction and defense. In the scope of food, citrus fruits are the rich sources of terpenes. The citrus fruit peel contains triterpenes (Limonene, citrol, etc.), leaves contain terpenoids (Linalool, β-elemene, etc.), and flowers contain triperpenes (Limonene).

④ Organosulphur compounds: Organosulfur compounds, such as Allicin, in Chives, garlic, leeks, onions, scallions provide significant amounts of Allicin. Indoles, also found as organosulfur compound. 3,3'-diindolylmethane (D)IM is found in substantial amounts in vegetables that are commonly consumed from the family Cruciferae particularly the genus Brassica which include broccoli, cauliflower, kale, cabbage brussels sprouts, turnips, kohlrabi, bokchoy, radishes, etc. It is now well established that Cruciferous vegetables contain a precursor phytochemical-Glucosinolate that undergoes hydrolysis by the plant enzyme myrosinase, yielding a bioactive compound known as indole-3-carbinol (I3C). I3C is chemically unstable in aqueous and gastric acidic environment, and is rapidly converted to numerous condensation products. A major condensation product of I3C in vivo is DIM. DIM has distinct pleiotropic effects on cancer cells resulting in inactivating survival signaling and simultaneously activating multiple death pathways.

⑤ Saponins: Saponins are compounds consisting of an aglycone (sapogenins) attached to one or more sugar moieties (sugars, uronic acids or other carboxylic groups). The sugars in the molecule of saponins often include glucose, galactose, rhamnose, arabinose, xylose or other pentose sugars. Saponins are a structurally diverse family of plant secondary metabolites. They are usually classified as triterpene (30 C-atoms) saponins and steroid (27 C-atoms) saponins based on their aglycones. Based on the biosynthesis of carbon skeletons of the aglycone, saponins can also be divided into 11 main classes, ie. dammaranes, tirucallanes, lupanes, hopanes, oleananes, taraxasteranes, ursanes, cycloartanes, lanostanes, cucurbitanes and steroids. Saponins are widely found in a variety of plant species like soybean (soyasaponins), chickpea, spinach, ginseng, sugar beet, sunflower, oats, Quillaja saponaria Molina tress, etc. The contents of saponins in different plant species vary from 0.1% to 10%. Saponins widely exist in the seed, root, stem, leaf, fruit, and bark of the plant. The steroid saponins mainly exist in Dioscoreaceae and Liliaceous plants whereas the triterpene saponins are primarily from Leguminosae, Caryophyllaceae, Campanulaceae and Araliaceae plants. The average daily dietary intake of saponins is estimated to be 10 mg which varies as the dietary habits and characteristics differ. For example, the population who likes eating soy foods has a dietary ingestion of more than 200 mg saponins per day.

The most important property of saponins is their ability to form very stable foam as a consequence of their surfactant ability. That is why the word "saponin" is derived from the Latin word "sapo", which translates to soap, and it refers to the interfacial activity.

⑥ Phytoestrogens: Phytochemicals structurally similar to human estrogen that weakly mimic or modulate estrogen's action in the body. Phytoestrogens include the isoflavones genistein, daidzein, and glycitein. Phytoestrogen supplements are ill-advised-especially for women with breast cancer and those with high risk factors-as phytoestrogens may promote the growth of estrogen-dependent tumors (such as breast cancer). The American Cancer Society recommends that women with breast cancer should consume only moderate amounts of soy as part of a healthy plant-based diet and should not intentionally ingest high levels of soy or supplements of phytoestrogens.

⑦ Phytic acid: Phytic acid, also known as inositol hexaphosphate (InsP6) is a naturally occurring compound and usually exists in its salt form phytate. It is widely distributed in the plant kingdom, especially in grains such as rice and corn. The content of phytic acids in grains and beans is as high as 1%—6%. Phytate is a storage form of phosphorus and minerals and contains about 75% of total phosphorus of the kernels. Phytic acid is also a component of mammalian cells with a concentration of 10—100 μm. Phytic acid is highly charged and shows an extremely high negative charge density. Therefore, it cannot cross the lipid bilayer of plasma membranes. However, recent investigations provided evidence to the gastrointestinal absorption of phytate in cell lines, rats and humans. The hydrolysis end-product of phytic acids in gastrointestinal tract is inositol and inorganic phosphate. The products may be mixtures of inositol monophosphate, diphosphate, triphosphate, tetraphosphate, and pentaphosphate if the phytic acids are not completely hydrolyzed.

Phytate is strong chelator of important minerals such as calcium, magnesium, iron, and zinc and can contribute to mineral deficiencies in human. Thus, phytate was often considered to be anti-nutrient. Recently, phytic acids have been found to have anticancer properties.

⑧ Phytosterols: Phytosterols are plant-derived steroid alcohols and have similar chemical structure to cholesterol. The difference to the structure of cholesterol is that the presence of one-or two-carbon, saturated or unsaturated, substituents in side chains at C-24 in the molecule of phytosterols. Phytosterols are mainly found in oilseeds, unrefined vegetable oils, wholegrain cereals, nuts, and legumes. They include sterols (sitosterol, campesterol, and stigmasterol) and stanols (sitostanol, campestanol, and stigmastanol). The absorption of phytosterol (0.6%—7.5%) is much lower than that of cholesterol (56% $\pm$ 12.1%) although they have similar chemical structures. The average amount of phytosterols in the Western diet is 150—400 mg/day according to the Scientific Committee on Food. The Chinese DRIs (2013 edition) suggest that the SPL and the UL for phytosterol is 0.9 g/d and 2.4 g/day, respectively.

(2) Bioactivity

Phytochemicals are increasingly accepted by researchers, industries, general society, and policy makers as health promoting, maintaining, and repairing agents to manage public health especially to fight against the NCDs, a current big public health issue world-widely. Although it is inconclusive, accumulated evidences have shown that phytochemicals have multiple biological activities.

① Cardiovascular protective effects: Cardiovascular diseases (CVDs) are still the leading causes of morbidity and mortality throughout the world. Animal, epidemiological and human population intervention studies show that phytochemicals play protective roles in the prevention and treatment of CVDs. Flavonoids compounds have been known for the bioactivities to decrease the atherosclerosis and coronary heart diseases. Tea polyphenols, quercetin and soy isoflavones can protect cardiovascular system through decreasing the TG, TC and LDL-C, inhibiting oxidized LDL (Ox-LDL), promoting nitric oxide (NO) production, and blocking platelet aggregation. Inflammation is an important mediator in the occurrence and development of CVDs. Polyphenols, saponins and lycopene can block the atherosclerosis-related inflammatory reactions, which help to reduce the accumulation of immune cells on the artery walls, prevent the formation of foam macrophages, and inhibit atherosclerotic plaques and thrombus. Dietary intake of 200 mg/day of proanthocyanidins has been suggested to reduce the risk of CVDs. Some phytochemicals (e. g. luten, puerarin, and ginsenoside) have been clinically used for treating CVDs.

② Anti-cancer effects: Numerous epidemiological studies find that dietary phytochemicals and other natural compounds are effective interventions in cancer development. It has long been shown that phytochemicals-rich vegetables and fruits can decrease the cancer incidence by approximate 50% in human populations. Sufficient evidence has proven that fresh vegetables and fruits are able to reduce the risk of tumors in gastrointestinal tract, lung, oral cavity and laryngeal epithelium. Drinking tea is dietary habit in many countries including China. The tea is rich in phytochemicals like catechin, epicatechin (EC), epigallocatechin (ECG), epi-gallocatechin-3-gallate (EGCG), catechingallate (CG), etc. A lot of epidemiological studies and meta-analysis show that drinking tea reduces the prostatic, breast and lung cancer, but not gastric and bladder cancer. It is well known that estrogen exhibit promotion effects in some cancers like breast cancer. Soy isoflavones ha ve anti-estrogen effects during the occurrence and development of breast cancer. This is probably because soy isoflavones increase the metabolism of estrogen into estradiol, which is anti-carcinogenic.

③ Anti-oxidative effects: Oxidative stress is a common pathogenic mechanism in many modern chronic diseases including aging, cancers, CVDs, diabetes, Alzheimer's disease (AD), Parkinson's disease (PD), etc. The anti-oxidative stress defense systems include anti-oxidant enzymes (superoxide dismutase, SOD; glutathione peroxidase, GSH-Px), endogenous antioxidants (uric acid, glutathione, alpha lipoic acid, coenzyme Q, etc.) and some anti-oxidative essential nutrients (vitamin E, vitamin C, etc.). In the past few decades, accumulated evidence has indicated that phytochemicals have anti-oxidative bioactivities. Moreover, the anti-oxidative abilities of some phytochemicals are much stronger than that of traditional anti-oxidative vitamins.

Polyphenols exhibit the strongest anti-oxidative abilities among all anti-oxidative phytochemicals. For example, the anti-oxidative ability of procyanidine is 50 times of that of vitamin E and 20 times of vitamin C. The reactive oxygen species (ROS) scavenging activity of anthocyanin is even stronger than that of common commercial anti-oxidants (butylated hydroxyanisole and vitamin E. The large quantity of hydroxyl groups located in the molecular structure contributes to the strong ROS scavenging activity of polyphenol compounds.

④ Anti-inflammatory effects: Excessive (chronic) inflammation has been linked with a variety of chronic diseases such as obesity, diabetes, cardiovascular disorders, some cancers. Phytochemicals has been shown to be effective in reducing excessive inflammation and preventing the development and progression of chronic diseases.

Soyasaponins and curcumins are reported to inhibit the production of pro-inflammatory cytokines (interleukin 1β, IL-1β; Tumor necrosis factor a, TNF-a), pro-inflammatory mediators (NO; prostaglandin E_2, PGE_2) as well as pro-inflammatory enzymes (nitric oxide synthase, iNOS; cyclooxygenase 2, COX-2).

⑤ Hypolipidemic and hypocholesterolaemic effects: Saponins, phytosterols, polyphenols and organosulphur compounds have been shown to be effective in reducing the lipids and cholesterol in blood. Clinical studies suggested that presence of saponins in food decreased blood lipids and reduced risk of coronary heart disease by lowering plasma cholesterol levels. Polyphenols like anthocyanin can enhance the biosynthesis of bile acids from endogenous cholesterol in liver and thus reduce the cholesterol in plasma. The hydroxyl-methyl-glutaryl coenzyme A (HMG-CoA) is the rate-limiting enzyme for the synthesis of cholesterol. Phytochemicals (eg. resveratrol, phytosterols) have also been shown to exhibit hypocholesterolaemic effects by direct inhibition of HMG-CoA.

⑥ Other effects: Besides the above-mentioned bioactivities, phytochemicals have also been shown to exhibit other effects such as antimicrobial and antivirus, immunomodulation, glucose improvement, vision protection.

Currently, our understanding about phytochemicals are far from complete and mature although there have been a lot of studies in this area. The phytochemicals are highly diversified. There are hundreds or thousands of compounds even in the same type of phytochemicals. Thus, the extraction, purification and identification of phytochemicals by using advanced analytical techniques should be continuously investigated. Most of the existing studies have been focused on the bioactivities of phytochemicals. However, majority of these studies are from cell and animal studies. There are to date relatively less human-based epidemiological or intervention studies which can provide high-quality evidences for our understanding about the bioactivities of phytochemicals. The Chinese DRIs (2013) have established the SPL and the UL of some phytochemicals based on the available scientific publications (as shown in Table 5. 7).

Table 5.7   The Specific Proposed Levels (SPL) and the Tolerable Upper Intake Level (UL) of
Some Phytochemicals Suggested by Chinese DRIs (2013)

Phytochemicals	SPL	UL
Phytosterol (g/d)	0.9	2.4
Phytosterol ester (g/d)	1.5	3.9
Lycopene (mg/d)	18	70
Lutein (mg/d)	10	40
Proanthocyanidins (mg/d)	—	800
Anthocyanin (mg/d)	50	—
Soy isoflavones (mg/d) *	55	120
Glucosamine (mg/d)	1000	—
Glucosamine sulfate or hydrochloride (mg/d)	1500	—

* : Postmenopausal women; — : Not established

5.2.4.2   Definition and Management of Functional Foods in Different Countries

It is an established fact that foods provide nutrients that nourish our body and keep our system in proper working conditions. However, from early civilization it was also known that certain foods confer additional health benefits to human beings such as prevention and treatment of various types of diseases. "Let food be the medicine and let your medicine be your food" is a popular quote from Hippocrates (460 BC—370 BC) that emphasizes the role of foods in disease prevention and recognizes a separate role for food in addition to being nutrient providers. Recently, scientists have become focused on the health-promoting effects of foods and there is now abundance evidence that support the role of various foods and their components in promoting human health.

In China, functional food is not completely equal to health food, but usually refers to health food (called Bao Jian Shi Pin). However, the research on functional food and its raw materials is very intense, and many of the research purposes are not only academic, but also hope to eventually develop health food for the market.

China has a long tradition of regimen. Regimen means the healthy ways to reduce disease, promote health, prolong life and improve life quality according to the law of life development. The ancient theory of 'drug homologous food' is actually the view of health foods. As the traditional medicine and culture regimen, the Chinese medicine is both an important theoretical basis and an effective material source for health foods development, as well as a unique advantage.

(1) Definition of functional foods: What are functional foods? A food can be regarded as 'functional' if it is satisfactorily demonstrated to affect beneficially one or more target functions in the body, beyond adequate nutrition, in a way that improves health and well-being or reduces the risk of disease. These definitions can be simply described as: foods that

may provide health benefits beyond basic nutrition; foods or food products marketed with the message of the benefit to health; everyday food transformed into a potential functional food by the addition of a functional ingredient; food and drink products derived from naturally occurring substances consumed as part of the daily diet and possessing particular physiological benefits when ingested; food derived from naturally occurring substances that can and should be consumed as part of the daily diet and that serve to regulate or otherwise affect a particular body process when ingested; food similar in appearance to conventional food, which is consumed as part of a usual diet and has demonstrated physiological benefit and/or reduces the risk of chronic disease beyond basic nutritional functions; food that encompasses potentially helpful products including any modified food or food ingredient that may provide a health benefit beyond that of the traditional nutrient it contains; food similar in appearance to conventional food that is intended to be consumed as part of a normal diet, but has been modified to subserve physiological roles beyond the provision of simple nutrient requirements.

Whatever definition is chosen, functional food is also a concept that belongs to nutrition and not to pharmacology. Functional foods are and must be foods, not drugs, as they have no therapeutic effects. Although functional food has a clear regulatory function, its function cannot replace drugs, not for the purpose of treating diseases, which is an important difference between functional food and drugs. Another difference is that drugs are allowed to have side effects, while functional foods are not allowed to have toxic side effects. Moreover, their role regarding disease will, in most cases, be in reducing the risk of disease rather than preventing it. At same time, functional food should be safe and non-toxic, without any acute, sub-acute or chronic harm to human body.

The idea of "functionality" reflects a major shift in attitudes to the relationship between diet and health. Nutritionists have traditionally concentrated on identifying a "balanced" diet, that is one ensuring adequate intakes of nutrients and avoiding certain dietary imbalances (for example, excessive consumption of fat, cholesterol and salt) which can contribute towards development of diseases. It is important that this lies behind all sound nutritional principles and guidelines. However, the focus is now on achieving "optimized" nutrition, maximizing life expectancy and quality by identifying food ingredients which, when added to a "balanced" diet, improve the capacity to resist disease and enhance health. Functional foods are one of the outcomes of this.

(2) Functional Food in Different Districts or Countries

Japan is the birthplace of the term "functional food". Moreover, that country has been at the forefront of the development of functional foods since the early 1980s when systematic and large-scale research programs were launched and funded by the Japanese government on systematic analysis and development of food functions, analysis of physiological regulation of function by food and analysis of functional foods and molecular design. As a result of a long decision making process to establish a category of foods for potential enhancing benefits as part of a national effort to reduce the escalating cost of health care, the concept of foods for specified health use (FOSHU) was established in 1991.

Functional food in Japan includes the following two categories. ① Specific health food: refers to the health food which is suitable for the specific population and has the function of regulating the body. ② Nutritional functional food: refers to the health functional food which aims to supplement specific nutritional components. In April 2015, the implementation of the Functional Marked Food System added functional labeled food. In 2009, Japan established the Consumer Affairs Office, which is responsible for the supervision and management of specific health food by the former Ministry of Health and Labor.

In the United States, functional foods are called dietary supplements. Dietary supplements, a more elaborate definition, covers "a product intended to supplement the diet and that bears or contains one or more of certain specified dietary ingredients (vitamins, minerals, herbs or other botanicals, amino-acids, a dietary supplement) to supplement the diet by increasing total dietary intake, a concentrate, metabolite, constituent, extract or combination. It is a tablet, capsule, powder, softgel, gelcap or liquid droplet or some other forms that can be a conventional food but is not represented as a conventional. " The United States enacted the "Dietary Supplement Health and Education Act" in 1994. The Food and Drug Administration (FDA) is responsible for the supervision and management of dietary supplements, including the supervision and management of raw materials, function claims, production and so on. However, the use of new dietary supplement ingredients other than those listed before the implementation of the "Dietary Supplement Health and Education Act" of October 15, 1994 should be submitted to the FDA at least 75 days before listing, and safety data should be submitted to show that the ingredients of the product are safe. At the same time, the manufacturer can also entrust FDA to invite relevant units to evaluate the safety of new dietary supplement ingredients. Although FDA does not register dietary supplements, it has the right to question the safety of dietary supplements.

In EU, a food can be regarded as functional if it is satisfactorily demonstrated to have beneficial effect to one or more target functions in the body, beyond adequate nutritional effects, in a way that is relevant to either improved stage of health and well-being. "Target function" refers to genomic, biochemical, physiological, psychological or behavioral functions that are relevant to the maintenance of a state of well-being and health or to the reduction of the risk of a disease. A functional food must remain food and it must demonstrate its effects in amounts that can normally be expected to be consumed in the diet: it is not a pill or a capsule, but part of the normal food pattern. The purpose of functional food or food supplement is to supplement the deficiency of normal diet supply, but cannot replace the normal diet. It is produced and sold in a certain dose and form. Its form should be tablets, capsules, drops and powder. The safety and function evaluation of food supplements is mainly carried out by the European Food Safety Agency (EFSA), and the specific supervision and management is carried out by the member states of the European Union. The main laws and regulations for functional claims in the EU region are the integration of the Food Supplementary Laws of Member States in the EU Regulations 1924/2006 and the EU Directive 2002/46. Food supplements shall be put on record before they are put on the market.

In Canada, functional foods are called natural health products. including herbs, homeopathic products, vitamins, minerals, traditional medicines, amino acids, probiotics and specific personal care products. Canada has enacted the Natural Health Products Regulations, which is supervised and administered by the Ministry of Health. Natural health products must meet the following two requirements: one is the efficacy of products; the other is the raw materials of products. Efficacy includes the following aspects: diagnosis, treatment, alleviation or prevention of symptoms such as human diseases and dysfunction; restoration or correction of human organ function; adjustment of human organ function to maintain or promote health. In the registration application, natural health products must provide relevant evidence of product validity. In terms of raw material management, Canada Ministry of Health has established a catalogue list of functional and non-functional ingredients that can be used in natural health products. Component catalogue (Table 5.8) and Natural Health Products monograph are included in the Natural Health Products Composition Database of the Canadian Ministry of Health for public inquiry.

Table 5.8   Raw Materials for Natural Health Products in Canada

No	Material Category
1	Raw materials from plants, algae, bacteria, fungi and animals
2	The extracts or isolates of the above raw materials which the main molecular structure is the same as that before extraction or separation
3	Any of the following vitamins: vitamin A, vitamin C, vitamin D, vitamin B_6, vitamin B_{12}, vitamin E. vitamin K_1, vitamin K_2, vitamin H (biotin), folic acid, nicotinic acid, pantothenic acid, riboflavin, vitamin B_1 (thiamine)
4	Amino acids
5	Esential fatty acid
6	Synthetic products of the above 2—5 components
7	Minerals
8	Probiotics

In China, according to the GB 16740—2014, National Food Safety Standard—"Health Foods", health foods are defined as claiming and having specific health functions, or aiming to supplement the vitamins and minerals. Health foods are suitable for specific population to consume and regulate body function, not intended to cure diseases, at same time the health foods have no any acute, subacute or chronic hazards to human body. In the "Food Safety

Law of the People's Republic of China", it is emphasized that based on science health foods can claim health function and cannot cause any hazards to human body.

According to the above definition, the health foods can be divided into two categories. The first category is nutrients supplement; including vitamins and minerals supplements, not including supplements that can provide energy to human body such as protein powder, fish oil. The roles of nutrients supplements are to supplement the inadequate dietary intake, to prevent nutritional deficiencies and reduce the risk of some chronic degenerative diseases. The second catergory is functional health food; refers to health foods that have one or several functional claims, such as enhancing immunity, alleviating physical fatigue, anti-oxidation action and so on.

In China, the following properties of heath foods are emphasized: a. Health food is a kind of special foods, which main character cannot be separated from food, but it is allowed to use capsules, tablets, granules, oral liquid and other pharmaceutical dosage forms; b. Health food must have efficacy; c. The suitable population of health food is different from general food, and it is only suitable for specific population to take; d. Health food is not designed for the treatment of diseases. Another difference between health food and medicines is that health food is not allowed to have side effects under the existing scientific and technological level, while medicines have clear side effects. Health food cannot replace reasonable diet, nor can it replace medicines.

(3) Functional Factors of Functional Food

Functional factors, also known as functional ingredients, are the key components of functional food to regulate the body's function. There are many kinds of functional factors.

① Functional carbohydrate: active polysaccharides include plant polysaccharides, algae polysaccharides, bacterial polysaccharides and fungal polysaccharides. Lentinus edodes polysaccharides, Ganoderma lucidum polysaccharides and Lycium barbarum polysaccharides are common. Most polysaccharides have immunomodulatory and anti-tumor effects. Some polysaccharides also have hypoglycemic effects. As a functional carbohydrate, dietary fiber has the functions of preventing obesity, lowering blood sugar, lowering blood lipid, moistening intestine and relieving stool, preventing colon cancer and improving intestinal flora.

② Proteins, active peptides and amino acids: proteins, active peptides and amino acids can be used as raw materials and functional ingredients of functional foods. They are mostly used in regulating immune function foods, especially essential amino acids. In addition, several amino acids with special physiological activities have also been widely used. Taurine can promote the growth and intellectual development of infants, protect the cardiovascular system, protect the retina and improve the immunity of the body. The taurine content of human breast milk is much higher than that of cow milk, so it is often used in infant formula food, health food and beverage. Arginine can enhance the activity of arginase in liver, alleviate hyperammonia and liver dysfunction. It also has the effects of immune regulation, inhibiting tumors and promoting wound healing. It can be used to prevent and treat mental symptoms caused by hepatic encephalopathy and other causes of elevated blood ammonia. It can also be used to develop functional food for immunoregulation and inhibiting tumors.

Active peptide refers to a kind of small molecular polypeptide with molecular weight less than 6 000 D, which is composed of no more than 10 amino acids in different composition and arrangement. It has many biological functions. In recent years, it has also been widely used in functional food. Some peptides are commonly used such as glutathione (GSH), casein phosphopeptide (which can promote calcium absorption, mostly used in functional food supplemented with calcium and iron), soybean oligopeptide (which can be used as protein source for allergic constitution and nutrition-related chronic diseases), high branched chain amino acid oligopeptide (mostly used in athletes' food), antimicrobial peptide, wheat oligopeptide, marine fish collagen peptide.

③ Functional lipids: functional lipids mainly include polyunsaturated fatty acids (linoleic acid, arachidonic acid, alpha-linolenic acid, eicosapentaenoic acid and docosahexaenoic acid), monounsaturated fatty acids (oleic acid, nervous acid), phospholipids and so on. These functional fatty acids can reduce blood lipids and prevent coronary heart disease.

④ Other plant active factors: flavonoids, saponins, alkaloids, carotenoids and allicin are also functional factors of many functional foods. These active factors are also the main active ingredients of traditional Chinese herbal medicine for both food and medicine in China.

⑤ Probiotics: the relationship between probiotics and health has become a hotspot in recent years. It has been found that probiotics are related to the occurrence and development of many human diseases and play an important role in health. The research and development of probiotic functional food has also become a hotspot, such as *Lactobacillus acidophilus*, *Lactobacillus casei*, *Lactobacillus bulgaricus*, *Bifidobacterium longum*, *Lactococcus*, *Streptococcus thermophilus* and so on.

(4) Functional (Health) Claims for Functional Food

According to the International Codex Alimentarius Commission, the definition of health claims are any text that indicates, prompts or implies the relationship between a food or ingredient and disease or health status in the food label. And health claims include the following types: a. Nutritional component functional claim: nutritional component function claims refer to the description of the physiological role of nutrients in the growth and development of the body and in the maintenance of basic functions; b. Other functional claims: other functional claims refer to descriptions of food or food ingredients that maintain or improve the function or physiological activity of the body, descriptions that promote the normal structure and function of the body; c. Reducing disease risk claims: reducing disease risk claims refer to the statement that food or food ingredients can reduce the risk of disease. Reducing disease risk usually refers to significantly antagonizing the major risk factors associated with disease.

Many functional foods contain more vitamins, minerals and other essential nutrients than ordinary foods. The health benefits of some of these nutrients have been demonstrated, and they can improve health to some extent. For example, folic acid can reduce neural tube deformities; polyunsaturated fatty acids can reduce the risk of heart disease, etc. In addition, functional foods may also contain other active substances such as phytochemicals, which have been shown to have certain physiological effects. For example, glycol can reduce the risk of dental caries; phytosterol/sterol esters can reduce LDL cholesterol; probiotics can reduce infant rotavirus infectious diarrhea, etc.

The opinion about claim of reducing disease risk is most controversial. A considerable number of countries remain cautious about whether such claims have sufficient scientific basis and are not allowed to mention any disease-related claims. Some countries, from the perspective of public health, allow the labeling of "Reducing Disease Risk Claim". However, the Codex Standards formulated by the Codex Alimentarius Commission on Nutrition and Special Dietary Food and many countries prohibit the use of "health claims" in infant and child foods.

Canada permits natural health products to have health claims, which must be declared simultaneously in the process of applying for licensing of natural health products. Health claims management focuses on the scientific and authentic evaluation including product safety. Applicants are required to provide relevant supporting evidence of safety and efficacy for the health claims of the applicant products in accordance with the regulations. Based on different classification criteria, modern health claims can be divided into three categories, namely: ① claims for different health states including severe, general and minor diseases; ② claims for different health functions namely for diagnosis, treatment, cure, risk reduction, prevention, general health maintenance/support/promotion and antioxidation; ③ claims for general health with low efficacy, namely source/provision/containment claim, component-based claim, claim of good health, general claim of helping/supporting/maintaining/promoting health, general claim of mechanism-based, alleviation of low efficacy impact and risk reduction of low efficacy impact.

The United States is one of the earliest countries to regulate health claims. FDA mainly regulates the format, content and health declaration on the labels. There are three types of claims allowed in traditional food and dietary supplements in the United States, namely health claims, nutrient content claims and structure/function claims. The approved claims have a Federal Rule Code (CFR) and are filed by the FDA. The claims of dietary supplements about solving nutrients deficiencies, improving health, or having specific functions such as immunomodulation and cardiovascular protection are allowed. However, the manufacturer should submit the scientific evidences of the claim to FDA. And these efficacy descriptions need to be noted later: "This efficacy statement has not been certified by the Food and Drug Administration. This product is not used to diagnose, treat, cure or prevent any disease".

In EU, functional claims mainly include "nutrition claims" and "health claims", in which "health claims" are further divided into "general health claims", "reducing disease risk claims", and "children's growth and development health claims". Relevant procedures and regulations have been formulated respectively. And EU has implemented the system of list record combined with administrative licensing. In addition to reducing disease risk claims and promoting health-related claims of adolescents and young children, administrative permission is required for other general claims. Under certain conditions, the technical information of the first applicant is protected for seven years.

In 1991, Japan regulated health claims in "Special Health Food" (FOSHU). In addition, 13 nutritional functional claims were approved and filed. The main claims of specific health food include regulating intestine and stomach, lowering cholesterol absorption, lowering blood pressure, inhibiting blood sugar rise, improving anemia, helping mineral absorption, and preventing dental caries. No specific functional evaluation criteria have been formulated, and the applicant enterprises conduct research by themselves.

In China, the nutrient supplements only claim to supplement the related nutrients, for example, one product containing calcium only claim that has the function of supplementing calcium. There are 27 functional claims of functional health foods permitted after registration now. Twenty-seven functional claims are listed in Table 5.9. In the registration ofhealth food, it is necessary to submit the safety and functional assessment data of qualified units. The label and instructions of health foods should not claim the function about diseases prevention and treatment. The contents should be real and consistent with filing and registration. Besides, the contents should clearly state the suitable and unsuitable for the consumption by specific population, function components or main components and its dosages. It also should claim "This product cannot replace drugs".

Table 5.9　Twenty Seven Functional Claims of Functional Health Foods in China

Animal Experiments Only Needed (7 Claims)	Human Trails Only Needed (5 Claims)	Both Animal Experiments and Human Trials Needed (15 Claims)
Enhancing immunity, improving sleep, increasing bone density, relieving physical fatigue, protecting against chemical liver injury, auxiliary protection against radiation hazards, enhancing hypoxia tolerance	Relieving asthenopia, dispelling acne, dispelling chloasma, improving skin moisture, improving skin oil	Auxiliary hypolipidemic effect, auxiliary hypoglycemic effect, anti-oxidation action, auxiliary memory improvement, promoting the excretion of lead, improving the function of pharynx, auxiliary function of lowering blood pressure, weight loss, improving growth and development, relieving nutritional anemia, regulating intestinal flora, promoting digestion, promoting the excretion of feces, auxiliary protective effect on gastric mucosa injury, promoting lactation

The new revision of "Food Safety Law of the People's Republic of China" passed on April 24, 2015 and implemented on Oct. 1, 2015. In this law document, the health food is considered as one kind of special foods also including foods for special medical purpose (FSMP) and infant recipe foods. All the special foods should be in strict supervision and management.

Health food raw materials refer to the initial materials related to the function of health food, and health food accessories refer to excipients and other additional materials used in the production of health food. The raw materials and excipients used in health food shall conform to the national standards and hygienic requirements.

According to the recent institutional reforms in China, the State Administration of Market Supervision and Administration is responsible for the supervision and management of health food. Recently, a draft consultation on functional claims and raw materials for health food filing has been issued.

(Sun Guiju, Pang Daohua, Qiu Lianglin, He Canxia, Tang Chunlan, Feng Dan, Zou Zuquan, Yang Danting, Ye Yang, and Zha Longying)

5.3　Life Cycle Nutrition

The life cycle is the age-related sequence of stages individuals pass through beginning with birth and ending with death. An individual's needs for nutrients, energy and concerns vary during different stages of life cycle. This chapter illustrates how nutrition impacts healthy people as they grow, develop, and function through the stages of life.

5.3.1　Nutritional Aspects of Pregnancy and Lactation

5.3.1.1　Nutrition During Pregnancy

Sufficient calories and nutrients are needed for a favorable pregnancy outcome owning that all parts of the infant-bones, muscles, organs, blood cells, skin, and other tissues are made from nutrients in the foods consumed by the mother. For most pregnant women, nutrient needs during pregnancy are higher than at any other time; however, only calories and the nutrients of particular importance during pregnancy are discussed in this chapter.

(1) Energy Needs During Pregnancy

A pregnant woman needs extra calories to support the growth of fetus tissue as well as to fuel the extra metabolic workload pregnancy putting on a woman's heart, lungs, and other organs. The intake of extra energy promotes the increase of body weight of pregnant woman, while maternal weight gain during pregnancy is linked closely to infant birth weight, which strongly indicates the health and subsequent development of the infant. Infants born to women who consumed insufficient calories are more likely to die soon after birth. Those who survive are likely born small and experiencing severe, lifelong consequences with a greater risk of developing heart disease, high blood cholesterol levels, diabetes, high blood pressure and impaired immune function. In contrast, women who gain excessively higher amounts than the recommendations typically give birth to very large babies and experience an increase in complications at delivery, infant mortality, and weight retention postpartum. The recommended intakes of energy and some important nutrients are summarized in Table 5. 10.

Table 5. 10   Recommended Energy or Nutrient Intake of Pregnant Women in China

Energy or Nutrient Intake	First Trimester	Second Trimester	Third Trimester
Energy (kilo calories)	+0	+340	+450
Protein (gram)	+0	+15	+30
Folate (micro gram)	+400	+400	+400
Calcium (mili gram)	+0	+200	+200
Zinc (mili gram)	+0	+2	+2
Iron (mili gram)	+0	+4	+9
Iodine (micro gram)	+0	+110	+110
VA (RAE)	+0	+70	+70

An underweight woman (BMI<19. 8) can improve her nutrient stores and pregnancy outcome by gaining weight before pregnancy or gaining extra weight during pregnancy. It is easy for a pregnant woman to meet the need for extra energy by choosing nutrient-dense foods like whole-grain breads and cereals, legumes, dark green vegetables, citrus fruits, low-fat milk and milk products, lean meats, fish, poultry and eggs. If a woman has not gained the desired weight by a given point in pregnancy, she should not try to gain the needed weight rapidly. Instead, she should slowly gain a little more weight than the typical pattern to meet the goal by the end of the pregnancy. Alternately, if a woman begins to gain too much weight during her pregnancy, she should slow the increase in weight by minimizing her intake of foods that provide unnecessary calories instead of losing weight. Pregnant women can develop significant amounts of ketones after only 20 hours of fasting, so eating regular meals and avoiding fasting for more than 12 hours are important. Table 5. 11 presents recommended weight gains for various pre-pregnancy weights in China.

Table 5. 11   Recommended Weight Gain of Pregnant Women Based on Prepregnancy Weight

Pre-pregnancy Weight	Recommended Weight Gain During Pregnancy
Underweight (BMI < 18. 5)	12. 5 to 18. 0 kg
Healthy weight (BMI 18. 5 to 24. 9)	11. 5 to 16. 0 kg
Overweight (BMI 25. 0 to 29. 9)	7. 0 to 11. 5 kg
Obese (BMI⩾30)	5. 0 to 9. 0 kg

It should be mentioned that the nutrient needs of a woman carrying multiple fetuses are higher than those of a woman carrying a single fetus. In addition, numerous previous pregnancies and/or closely spaced pregnancies (less than 1 year apart) may deplete a woman's nutrient stores, which increases the risk that a subsequent pregnancy will result in a preterm birth, low birth weight infant, or small for gestational age infant.

(2) Nutrients Needs During Pregnancy

① Carbohydrate: Sufficient carbohydrate ensures that the protein needed for growth will not be broken down and used to make glucose. Ketosis can result from restricting carbohydrate intake or fasting and is not desirable for the growing fetus. Ketone bodies are thought to be poorly used by the fetal brain and may slow its development. Ample carbohydrate (at least above 175 g to prevent ketosis) is necessary to fuel the fetal brain. A good choice for pregnant women is to select whole-grain breads and cereals, legumes, dark green vegetables, citrus fruits, because these foods can provide carbohydrate and phytochemicals, along with dietary fiber which is helpful to alleviate the constipation that many pregnant women experiences.

Gestational diabetes develops in approximately 4% of women who entered pregnancy without diabetes often between 24 to 28 weeks of pregnancy due to the hormones synthesized by the placenta. Uncontrolled diabetes can cause the fetus to grow quite large. The oversupply of glucose from maternal circulation signals the fetus to increase insulin production, which causes fetal tissues to readily use glucose for growth. Another threat is that the infant may have low blood glucose at birth because of the tendency to produce extra insulin that began during gestation. Other concerns are the potential for preterm delivery and increased risks of birth trauma and malformations. Infants born to mothers with gestational diabetes also may have higher risks of developing obesity and type 2 diabetes as they grow to adulthood. Untreated gestational diabetes can severely deplete fetal iron stores. The abnormally high blood glucose levels caused by gestational diabetes often return to normal after giving birth; however, the mother's risk of developing diabetes later in life will rise, especially if she is obese. Exercise and a diet that distributes low glycemic load carbohydrates throughout the day are important to keep gestational diabetes under control. Some women may need insulin therapy.

② Protein: Pregnant women can easily meet their protein needs (table 5.6) by selecting meats, milk products, and protein-containing plant foods such as legumes, nuts and seeds. The use of high-protein supplements during pregnancy may be harmful to the infant's development; therefore, protein supplements are neither needed nor recommended during pregnancy.

③ Essential fatty acid: The high nutrient requirements of pregnancy leave little room in the diet for excess fat, but the essential long-chain polyunsaturated fatty acids are particularly important to the growth and development of the fetus. The brain is largely made of lipid material, and depends heavily on the long-chain omega-3 and omega-6 fatty acids for its growth, function and structure. The recommended foods are fish, marine products and nuts.

④ Folate and vitamin B12: As the fetus grows and develops, new cells are laid down at a tremendous pace. All nutrients are important in these processes, but for folate, vitamin B12, iron and zinc, their needs are especially great due to their key roles in the synthesis of DNA and new cells.

Folate and vitamin B12, two vitamins famous for their roles in cell reproduction, are needed in increased amount during pregnancy. The sufficient folate from a combination of supplements, fortified foods, and a diet that includes fruits, juices, green vegetables and whole grains is known as vital to prevent neural tube defect. Pregnant woman also needs a greater amount of B12 to assist folate in the manufacture of new cells. Generally, even modest amounts of meat, fish, eggs, or milk products together with body stores easily meet the need for vitamin B12. Vegans who exclude all foods of animal origin, however, need daily supplements of vitamin B12 or vitamin B12-fortified foods to prevent the neurological complications of a deficiency.

⑤ Iron: A pregnant woman needs iron to support her enlarged blood volume and to provide for placental and fetal needs. The developing fetus draws on mother's iron stores to create a sufficient supply of iron to last through the first four to six months of life. Even a woman with inadequate iron stores transfer significant amounts of iron to the fetus, suggesting that the iron needs of the fetus have priority over those of the mother. In addition, blood losses are inevitable at birth, especially during a cesarean section, and further draining the mother's iron supply.

In fact, maternal body makes several adaptations including the increase in iron absorption of up to threefold and blood transferrin (iron-absorbing and iron-carrying protein) level as well as cease of menstruation to meet the exceptionally high need for iron of infants. Without sufficient intake, though, iron deficiency is common among pregnant women. Therefore, for all pregnant women, the only supplement needed is iron during the last 2 trimesters. For this reason, most prenatal supplements provide standard dose of 30 mg of iron maybe prescribed when a low hemoglobin or hematocrit is diagnosed. To enhance iron absorption, the supplement should be taken between meals or at bedtime and with liquids other than milk, coffee, or tea, which inhibit iron absorption. Vitamin C enhances iron absorption by converting iron from ferric to ferrous, it is also helpful in preventing the premature rupture of amniotic membranes.

⑥ Zinc: Zinc is vital for DNA, RNA and protein synthesis, as well as cell development. Typical zinc intakes for pregnant women are lower than recommendations, but fortunately, zinc absorption increases when zinc intakes are low. Zinc is abundant in protein-rich foods such as shellfish, meat, and nuts, thus routine supplementation is not advised. However, women taking iron supplements (more than 30 mg per day), may need zinc supplementation, since large doses of iron can interfere with the zinc absorption and metabolism.

⑦ Vitamin D and calcium: Pregnancy is not a time to self-prescribe medications or vitamin and mineral supplements. For example, although vitamin A is a routine component of prenatal vitamins, it is important to note that intakes over 3 times the RDA can have toxic effects on the fetus. However, vitamin D and the bone-building mineral (calcium, phosphorus, magnesium, and fluoride) are in great demand during pregnancy. Insufficient intakes may produce abnormal fetal bones and teeth development.

Vitamin D plays a vital role in calcium absorption and utilization, severe maternal vitamin D deficiency interferes with normal calcium metabolism, which may cause osteomalacia in the mother, and rickets in the infant in rare cases. Regular exposure to sunlight and consumption of vitamin D-fortified milk are usually sufficient to provide the recommended amount of vitamin D during pregnancy. Vegans who avoid milk, eggs, and fish may receive enough vitamin D from regular exposure to sunlight and fortified soy milk.

Calcium absorption and retention increases dramatically early in pregnancy, helping the mother to meet the calcium needs of pregnancy. During the last trimester, as the fetal bones begin to calcify, the mother's bone calcium stores are mobilized, there is a dramatic shift of calcium across placenta. In the final weeks of pregnancy, over 300 mg per day are transferred to the fetus. Recommendations to ensure an adequate calcium intake during pregnancy are aimed to conserve the mother's bone mass when supplying fetal needs.

(3) Dietary Guidelines for Pregnant Women

The Dietary Guidelines provides evidence-based food and beverage recommendations. Public health agencies, health care providers, and educational institutions all rely on Dietary Guidelines recommendations and strategies. Dietary guidelines for pregnant women by CNS (2016) add the following five items to the Guidelines for the general population:

① Supplement folic acid, often consume iron-rich food, choose iodized salt.

② If the pregnancy and vomiting is serious, women can consume a small amount of meals to ensure the intake of food containing the necessary amount of carbohydrates.

③ In the middle and third trimester of pregnancy, the intake of milk, fish, poultry, eggs and lean meat should be increased.

④ Appropriate physical activity to maintain proper weight gain during pregnancy.

⑤ No smoking and alcohol, happy to give birth to a new life, actively prepare for breastfeeding.

5.3.1.2　Nutrition During Lactation

Breastfeeding is the perfect way to nourish a baby for its first 6 months of life, offers many health benefits to both mother and infant (Table 5.12), and every pregnant woman should seriously consider whether to feed her infant with breast milk, infant formula, or both as the time of childbirth nears.

Table 5. 12   Benefits of Breastfeeding

For infants:

Provide the appropriate composition and balance of nutrients with high bioavailability

Provide hormones that promote physiological development

Improve cognitive development

Offer immunological protection

May protect against some chronic diseases, such as diabetes, obesity, atherosclerosis, asthma, and hypertension, later in life

Protect against food allergies

For mothers:

Contract the uterus

Delay the return of regular ovulation, thus lengthening birth intervals

Conserve iron stores

May protect against breast and ovarian cancer and reduce the risk of type 2 diabetes

Others:

Cost saving from not needing medical treatment for childhood illnesses or time off work to care for them

Cost saving from not needing to purchase formula

Environmental savings to society from not needing to manufacture, package, and ship formula and dispose of the packaging

Convenience of not having to shop for and prepare formula

Promote mother-infant bonding

(1) Lactation: A Physiological Process

During pregnancy, hormones promote the growth and branching of a duct system in the breasts and the development of the milk-producing cells. The infant's sucking stimulates the release of prolactin and oxytocin, these hormones finely coordinate mammary glands to supply milk. Prolactin is responsible for milk production, while the oxytocin causes the mammary glands to eject milk into the ducts, and secret of milk from mother's mammary glands to nourish the infant.

(2) Maternal Energy and Nutrient Needs during Lactation

A nursing mother produces about 25 ounces of milk per day, with considerable variation from woman to woman and in the same woman from time to time. The volume produced depends primarily on the infant's sucking. Ideally, the mother who chooses to breastfeed her infant will continue to consume nutrient-dense foods throughout lactation.

① Energy intake: Producing an adequate supply of milk almost costs a woman 500 kcal a day above her regular need during the first six months of lactation. To meet this energy need, womenare advised to consume an extra 330 kcal from foods each day. The other 170 kcal can be drawn from the accumulated fat which she reserves during pregnancy.

② Macronutrients: During lactation, recommendations for protein and fatty acids intakes remain the same as during pregnancy, but needs for carbohydrates and fibers increase. Nursing mothers need additional carbohydrate to synthesize lactose in breast milk.

The fiber recommendation is 1 gram higher with the increase of energy intake during lactation.

③ Vitamins and minerals: In general, nutritional inadequacies of mother reduce the quantity not the quality of breast milk. Women can produce milk with adequate protein, carbohydrate, fat and most minerals, even when their own supplies are limited at the expense of maternal stores. This is most evident in the case of calcium: dietary calcium has no effect on the calcium concentration of breast milk, but maternal bones lose some density during lactation if calcium intakes are inadequate. Most lactating women can obtain all the nutrients they need from a balanced diet. However, some may need iron supplements so as to refill their exhausted iron store which is caused by mother supplying the developing fetus with enough iron to last through the first four to six months of the infant's life. Furthermore, childbirth may have incurred blood losses. Therefore, a woman may need iron supplements during lactation.

Nutrients in breast milk that are most likely to decline in response to prolonged inadequate intakes are the vitamins-especially vitamins B6, B12, A, and D. Vitamin supplements appear to help normalize the vitamin concentrations in the milk of undernourished women.

④ Water: Breast milk contains lots of water, so a lactating woman needs to drink plenty of fluids to preventdehydration. Nursing woman is advised to take a glass of milk, juice, or water at each meal and each time the infant nurses.

(3) Dietary Guidelines for Lactating Women

Dietary guidelines for lactating women by Chinese Nutrition Society (2016) add the following five items to the guidelines for the general population:

① Increase the animal food and seafood rich in high quality protein and vitamin A, opt for iodized salt.

② Do not overeat the food during the puerperal period, attach importance to the nutrition of the whole lactation period.

③ Enjoy the mood, get enough sleep and promote the secretion of milk.

④ Insist on breastfeeding, moderate exercise, gradually restore appropriate weight.

⑤No tobacco and alcohol, avoid strong tea and coffee.

5.3.2　Nutrition During the Growing Years-Infancy, Childhood, and Adolescence

5.3.2.1　Nutrition During Infancy

(1) Energy and Nutrients Need

The period from birth to 12 months of age, known as infancy, is a time of phenomenal growth and development. An infant generally grows about 10 inches in length and triple in weight, that growth rate more rapid than will ever occur again. Infants' rapid growth and development depend on adequate energy and nutrient supply. Breast milk is a naturally well-nourished food for infants. According to WHO recommendations, exclusive breastfeeding is recommended as optimal feeding for infant during their first 6 months of life, and subsequently nutritionally adequate and safe complementary feeding starts from the age of 6 months with continued breastfeeding for at least the first year of life, and if possible, up to 2 years of age or beyond.

① Energy and macronutrients: Most of energy intake during infancy is used to support growth and development. In the first few months, eating and sleeping are infants' main activities. During 6 to 12 months of life, infants begin some activities such as rolling over, sitting up, crawling, standing, and finally taking the first few wobbly steps. The babies' basal metabolic rates are high during infancy, in part because the growth of brain is higher than at any other time, and body surface area is larger compared to their body size. According to the DRIs from Chinese Society of Nutrition, during the first 6 months, a healthy infant generally needs about 90 kilocalories per kilogram of body weight per day (kcal/kg/d), whereas most adults need fewer than 40. After 6 months, the infant's energy needs decline to 80 kcal/kg/d as the growth rate slows down, but some of the energy saved by slower growth is spent in increased activity.

No single nutrient is more essential to growth and development for infants than protein, which is the basic building material of the body's tissues and organs. An adequate intake (AI) for protein is set at 9 g/d for infants 0 to 6 months of age, while recommended nutrient intake (RNI) is set at 20 g/d for infants 7 to 12 months old. Breast milk and infant formula provide enough high-quality protein to meet infants' needs.

Carbohydrate provides energy to all the cells in the body, especially those in the brain, which depend primarily on glucose to fuel themselves. Carbohydrates from breast milk can satisfy the infants' needs. Based on the data of carbohydrate concentration in the breast milk from Chinese population, the AI for carbohydrate for infant aged 0 to 6 months and infant 7 to 12 months old is set at 60 g/d, and 85 g/d respectively.

The recommendation for total lipids for infants aged 0 to 6 months is 48% of total energy, for infants 7 to 12 months old is 40%. The percentage of energy providing by fat to total energy (about half) in breast milk is well ideal. In addition, breast milk is an excellent natural source of essential fatty acids, such as docosahexaenoic acid (DHA) and arachidonic acid (AA), which are essential for the rapid growth and nervous system development of infants at their 0 to 2 years of life. The AI for DHA for infants is 100 mg/d. The AI for AA for infants 0 to 6 months old is set at 150 mg/d.

② Vitamins and minerals: The DRIs for selected micronutrients for Chinese infants' listed in Table 5.13. Infants need micronutrients to meet their rapid growth and development. Among them, iron, zinc, fluoride, iodide and vitamin D are of special concern. The mineral iron concentration is relatively low in breast milk, but healthy full-term infants are born with enough iron stores to satisfy their needs until 6 months old. Iron need increases dramatically to 10 mg/d for infants 6 to 12 months old. Thus, the complementation of iron-rich foods is recommended for infants 6 months old. Vitamin D could not be efficiently transferred through mammary glands to breast milk, infants need sunlight exposure to generate endogenous vitamin D, if this is not possible, exclusive breast-fed infants are recommended to be given 10 μg (400 IU) of vitamin D supplement each day within the first few days after birth. Moreover, all infants are routinely given an injection of vitamin K shortly after birth. This is helpful for infant until vitamin K producing by healthful bacteria can be developed in infants' intestine.

Table 5. 13   AI for Selected Micronutrients During Infancy

Micronutrients	Birth—6 Months	6—12 Months
Calcium (mg/d)	200	250
Iron (mg/d)	0. 3	10
Zinc (mg/d)	2	3. 5
Fluoride (mg/d)	0. 01	0. 23
Iodine (μg/d)	85	115
Vitamin A (μgRAE/d)	300	350
Vitamin D (μg/d)	10	10
Vitamin K (μg/d)	2	10

③ Water: Fluid is critical for everyone, especially infants. The younger the infant, the greater the percentage of body weight is water. During early infancy, breast milk or infant formula normally provides enough water to replace fluid losses of a healthy infant. The supplement of water is necessary under the conditions of rapid fluid loss, such as fever, diarrhea or vomiting in order to prevent dehydration.

(2) Nutritional Quality of Breast Milk

Breast milk serves as an ideal source of nutrients for infants for the first 6 months of life, including proteins, carbohydrates, fats, vitamins, minerals and water; thus, infants under 6 months can receive only breast milk without liquids or solids, even water. Furthermore, breast milk contains bioactive factors that improve the infant's immature immune system, and protect against a variety of infectious and other diseases.

① Protein: The amount and type of protein in breast milk are ideal for the infant growth. The lower concentration of protein in breast milk compared with animal milk and infant formula doesn't overload the infants' immature kidneys with waste nitrogen products. About 80% of protein in colostrum is the easily digested whey, while the remaining is the curd-forming casein which is harder for infant to digest. The whey-to-casein ratio makes human milk ideal for infants' immature gastrointestinal tracts, with lower risk for gastric distress. In contrast, casein is the main protein in cow's milk. Furthermore, colostrum contains high levels of antibodies and immunoglobulin, especially secretory immunoglobulin A (sIgA), which can be absorbed by infants' immature digestive tract and defend against infectious disease.

② Carbohydrate: The primary carbohydrate in human milk is lactose, which is a disaccharide composed of glucose and galactose. Breast milk contains more lactose than cow's milk, which provides energy for infant and prevent from ketosis. Breastfeeding promotes growth of *lactobacillus bifidus* in an infant's gastrointestinal tract, these bacteria could aid in lactose digestion and control the growth of potential harmful bacteria. Breast milk also contains oligosaccharides, which act as natural prebiotics by promoting the growth of the beneficial bacteria in the large intestine, and provide important protection against intestinal infections during infancy.

③ Fat: The amount and type of fat in breast milk are greatly suitable for the human infant growth. The high concentration of fat in breast milk (3. 5 g per 100 mL), in contrast to cow milk, can provide about 48% of the energy of the breast milk. More interestingly, the amount of fat changes as the feeding processing. At the beginning of the session, the mother's milk, known as foremilk, is watery and low in fat, which is helpful to rapidly satisfy the infants' initial thirst. As the feeding progresses, the milk acquires more fat and becomes more like whole milk. Finally, the higher fat content of hind milk satiates the infant and as a result, discontinues feeding. Babies who do not suckle long enough to receive the hind milk may become hungry soon after the feeding, so mothers are suggested to let baby drain one breast before moving to the other. Furthermore, breast milk contains relatively high level of essential fatty acids and cholesterol.

④ Vitamins and minerals: Generally, the vitamin content of breast milk depends on the maternal intake. For most lactating women, breast milk contains sufficient vitaminsfor infants, unless the mother herself is deficient. The exception is vitamin D and iron, where both are relatively low in breast milk.

⑤ Fluid: Another important aspect of breastfeeding is the fluid it provides. In order to supply enough fluid and prevent dehydration, feeding must be consistent and frequent.

(3) Complementary Foods

Complementary foods are mashed, pureed (ground up, moistened, and blended), or solid foods as well as beverages other than breast milk or infant formula. The primary food for infants during the first 12 months is either breast milk or iron-fortified formula. Infants gradually develop the ability to chew, swallow, and digest, thus they are developmentally ready for complementary foods at about four to six months of age. Caregivers should notice the signs indicating that an infant is ready for complementary foods. The child: ① can sit with some back support; ② has lost the extrusion reflex; ③ can hold its head up steady and straight; ④ shows interest in consuming foods that adult caregivers and older children eat; ⑤ opens his or her mouth when he or she sees food. Solid foods should be introduced no later than 8 months old.

The main purpose of complementary foods is to provide needed nutrients that are no longer supplied adequately by breast milk or formula alone. Iron-fortified cereals for infants are often the first food introduced for two reasons. Firstly, rapid growth of infants demands iron, while infant iron stores are depleted at about six months of life. Secondly, rice cereal rarely provokes an allergic reaction and is easy to digest. The disadvantage of iron-fortified cereals is poor bioavailability, therefore, serving vitamin C-rich foods with meals is necessary to enhance iron absorption from iron-fortified cereals. It is noteworthy to introduce one new food at a once, in a small portion, and wait for 4 to 5 days before introducing the next new food, so that parents can watch for signs of allergies. A variety of foods should be gradually introduced by the end of the first year. By one year, they can eat many kinds of foods as the rest members of the family. Some foods should never be offered to an infant, including foods that can cause choking, honey, goat's milk and cow's milk, unpasteurized milk, too much salt and sugar.

(4) Infant Feeding Guideline in China (2016)

① Birth to 6-month-old.

- Baby starts sucking after birth, the newborn's first food is breast milk;
- Exclusive breastfeeding for the 6 months of life;
- Transfer from feeding on demand to regular feeding;
- Supplement vitamin D from several days after birth, no need to supplement calcium;
- Infant formula is the alternative to exclusive breastfeeding;
- Monitor anthropometric indicators and maintain healthy growth.

② 6-month-old to 24-month-old.

- Continue to breastfeed and introduce solid foods around 6 months;
- Start with iron-rich mashed foods, progressing to variety of healthy foods;
- Responsive feeding, no force feeding;
- Complementary food cooking without condiments, minimize the consumption of sugar and salt;
- Pay attention to food hygiene and safety;
- Regularly monitor anthropometric indicators and maintain healthy growth.

5.3.2.2　Nutrition During Childhood

Childhood covers the period from infancy to puberty. Toddler refers to children between age 1 and 3 years old. Children between age 4 and 6 years old usually are called aspreschool-age child. School-age child refers to child between 7 and 10 years old.

(1) Toddler Nutrition

The rapid growth rate in the first 12 months tapers off quickly during toddler to school age years. During toddler, a child typically grows taller by 2 to 3 inches and heavier by 5 to 6 pounds per year. A child's height and weight should continue to be monitored during routine medical checkups as important indicators of nutrition status.

The toddler period is a time of physical and nutritional transition. At age one year, children can stand alone and are beginning to toddle; by two years, they can walk and learn to run, most have a full set of teeth which makes chewing easier; and by three years old, they are more confident in jumping and climbing, most can feed themselves with a fork or spoon. Bones and muscles increased in mass and density to make these accomplishments possible. Thus, children must be provided adequate energy and nutrients to support their growth and development.

① Energy and macronutrients: Although a child's energy needs per kilogram of body weight is slight less than infants, total energy requirements are higher because toddlers are much more active than infants. The amount of calories a toddler needs varies by age and gender. At age 1 year old, the estimated energy requirement (EER) for boy is 900 kcal/d, for girl is 800 kcal/d. At age 2 years old, the EER for boy is 1,100 kcal/d, for girl is 1000 kcal/d. At age 3 years old, the EER for boy is 1,250 kcal/d, for girl is 1,200 kcal/d.

Toddler's protein needs increase modestly. The RNI for protein for age 1 and 2 is 25 g/d, for age 3 is 30 g/d. Thus, toddlers should continue to keep the habit of drinking milk and increase other high-quality protein food source, such as tofu and meat.

Fat intake is important for toddlers, it can provide a concentrated source of energy in a relatively small amount of food. Children who eat low-fat diets tend to have low intakes of some vitamins and minerals. In addition, sources of essential fatty acids, such as flaxseed oil, nuts, fish or supplement, are beneficial to continuously developing nervous system of toddlers. Thus, the recommendation of total fat intakes for a healthy toddler with appropriate body weight is 35% of total energy. Toddlers' AI for linoleic acid and α-linolenic acid are 4% and 0.6% of total energy. The AI for DHA is 100 mg/d.

The EAR for carbohydrate is 120 g/d, should account for about 50%—65% of total energy intake. Complex carbohydrate from whole-grain breads and cereals, fresh fruits and vegetables are helpful food choices for toddlers. In contrast, refined carbohydrate resource such as candies, desserts and snacks should be avoided as possible.

② Vitamins and minerals: The vitamin and mineral needs of toddlers increase with their age. Adequate intake of calcium, iron and vitamin D is of concern to toddlers. Calcium is necessary for toddlers to obtain optimal bone mass, which continuously accumulates until early adulthood. The RNI for calcium is 600 mg/d. Dairy products are excellent source of calcium. Consuming 300—400 mL milk or milk product per day could meet the calcium requirement of toddlers. At 1 year of age, whole cow's milk can be given to toddlers; however, reduced-fat milk should not be given until age 2 due to their high need for energy. A balanced and nutritious diet can meet children's needs for these nutrients, with the notable exception of iron. During the second year of life, the diet of toddlers changes from a diet of iron-rich infant foods including iron-fortified formula or cereal to a diet of adult foods and iron-poor cow's milk. Iron deficiency anemia is the most common nutrient deficiency disease in young children especially toddlers 1 to 2 years of age in the world. Toddlers' RNI for iron is 9 mg/d. Lean meats, fish, poultry are good source of heme iron, whereas eggs, green vegetables and fortified cereal provide non-heme iron. The iron absorption of non-heme iron is much less than heme iron, serving vitamin C-rich foods, such as fresh vegetables and fruits with meals can enhance non-heme iron absorption. In order to obtain adequate vitamin D, toddlers are suggested to spend one hour a day on outside activities. If not possible, they are suggested to take 10 μg/d vitamin D supplements.

③ Fluid: Compare to infants, toddlers loss less fluid from evaporation, and their mature kidneys can concentrate urine. However, physical activity causes them to loss significant fluid through sweat, especially in hot weather. An active toddler needs to drink enough water. 1300—1600 mL of water (including plain water, milk, soy milk, and soup) per day is recommended for toddlers.

(2) Nutrition for Preschool and School-Age Children

During the preschool and school-age years, children become even more active, but their growth rate slows down. Children grow at a slow and steady pace with an annual increase by 2 to 4 inches in height.

① Energy and macronutrients: The need for energy of kids throughout the childhood continues to increase owning to the increasing body size and higher level of physical activity. Parents should provide diet that allow for normal growth and support physical activity while minimizing the risk for excessive weight gain. The number of calories a child needs varies by age and gender. Table 5. 14 lists the Chinese DRIs for children's energy intake.

Table 5. 14   RNIs for Energy Needs During Preschool and School Age Children(kcal/d)

Age	Estimated Energy Requirement	
	Boy	Girl
4—	1,300	1,250
5—	1,400	1,300
6—	1,600	1,450
7—	1,699	1,511
8—	1,850	1,699
9—	2,000	1,800
10—	2,051	1,900

Although the protein needs per kilogram body weight for children aged 4 to 13 years is lower than that of toddlers, the total protein intake of school-age children is higher due to their higher body weight. The RNI for protein for children ages 4—5 is 30 g/d, for age 6 is 35 g/d, for ages 7—8 is 40 g/d, for age 10 is 50 g/d. Lean meats/fish/poultry, dairy products, soy-based foods are good source of protein that can be served to children of all ages.

Although dietary fat remains a key macronutrient in the preschool and school years, in order to prevent the risk of obesity and overweight caused by fat over consumption, total fat intake should gradually be reduced to a level identical to that of an adult, 20%—30% of total energy. A diet providing fewer than 20% of calories from fat is not recommended for children, as they are still growing, developing, and maturing. Furthermore, children should limit the unhealthy fat intake, for example, saturated fat intake should be less than 8% of total energy per day, trans fatty acids should be less than 1% of total energy per day.

One easy way to start reducing unhealthy dietary fat is to gradually introduce lower-fat dairy products, such as 2% or 1% milk, and to minimize the intake of fatty meat, fried foods, baked foods, cream cake, etc. On contrary, the intake of healthy essential fatty acids, including linoleic acid and α-linolenic acid should achieve the recommended 4% and 0. 6% of total energy. Parents should guide children to categorize the food source of unhealthy and health fats, encourage children to take foods with healthy fats.

The AMDR for carbohydrate for children is 50%—65% of total daily energy intake. Complex carbohydrate from whole grains, fruits, vegetables, and legumes should be emphasized. In order to prevent the risk of dental decay and obesity, children should limit the refined sugar intake less than 10% of total energy.

② Vitamins and minerals: The needs for most micronutrients also increase slightly for children because of their increasing size and transition into full adolescence; this increase is due to the beginning of sexual maturation and preparation for the impending adolescent growth spurt. The intakes of some minerals like calcium, iron, zinc and vitamin D are still of concern.

③ Fluid: The level of physical activity and the weather condition determine the exact amount of fluid a child need. The fluid intake recommended for children generally is 800—1,000 mL.

(3) Dietary Guideline for Preschool Children in China (2016)

① Children feeding themselves without picking eating, develop regular and good eating habits.

② Drink milk and plenty of water every day, choose healthy snacks.

③ Cooking foods with rational methods and eating more digestible foods, minimize condiments and fried foods.

④ Participate in food selection and preparation to enhance the knowledge and love for foods.

⑤ Regular outdoor activities to ensure healthy growth.

5. 3. 2. 3　Nutrition during Adolescence

There is no consensus on the exact age range for adolescence. This life stage generally starts from the onset of puberty, when secondary sexual characteristics develop and reproduction capability gradually mature. In this chapter, we refer to children who are 11 to 17 years of age as adolescents.

Adolescence is the second most rapid period of physiological growth after infancy during the whole life, referred as "the adolescent growth spurt". During the adolescent growth spurt, the growth patterns between boys and girls become distinct. Firstly, the adolescent growth spurt can begin as early as 9 to 10 years of age for girls and 10 to 11 years for boys. It lasts about two and a half years until emerging of adulthood. Secondly, hormonal changes, including increased level of testosterone for boys and estrogen for girls, directly influence the intensity of the growth spurt, profoundly affecting every organ including the brain. Thirdly, significant differences between boys and girls appear in the skeletal system, lean body mass, and fat stores. The average weight gain by girls and boys during adolescence is 39 and 52 pounds, respectively, but the composition of weight gained is considerably different. Girls tend to gain significantly more body fat, while boys gain significantly more lean body mass, principally muscle and bone. On average, boys grow 8 inches taller, and girls, 6 inches taller.

On account of gender difference, the amount of energy and nutrients required during adolescences for boys and girls depend on the individual stage of growth and level of physical activities.

(1) Energy and Macronutrients

Energy and nutrient needs rise throughout childhood, and peak in adolescence. To support their rapid growth and maturation, and fuel their physical activity, adolescents need very high level of energy. The energy needs vary greatly depending on growth stage, gender, body composition, and physical activity. For example, an exceptionally active boy of 15 whose growth spurt begins may need 3,200 kcal energy a day just to maintain his weight, while a sedentary girl aged 15 whose growth rates low may need fewer than 2,000 kcal a day to avoid excessive weight gain. Thus, to meet their nutrient needs without exceeding their energy needs, adolescent girls need to pay special attention to being physically active and selecting foods of high nutrient density. Table 5.15 lists the Chinese DRIs for adolescents' energy intake.

Table 5. 15   RNIs for Energy Needs During Adolescence (kcal/d)

Physical Activity Level	11—13 ages		14—17 ages	
	Boy	Girl	Boy	Girl
Light	2,051	1,800	2,500	2,000
Medium	2,349	2,051	2,849	2,299
Heavy	2,600	2,299	3,200	2,550

As for macronutrients, the RNI for protein is similar to that of adults, is 60 g/d for boys of 11—13, 55 g/d for girls of 11—13, increasing to 75 g/d for boys of 14—17 and 60 g/d for girls of 14—17. The AMDR for fat for adolescents is 20%—30% of total energy, adolescents should consume no more than 8% of total energy from saturated fat sources. The AMDR for carbohydrate is 50%—65% of total energy, and most carbohydrate should come from complex sources. Limiting the refined sugar intake less than 10% of total energy.

(2) Vitamins and Minerals

For adolescents, the RNI for all minerals and most vitamins are higher than school age children. Adequate calcium and vitamin D intakes are critical to achieve peak bone density. Adolescence is a crucial time for bone development, and the requirement for calcium reaches its peak during these years. During puberty, both the absorption of calcium and the activation of vitamin D are enhanced to support the intense skeletal growth of adolescents. The RNI for calcium for adolescents aged 11—13 years is 1,200 mg/d, for aged 14—17 years is 1,000 mg/d. Adolescents' RNI for vitamin D is 10 μg/d. However, most foods are naturally deficient in vitamin D; thus, enough sunlight exposure or supplement is important source of vitamin D.

In adolescence, the iron needs increase for both girls and boys, but for different reasons. Iron is blood lost during menstruation in girl and used to support the growth of lean body mass in boys. Hence, the RNI for iron for boys and girls is 15—16 mg/d and 18 mg/d, respectively. Iron intakes often fail to keep pace with increasing needs, especially for girls, who consume less food rich in heme iron such as lean meat/fish/poultry. Not surprisingly, iron deficiency is the most prevalent among adolescent girls.

Vitamin A is critical to support the rapid growth and development in adolescence. The RNI for vitamin A is 670 μg RAE/d and 820 μg RAE/d for boys ages 11—13 years and boys ages 14—17 years, 630 μg RAE/d for adolescent girls. Naturally vitamin A enriched foods are animal liver, meat, green and orange vegetables, and fruits.

(3) Fluid

The fluid needs of adolescents are higher than children due to their higher physical activity level and the extensive growth and development. They need to drink about 1,100— 1,400 mL water daily. Particularly, boys require more fluid intake because they are generally more active than girls and have more lean tissue. Highly active adolescents should be encouraged to drink often to quench their thirst and avoid dehydration.

Dietary guideline for teenagers in China (2016).

① Get to know food, learn cooking, and improve nutrition science literacy.

② Keep healthy eating behavior with reasonable and regular meals.

③ Choose healthy snacks, drink plenty of water and avoid sugar-sweetened beverages.

④ No picky or on a diet, no overeating, keep a proper weight gain.

⑤ Increase outdoor activities, assure at least 60 minutes physical activity per day.

5.3.3　Adulthood and the Later Years

Aging is defined as the time-dependent physical and physiological decrease of body structure and function which work normally in adulthood. The pace of aging in the elderly is personalized and determined by many factors like heredity, lifestyle which includes nutrition, and environment. Especially, nutrition has many documented roles that are critical to slowdown the aging process.

5.3.3.1　Age-Related Physiological Changes

As aging advances, inevitable changes in each body's organ systems induce the decline of body's function. These physiological changes influence nutrition status, just as what growth and development do in the earlier stages of the life cycle.

(1) Body Composition

With aging, the number of human cells and the weight of muscle tissue decreases and muscle atrophy occurs. The adipose tissue in the body increases gradually, and the distribution of fat in the body storage site also changes. There is a trend of centripetal distribution, that is, the body fat gradually turns from the limbs to the trunk.

Typically, bone minerals, bone matrix and bone density decrease with age. In women, loss rises significantly in the first 5 to 10 years after menopause, which may lead to osteoporosis.

The decrease of intracellular fluid is a main factor causing the reduction of total amount of water in the human body. The latter elevates the risk of dehydration and decreases the body's ability to regulate its internal temperature.

(2) Digestive System

Significant changes occur in the mouth, stomach, intestinal tract, and related organs with aging. The elderly is more likely to suffer from tooth loss or gum disease, which tends to limit their food choices on soft foods. Salivary production declines with age, thereby reduces taste perception, increases tooth decay, and makes chewing and swallowing more difficult. Along with the deterioration of swallowing function, choking may easily occur during drinking water. Consequently, the person may eat less food and drink fewer beverages, resulting in weight loss, malnutrition, and dehydration.

Older adults also have a risk of lack of gastric acid and intrinsic factor. The reduced gastric acid secretion limited the absorption of some nutrients, most notably, vitamin B12, folate, calcium, iron, and zinc. A lack of intrinsic factor greatly reduced the absorption of vitamin B12. Reduced secretion of digestive enzymes may impair the digestion and absorption of macronutrients.

With aging, the intestinal wall gradually loses strength and elasticity, and hormone secretions decline, which leads to slow motility. Constipation is much more common in the elderly than in the young individuals. Decreased secretion in gastrointestinal tract hormone that regulates appetite reduces energy intake and elevates the risk for nutrient deficiencies.

(3) Immune System

Thymus atrophy, weight loss and significant reduction of T lymphocytes number occur in the elderly. Nutrient deficiencies may aggravate the functionally decreasing of the immune system. In addition, the elderly is more sensitive to food intake adverse effects. Thus, the combination of age and malnutrition makes older people vulnerable to infectious diseases and foodborne diseases. Adding insult to injury, antibiotics often are not effective against infections in people with compromised immune systems.

(4) Sensory Losses

For most individuals, eating is a complicated process, since the sights, sounds, odors, and texture stimulate one's appetite. But the process of aging, sense of smell, touch, taste, and vision decline and negatively influence the food intake and the nutritional status of the elderly. Loss of vision and hearing may contribute to social isolation, and eating alone may lead to poor food intake. Subsequently, weight loss and nutrient deficiencies may follow.

(5) Endocrine System

There is a gradual decrease in synthesis, release of hormone, or sensitivity to hormones during old age. Reduced insulin sensitivity means that it takes longer for blood sugar to return to normal after a meal. A decrease in thyroid hormones slows metabolism and reduces the need for calories. A decrease in growth hormone leads to a decrease in lean tissue and an increase in adipose tissue, both of which reduce metabolic rate and calorie demand. Decline in growth hormone also causes thinning of the skin. Female, whose estrogen levels drop after menopause, are more likely to develop osteoporosis than male.

(6) Cardiovascular and Respiratory Systems

The ability of delivering the blood, which is rich in oxygen and nutrient, to body cells and removing metabolic wastes of the heart and lungs gradually decreases, meanwhile, the blood pressure rises. It is better for older adults to consume more foods which are low in fat and high in antioxidants.

(7) Urinary System

The kidneys are less efficient in filtering waste, concentrating and excreting urine, and the muscles that control urination are weaker in progress. Decreased renal function may impair the reabsorption of glucose, amino acids, and vitamin C, and even impede the activation of vitamin D.

(8) Other Changes

In addition to the physiological changes that accompany aging, psychological changes such as depression, economic changes such as loss of income, and less social communication such as loneliness contribute to poor food intake, thereby influence the nutrition status of the elderly.

5.3.3.2　Energy and Nutrient Needs

Although many nutrients requirements for older adults are the same as young and middle-aged adults, some nutrients requirements increase, and others decrease. Clearly, that balanced diet contributes in substantial ways is helpful to improve the quality of life in old age.

(1) Energy and Macronutrients

① Energy: With aging, lean body mass and thyroid hormones diminish, and basal metabolic level gradually declines at the pace of 2% per decade in adulthood after age 30, and more after menopause. Occupational activity and physical activity decrease and energy expenditure cut down gradually with increasing age. As a result, average energy need declines 5% per decade. The lower energy expenditure of older adults means that the elderly should eat less food to maintain their weights. Upon limited energy allowances, nutrient-dense foods are the best choice for the elderly.

In China, intake energy for elderly people over 65 years old with light physical labor intensity is set at 2,050 kcal/d (male) and 1,700 kcal/d (female). The energy intake is established for the elderly over 80 years old with light physical labor intensity at 1,900 kcal/d for male and 1,500 kcal/d for female. In U.S.A, the intake energy recommendations for adults over 50 years old are set at 3,067 kcal/d for male and 2,403 kcal/d for female.

② Protein: Although energy need decreases, older adults still need adequate protein to help minimizing the loss of muscle and lean tissue, maintaining immunity, preventing excessive bone loss, and optimizing healing after injury or disease. The DRI for protein is the same for adults of all ages: 0.8 g/kg of body weight daily in U.S.A; 65 g/d (male) and 55g/d (female) in China. It is good choice for the elderly to obtain protein from foods with low-calorie, high-quality protein, such as lean meats, poultry, fish, and eggs; fat-free and low-fat milk products; and legumes. High quality protein should account for 50% of total protein intake.

③ Carbohydrate and fiber: In addition to the slow gastrointestinal movement caused by hormonal changes, low dietary fiber intake is also a common cause of constipation in the elderly. Majority of older adults fail to obtain their recommended 25 or so grams of fiber each day. Eating high-fiber foods and drinking water can alleviate constipation.

Carbohydrate food is the main energy source for the elderly. It is appropriate that the energy supplied by carbohydrate accounts for 50%—65% of the total energy daily. In order to meet the needs of cerebral nervous system for glucose, the elderly should consume at least 100 to 150 g of carbohydrates per day. In the United States, it is recommended that older adults consume 130 grams of carbohydrates per day. Sources of complex carbohydrates such as legumes, vegetables, whole grains, and fruits, which are rich in fiber and essential vitamins and minerals, are suitable to older adults.

④ Fat: To reduce the risk of heart disease and other chronic diseases, total fat intake should be controlled within 20%—30% total daily energy intake. It is important to control the intake of saturated fatty acids in the diet for improving blood lipids and reducing the risk of cardiovascular and cerebrovascular diseases. Therefore, it is proposed that the energy provided by saturated fatty acids should not exceed 10% of the total energy per day for the elderly. The elderly should pay attention to the content of trans-fatty acids indicated in nutrition labels, and the energy provided by dietary trans fatty acids should be less than 1% of the total energy daily. Nuts and cooking oil are the main sources of unsaturated fatty acids. The elderly is advised to consume nuts in moderation, with an average intake of about 10g per day. Elderly people should be encouraged to consume non-fried fish more than twice a week, and pay attention in choice of fish with less spines or large spines. Poultry (such as chicken) is a better choice with chicken containing less fat than livestock.

However, severely limited fat stores may lead to nutrient deficiencies thereby bring about greater health risk in the elderly. Epidemiological studies have found that older adults who are slightly obese (with a BMI at or above the upper limit of a healthy weight) have lower mortality rates, supporting that being slightly obese may be better for the elderly's health. In principle, the BMI of the elderly should be no less than 20. 0kg/m² and no more than 26. 9 kg/m².

(2) Vitamins and Minerals

Most people can achieve adequate vitamins and minerals through a balanced diet to meet their physiological needs. But older adults tend to omit vegetables and fruits and consume fewer dairy products. This will lead to malnutrition and also aggravate the decline in physiological function brought about by aging. Most of the research findings point toward the need for nutrients of elder people, with an increased emphasis on micronutrient intake levels. Diet high in fruit and vegetables, the major sources of carotenoids and other beneficial phytochemicals, is consistently shown to be protective against a wide variety of age-related conditions.

① Vitamin B: Older adults need to pay close attention to vitamin B, especially vitamin B12, vitamin B_6 and folate. About 30% of adults over than 50 cannot absorb vitamin B12 due to low production of gastric acid and intrinsic factor. Vitamin B12 deficiency is associated with the poor cognition, anemia, and devastating neurological effect, thereby an adequate intake vitamin B12 is imperative. The RNI for older adults is the same as younger adults. The bioavailability of vitamin B12 from fortified foods and supplements is better than from foods. Therefore, it is recommended that the older adults should choose appropriate vitamin B12 fortified foods and supplements.

② Calcium and vitamin D: Aging reduces the skin's capacity to make vitamin D and the kidneys' ability to convert it to its active form, moreover widespread use of sunscreen blocks the sunlight needed for vitamin synthesis in the skin. Vitamin D deficiency is a frequent problem among older adults. In addition, the calcium absorption is declined in the elderly. The deficiency of Vitamin D and calcium can further aggravate the decline in bone density in older adults. Therefore, the requirements for both vitamin D and calcium are higher. In China, the RNI of vitamin D for the aged over 65 is 15 μg/d, and the RNI of calcium for the aged over 50 is 1000 mg/d. In the United States, the RDA of vitamin D is 15 μg/d for the adults above 50 years old and 20 μg/d for the adults above 80 years old. The RDA of calcium is 1200 mg/d for female over the age of 50 and male over the age of 70 in USA. In addition to intake vitamin D through food supplements, such as the choice of some vitamin D-fortified foods or vitamin D supplements, the elderly is advised to have frequent exposure to sunshine in order to promote the synthesis of vitamin D by skin. Considering that the elderly is more likely to have lactose intolerance, it is recommended that the elderly choose calcium-fortified foods, cheese, yogurt and dark leafy green vegetables to meet their calcium needs.

③ Carotenoids: Dietary intakes of certain carotenoids have been shown to have a variety of important anti-aging and health protective effects. Specifically, lutein and zeaxanthin are associated with the prevention of cataracts and age-related macular degeneration. Some studies suggest that a diet high in foods that provide ample antioxidants—carotenoids, vitamin C, and vitamin E can reduce the risk of early onset and progression of cataracts.

④ Iron: The iron status generally improves in women's later life, especially in women after menstruation ceases, and those who take iron supplements, consume red meat regularly, and include vitamin C-rich fruits in their daily diet. Nevertheless, iron deficiency may develop in older people, especially those with decreased chewing function, insufficient animal foods, chronic blood loss from diseases and medicines, and poor iron absorption due to reduced stomach acid secretion or antacid use. Iron deficiency impairs immunity causes older people vulnerable to infectious diseases. It is better for the elderly people to consume lean meat in an appropriate amount. Lean meat has less fat, higher protein and iron with higher absorption rate.

⑤ Sodium: Salt is the main source of sodium. Older people have fewer taste buds and a diminished sense of taste, so they tend to consume more saltier foods. Older adults, especially those with familial hypertension, overweight and obesity, are more sensitive to salt. High-salt diet also influences the cardiac rhythm of blood pressure, switching it from a normal pattern that blood pressure is high in the daytime and low at night to a abnormal patter that blood pressure is steadily high during the whole day, thereby greatly increasing the risk of cardiovascular and cerebrovascular accidents in the elderly. Therefore, it is recommended that elderly should consume less than 5 grams of salt per day.

⑥ Zinc: As aging, intake of zinc in the elderly is often inadequate and absorption is poor, however, the body requirement for zinc increases with aging. Some medications may interfere with its absorption. Zinc deficiency can depress the appetite and blunt the sense of taste, thereby reducing food intake and further exacerbating zinc deficiency. Zinc deficiency is known to impair immune function and even increase the likelihood of infectious diseases, such as pneumonia.

(3) Water

Kidney function changes with age, and the thirst mechanism can be impaired. These changes can lead to chronic dehydration. Some elderly intentionally limits fluid intake because they have urine incontinence or do not want to be awakened by midnight urine. In fact, some old adults, who take diuretics and laxatives because of illness, may increase fluid output. However, this may raise the risk of dehydration. Dehydrated older adults seem to be more susceptible to urinary tract infections, pneumonia, and pressure ulcers. To prevent dehydration, elderly people living in mild climate and having light physical activity should drink water at least 1,200 mL per day, and it is a better choice to drink 7—8 cups (1,500—1,700mL) one day. It is suggested that the elderly should drink a small amount of water in many times, and 200 mL each time is advised. The elderlywith liver, kidney and heart diseases may suffer from serious consequences if they drink too much water in a short period of time.

Dietary guideline for the elderly in China(2016):

① Have a small number of soft meals and prevent nutritional deficiencies.

② Drink plenty of water and take outdoor actives in positively.

③ Delay muscle attenuation and maintain an appropriate body weight.

④ Intake adequate food and encourage dining companions.

5.4   Public Nutrition

Nutritional problems include many aspects such as protein-energy malnutrition, vitamin and mineral deficiency, suboptimal growth, infection, and chronic disease. They may happen at individual, community, and national levels. The term "public nutrition" first appeared in 1996 in a letter to the editor of the American Journal of Clinical Nutrition. In 1997, the 16th International Congress of Nutrition decided to use the concept of public nutrition which has previously been called public health nutrition, society nutrition, or community nutrition.

Public nutrition is a branch of nutrition. It is a broad-based, problem-solving approach to addressing nutritional problems of populations or communities. The core mission of public nutrition is to achieve high health outcomes including lifespan extension and life quality improvement. The content of public nutrition mainly includes nutrition survey, nutrition surveillance, formulation and revision of dietary reference intakes and dietary guidelines, public health-related scientific researches, technical consultation for national policy and regulations of food and nutrition, nutrition education and food insecurity management.

5.4.1   Nutrition Survey and Nutrition Surveillance

The nutritional status of individual is often influenced by the adequacy of food intake and physical health. The nutritional status of a community or nation is theoretically the sum of nutritional status of the individuals who form that community or nation. Nutrition survey refers to obtaining precise information on various nutritional indexes of a given individual or community and identifying their nutritional and health status. Nutrition survey is mainly used to identify groups at risk of nutritional problems based on obtaining information about the energy and nutrient intakes of populations with different geographic distribution, age and sex, and on the etiology and influencing factors of nutrition-related diseases. Moreover, nutrition survey helps to monitor the changes and development tendency of dietary pattern and thus to provide data for establishing intervention programs and forming policies and regulations of nutrition and food.

The methods used for nutrition survey include assessment of dietary intake, anthropometry, biochemical evaluation and clinical examination. These methods are usually performed simultaneously in the same nutrition survey. Furthermore, nutrition survey should be synchronously done with health survey in order to obtain comprehensive information on the causative relationship between nutrition and health as well as their affecting factors, which help to improve the precision and effectiveness of nutrition intervention.

(1) Assessment of Dietary Intake

Direct assessment of food consumption or dietary survey acquire the information on intakes of energy and various nutrients both in quantity and quality, which is the basis for understanding whether and what extent the respondents' intakes of energy and nutrient meet the dietary reference intakes. Dietary survey may be household inquiries or individual food consumption survey through available well-organized survey methods.

The assessment of dietary intake may be carried out by one of the following methods: ① Food weighing: This method is practicable and considered fairly accurate for survey on individuals, households and collective units. All food that is going to be cooked and eaten as well as that which is wasted or discarded must be weighed. The duration of the survey is often 7 days (the so-called "one dietary cycle") although it may vary from 1 to 21 days. The results should be standardized if the respondents differ greatly in their ages, sex and labor intensity. ② Bookkeeping: This method is simple, manpower-& materials-sparing and cost-effective. The survey team visits the collective units, and checks in detail the bookkeeping of total food consumption and the corresponding number of diners in a period of time. The average food consumption for each people per day is thus calculated. The food consumption of one month is commonly checked and statistically counted. The survey is usually done once a season. ③ Dietary recall: This method is also known as twenty-four-hour (24 h) dietary recall. The principle of a 24 hours dietary recall is that a participant recalls actual food and beverage consumption for the past 24 hours or the preceding day. Three days (two continuous working days and one weekend day) dietary recalls are usually needed. The method is useful in carrying out a diet survey of a large number of people in a short time and is easy and practicable. However, this method is not suitable for younger than around 7 years and persons with impaired short-term memory. Generally, this method can give reliable results if the oral questionnaire is well carried out by the help of food models and pictures. The method is often used for national food consumption surveys. For example, in Europe it is the recommended method by European Food Safety Authority (EFSA) for that purpose in adults. ④ Food frequency questionnaires (FFQ): The FFQ is a preprinted list of foods on which subjects are asked to estimate the frequency and also the amount of habitual consumption during a specified period. FFQ estimates the food and nutrient intake of an individual in a long period of time. Nowadays, the online web-based FFQs are also common. The quality of FFQ is up to the development of the questionnaire. The foods listed, length of the reference period, response intervals for specifying frequency of use, procedure for estimating portion size (pictures, household measures, units) and manner of administration all influence the data accuracy and completeness. ⑤ Chemical analysis: This is a method by using the chemical detection to analyze the nutrient contents in all food (staple and non-staple food) after collecting one day diet of the respondent. The method includes "The

Duplicate Portions of Meals Study" and "The Duplicate Portions of Food Raw Materials Study".

(2) Anthropometry

Anthropometric measurements such as body weight, height, skinfold thickness and arm circumference are valuable indicators of nutritional status of individuals and populations. Anthropometric measurements over a period of time can reflect the patterns of growth and development and tell the deviation of an individual from the average levels of the particular population.

① Body mass index: The body mass index (BMI) is currently the most widely used method for measuring nutritional status. It is measured as weight (in kg) divided by the square of height (in meters). The suggested standards for evaluating optimal body weight are listed in Table 5.16. Because both sex and pubertal development are associated with dramatic changes in body composition, the BMI values may require adjustment as per the sexual maturity especially when it is used for measurement in children. For this purpose, the BMI cut-offs for children (WHO BMI reference charts from 0—19 years, and the BMI for age index for both boys and girls from birth to 5 years) is available on WHO website.

② Ideal body weight: Ideal body weight (IBW) is also widely used for measuring the optimal body weight. The first person to focus on IBW was Paul Broca (a French Army doctor) who had to establish the IBW weight for soldiers. The Broca index is height (cm) minus 100. For example, if a person's height is 170 cm, his ideal weight is (170−100)=70 kg. China uses the Broca modified formula [IBW (kg)=body height (cm)−105] for the calculation of IBW. The standards are shown in Table 5.17.

Subsequent formulas like the Devine formula, the Robinson formula, the Miller formula, the Hamwi formula and Lemmens formula were built on or adapted from the Broca index.

Table 5.16　Standards of Optimal Body Weight by Using Body Mass Index (BMI)

Category	BMI (kg/m^2)		
	WHO	Asia	China
Underweight	BMI<18.5	BMI<18.5	BMI<18.5
Normal (healthy) weight	18.5≤BMI<25	18.5≤BMI<23	18.5≤BMI<24
Overweight	25≤BMI<30	23≤BMI<25	24≤BMI<28
Obese (Class Ⅰ)	30≤BMI<35	25≤BMI<30	BMI≥28
Severe obese (Class Ⅱ)	35≤BMI<40	BMI≥30	BMI≥30
Morbidly obese (Class Ⅲ)	BMI≥40	BMI≥40	BMI≥40

Source: PARK K. Preventive and Social Medicine [M]. 19th ed. Jabalpur: M/S Banarsidas Bhanot, 2007.

Table 5. 17   Standards of Optimal Body Weight by Using Ideal Body Weight (IBW)

Category	Actual body weight (kg)
Severely underweight	$\leqslant -20\%$ IBW
Underweight	$-10\% - -20\%$ IBW
Normal (healthy) weight	$10\% - -10\%$
Overweight	$10\% - 20\%$ IBW
Obese	$\geqslant 20\%$ IBW
Mild obese	$20\% - 30\%$ IBW
Severe obese	$30\% - 50\%$ IBW
Morbidly obese	$\geqslant 50\%$ IBW

Source: SUN C H, LING W H, HUANG G W, et al. Nutrition and Food Hygiene[M]. 8th ed. Beijing: People's Medial Publishing House, 2018.

③ Weight-for-age, height-for-age and weight-for-height: Weight-for-age, height-for-age and weight-for-height is a group of indexes mainly used for measuring the growth and development and nutritional status in children. Weight-for-age is often used to classify malnutrition and determine its prevalence in infants. 80% of the median weight-for-age of the reference is the cut-off point below which infants could be considered malnourished. Height is a stable measurement of growth as opposed to body weight. The length of baby at birth is about 50 cm, increases by about 25 cm during first year and by another 12 cm during the second year. The use of growth (height) centile chart is particularly valuable in studying the trend of height curve. Low height-for-age is known as nutritional stunting or dwarfing. Body weight and height are interrelated. Weight-for-height helps to determine whether a child is within range of "normal" weight for his height. Low weight-for-height is known as nutritional wasting or emaciation (acute malnutrition).

④ Waist Circumference, hip circumference and waist-to-Hip ratio: Waist circumference (WC), hip circumference (HC) and waist-to-hip ratio (WHR) are important indexes for assessing nutritional status. When measuring, the subject should keep empty stomach, stand up with hands straight and droop naturally, spread feet 25—30 cm apart, and breathe steadily with no breath holding or abdomen in. The measurement site is the midpoint between the lower border of the rib cage and the iliac crest, and 1 cm above the umbilicus. The HC is the horizontal circumference of the widest part of your buttocks. WHR is the ratio of WC (cm) to HC (cm). WC is a convenient and simple measurement that is unrelated to height but an approximate index of intra-abdominal fat mass and total body fat. The excess abdominal body fat accumulation is related to increased risk for chronic diseases. WC are useful for predicting risk for non-communicable diseases, including hypertension, type 2 diabetes, dyslipidaemia and coronary heart disease. In order to define individuals at different degrees of metabolic risk, the gender-specific WC cut-offs have already been established. These cut-offs have been revised downwards for individuals from Asian backgrounds (Table 5. 18). In public health and clinical practice, WC and BMI are usually measured together, and between the two indices a level of risk can be established (Table 5. 19).

Table 5. 18　International Diabetes Federation Criteria for Ethnic or Country-specific Values for WC

Country/ethnic group	Sex	WC (cm)
Europid	Male	>94
	Female	>80
South Asian, Chinese, Japanese	Male	>90
	Female	>80

Source: BUTTRIS J L, Welch A A, KEARNEY J M, et al. The Public Health Nutrition [M]. Chichester: John Wiley & Sons, Inc. , 2017.

Table 5. 19　Combined Recommendations of BMI and WC Cut-off Points Made for Overweight or Obesity, and Association with Disease Risk

Category	BMI (kg/m²)	Disease Risk (Relative to Normal Weight and WC)	
		Men<102 cm Women <88 cm	Men > 102 cm Women > 88 cm
Underweight	<18. 5		
Normal	18. 5—24. 9		
Overweight	25. 0—29. 9	Increased	High
Obesity Ⅰ	30. 0—34. 9	High	Very high
Obesity Ⅱ	35. 0—39. 9	Very high	Very high
Obesity Ⅲ	≥40. 0	Extremely high	Extremely high

Source: NHLBI Obesity Education Initiative Expert Panel (2000).

⑤ Skinfold thickness: A large proportion of total body fat is distributed just under the skin. Skinfold thickness is a rapid and "non-invasive" method for predicting body fat levels by using callipers in both clinical (individual) and public health (populations) practice. The measurement may be taken at all the four sites mid-triceps, biceps, subscapular and suprailiac regions. Standards for subcutaneously fat do not exist for comparison. It tends to be less routinely employed in contemporary public health nutrition practice because of its poor validity and repeatability. However, the technique can still be favored in some assessment contexts, such as in health clubs and for weight management programs due to the relative low cost of callipers, their portability and perceived ease of operation. In the technique, training the measurer is essential.

⑥ Upper Arm circumference and upper arm muscle circumference: Upper arm circumference (UAC) is to measure the circumference of the mid-upper arm (between the shoulder and elbow). UAC should be measured on the left upper arm by using a flexible measuring tape while the arm is hanging down the side of the body and relaxed. UAC is used for rapid screening of acute malnutrition in the age group of 1—5 years. Age specific cut-offs for UAC have been released by the WHO. In Chinese 1—5 years old children, UAC less than 12.5 cm is considered as malnutrition, between 12.5 cm and 13.5 cm is moderate, and above 13.5 cm is good nutritional status. Upper arm muscle circumference (UAMC)= UAC—3.14×skinfold thickness of triceps muscle. The reference standard for adults is 25.3 cm in males and 23.2 cm in females.

(3) Biochemical Evaluation

With the increasing knowledge of the metabolic functions of nutrients, biochemical evaluation may be more and more widely used to provide precise evaluation on nutritional status such as low nutrient storage, under nutrition, and over nutrition. The samples of blood, stools and urine are usually collected and analyzed by laboratory instruments. Biochemical tests are not applied on a large scale because they are time-consuming and expensive.

(4) Clinical Examination

Clinical examination is to assess levels of health of individuals or of population groups in relation to under-or over-nutrition based on clinical syndromes and signs. It is an essential feature of all nutrition surveys and the simplest and the most practical methods of ascertaining the nutritional status of a group of individuals. Some specific, e.g. Pitot's spots with vitamin A deficiency, pellagra inflammation with niacin deficiency and many non-specific, e.g. anemia with possible deficiency of protein, ion, vitamin B12, vitamin B_6, or vitamin C physical signs have been known to be associated with states of malnutrition. Clinical signs have several drawbacks in nutrition survey. First, malnutrition cannot be quantified on the basis of clinical signs. Second, many deficiencies are unaccompanied by physical signs. Third, most of the physical signs are lack of specificity and have subjective nature. Standard survey forms or schedules are always needed to minimize subjective and objective errors in clinical examination.

Nutrition surveillance is a system established to continuously monitor the dietary intake and nutritional status of a population or selected population groups using a variety of data collection methods whose ultimate goal is to lead to policy formulation and action planning.

The information obtained through nutrition surveillance is used for three main objectives: ① to aid long-term planning in health and development; ② to provide input for program management and evaluation; ③ to give timely warning and intervention; ④ to prevent short-term food consumption crises.

Nutrition surveillance is also called food and nutrition surveillance since it also collects information on food. A nutrition surveillance system obtains nutrition information along that continuum from food supply to health. It ideally collects data on food production, food supply and availability for consumption (national and household), food consumption patterns, dietary composition of foods, nutrient intake, nutrient utilization, and nutritional status. It also includes variables that may influence these processes, such as food culture, food security, lifestyle, knowledge, attitude and behavior toward food, and socio-demographic factors. The core of a nutrition surveillance system is the collection of dietary intake patterns because they provide a basis for nutritional risk assessment. These dietary data can be obtained from the national food supply and from food consumption by households and by individuals.

The United States has the most extensive and comprehensive nutrition surveillance system in the world. Food consumption surveys were initiated in the 1930s and the surveillance system has expanded since then to include many cross-sectional and longitudinal surveys and surveillance systems. China initiated its nutrition surveillance system in 1988. In 2010—2012, China completed the first nation-wide regular nutrition surveillance.

5.4.2   Recipe Design

(1) Concept of Recipe Design

Generally, recipe design refers to different food preparation and cooking methods. A narrow concept of recipe design is the specific design of diet based on the principle of nutrient balance for different individuals or populations. The recipe can be designed for the food consumption of individuals or populations in one day, one week or longer period of time.

(2) Scientific Basis for Recipe Design

Dietary guidelines provide scientific basis for recipe design. Specifically, the requirement of energy and nutrients is based on the DRIs. At the same time, the physiological status of the subjects must primarily be taken into account. For example, the characteristic of development and growth must be considered if the recipe is designed for children. The balance diet pagoda gives practical suggestions for the use of designed recipe.

(3) Principles of Recipe Design

The design of nutrition recipe should follow the following principles.

① Ensure adequate nutrition and balance. The primary requirement of recipe design is to ensure adequate nutrition and balance for targeted individual or population. According to the dietary guidelines, recipe must provide adequate amount of energy, protein, lipids, carbohydrates, vitamins and minerals to meet the physiological requirement for individual. The most important is to provide sufficient energy which can be supplied by carbohydrates, lipids and protein. For Chinese adults, the appropriate proportion of energy supplied by carbohydrates, lipids and protein to total energy has been suggested to be 50%—65%, 20%—30%, and 10%—15%, respectively.

② Include a variety of foods. The diversified foods are an important principle of nutrition recipe design. It is known that various foods differ in their nutrient-containing characteristics. Cereals-based foods are important prerequisites of balance diet. Animal-derived foods that usually contain high-quality proteins, lipids, fat-soluble vitamins, vitamin B family and minerals should be properly selected. Vegetables and fruits are important parts of a nutrient recipe. Choosing different types of cooking oil helps to keep fatty acids balanced and also to improve the palatability.

③ Keep reasonable distribution of energy in three meals. The reasonable distribution of total energy to three meals in one day should be carefully considered.

④ Pay attention to eating habits and palatability. Eating habits and palatability are also important principle of recipe design. A good nutrition recipe must take palatability and likes or dislikes into account to ensure the deliciousness.

⑤ Take into account the season and food market supply and financial situation. The food market supply varies along with the season which further affects the food prices. Food consumption must be compatible with the living standard. Cost saving must be advocated after ensuring the diet to meet all requirements by DRIs.

⑥ Good food hygiene. The food materials used in recipe preparation should be fresh with no tainting or spoilage.

(4) Methods for Recipe Design

The nutrition recipe is usually made by using methods of calculation or food exchange scheme.

As for calculation method, the average daily energy requirement is firstly determined based on the sex, age and labor intensity of the eating subjects. The energy supplied by macronutrients (carbohydrates, lipids and protein) and the daily requirements (in grams) of these three energy-yielding nutrients are correspondingly calculated. Next, the requirement of carbohydrates, lipids and protein are reasonably distributed over breakfast, lunch and dinner. Upon these, the recipe is preliminary made and needs further evaluation and adjustment to ensure the scientific rationality.

Food exchange scheme is another method for designing recipe. It is first introduced by the American Diabetes Association, in conjunction with the U. S. Public Health Service in the 1950s. The "food exchange scheme" categorizes foods into food groups such as fruits, starches, proteins and vegetables. Each group includes appropriate serving sizes with similar contents of nutrients. Therefore, one serving of any food in this group is considered "equal" to one serving of any other food in the same group. For example, one may change one slice of bread with three quarters of a cup of cold cereal. Both of these foods belong to the "starch" group and have the same nutritional value.

5.4.3 Dietary Guidelines

Dietary guidelines illustrate food choices that will meet nutritional needs within appropriate energy allowances and include a variety of foods to accommodate personal preferences. Dietary guidelines are evidence-based and timely reflect the body of nutrition science. A large number of countries, both industrialized and developing countries, have authoritative sets of dietary guidelines.

(1) The Dietary Guidelines for Americans

The Dietary Guidelines for Americans was first released in 1980. In 1990, Congress passed the National Nutrition Monitoring and Related Research Act, which mandates in Section 301 that The U. S. Department of Health and Human Services (HHS) and the U. S. Department of Agriculture (USDA) jointly review, update, and publish the Dietary Guidelines every 5 years. The Dietary Guidelines provides evidence-based food and beverage recommendations for Americans ages 2 and older. These recommendations aim to promote health, prevent chronic disease and help people reach and maintain a healthy weight.

The 2015—2020 Dietary Guidelines, the latest edition, is designed to help Americans eat a healthier diet. It outlines how people can improve their overall eating patterns. It offers 5 overarching Guidelines and a number of Key Recommendations with specific nutritional targets and dietary limits as follows.

① Follow a healthy eating pattern across the lifespan. All food and beverage choices matter. Choose a healthy eating pattern at an appropriate calorie level to help achieve and maintain a healthy body weight, support nutrient adequacy, and reduce the risk of chronic disease.

② Focus on variety, nutrient density, and amount. To meet nutrient needs within calorie limits, choose a variety of nutrient-dense foods across and within all food groups in recommended amount.

③ Limit calories from added sugars and saturated fats and reduce sodium intake. Consume an eating pattern low in added sugars, saturated fats, and sodium. Cut back on foods and beverages higher in these components to amounts that fit within healthy eating patterns.

④ Shift to healthier food and beverage choices. Choose nutrient-dense foods and beverages across and within all food groups in place of less healthy choices. Consider cultural and personal preferences to make these shifts easier to accomplish and maintain.

⑤ Everyone has a role in helping to create and support healthy eating patterns in multiple settings nationwide, from home to school to work to communities.

The Key Recommendations provide further guidance on how individuals can follow the five guidelines. The Dietary Guidelines' Key Recommendations for healthy eating patterns should be applied in their entirety, given the interconnected relationship that each dietary component can have with others.

The Dietary Guidelines is developed and written for a professional audience. Therefore, its translation into actionable consumer messages and resources is crucial to help individuals, families, and communities achieve healthy eating patterns. MyPlate is one such example (Figure 5. 6). MyPlate is used by professionals across multiple sectors to help individuals become more aware of and educated about making healthy food and beverage choices over time. Created to be used in various settings and to be adaptable to the needs of specific population groups, the MyPlate symbol and its supporting consumer resources at ChooseMyPlate. gov bring together the key elements of healthy eating patterns, translating the Dietary Guidelines into key consumer messages that are used in educational materials and tools for the public. MyPlate serves as a reminder to build healthy eating patterns by making healthy choices across the food groups.

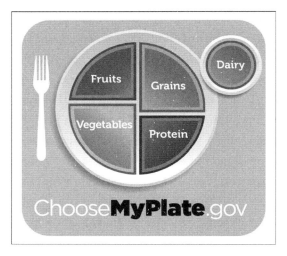

Figure 5. 6　The MyPlate in Dietary Guidelines for Americans

Source: 2015—2020 Dietary Guidelines for Americans.

(2) Chinese Dietary Guidelines

Chinese Dietary Guidelines was first released in 1989. It has been revised twice in 1997 and 2007 respectively. In May 2016, the latest edition was released. It includes the Dietary Guidelines for general population, the Dietary Guidelines for special population (pregnant and lactating women, infants, adolescent, elderly and vegetarian) and Balanced Dietary Pattern and its practice.

Chinese Dietary Guidelines (2016) outlines six key recommendations for general population.

① Eat a variety of foods, cereal based. Each day's diet should include grains and tubers; vegetables and fruits; livestock, poultry, fish, eggs and dairy products; and soybeans and nuts. Eat at least 12 kinds of foods each day and 25 kinds each week. Consume 250—400 g cereals and tubers each day, which contains 50—150 g whole grains and mixed beans and 50—100 g tubers. The important characteristic of balanced diet pattern is eating a variety of foods, cereal based.

② Be active to maintain a healthy body weight. All age stages of people should do exercise every day and keep healthy body weight. Keep energy balance by not overeating and controlling the total intake of energy. Stick to routine physical activities. Perform at least 5 days moderate intensity exercises with an accumulation time of more than 150 minutes weekly. Carry out active physical activities of at least 6,000 steps daily. Reduce sedentary times and get moving every hour.

③ Eat plenty of vegetables, fruits, dairy products and soybeans. Vegetables and fruits are important components of balanced diet. Dairy products are rich in calcium. Soybeans contain high-quality proteins. Include vegetables in every meal and ensure a daily intake of 300—500 g with half of them are in dark color. Eat fruits every day and ensure the daily intake of 200—350 g fresh fruits. Fresh fruits cannot be replaced by fruit juices. Eat a variety of dairy products with equal amount to 300 g liquid milk each day.

④ Eat moderate amount of fish, poultry, eggs and lean meats. The intake amount of fish, poultry, eggs and lean meats should be moderate. Eat 280—525 g fish, 280—525 g livestock and poultry meats, and 280—350 g eggs each week with a daily total intake of 120—200 g. Consider fish and poultry the prior choice. Do not discard egg yolks when eating eggs. Consume less fatty meats, smoked and salted meat products.

⑤ Limit salt, cooking oil, added sugar and alcohol. Develop the habits of eating light and healthy, and eat less salty foods and fried foods. The daily intake of salt for an adult is not more than 6 g and that of cooking oil not more than 25—30 g. Control added sugar. The daily intake of added sugar is not more than 50 g and the best is less than 25 g. The daily intake of trans-fatty acids is not more than 2 g. Drink plenty of water. The adult drinks 7— 8 cups (1,500—1,700 mL) of waters each day. Drink the plain boiled water, and do not drink or drink less sugared beverages. Children, pregnant women and lactating women should not drink alcohol. Daily intake of alcohol should not be more than 25 g for male adult and 15 g for female adult.

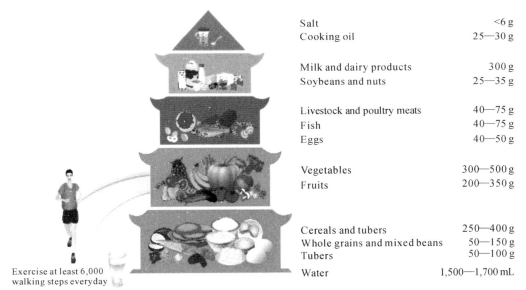

Salt	<6 g
Cooking oil	25—30 g
Milk and dairy products	300 g
Soybeans and nuts	25—35 g
Livestock and poultry meats	40—75 g
Fish	40—75 g
Eggs	40—50 g
Vegetables	300—500 g
Fruits	200—350 g
Cereals and tubers	250—400 g
Whole grains and mixed beans	50—150 g
Tubers	50—100 g
Water	1,500—1,700 mL

Exercise at least 6,000 walking steps everyday

Figure 5. 7   The Chinese Food Guide Pagoda

Source: Chinese Nutrition Society, 2016.

⑥ Develop healthy eating habits, avoid food waste. Cherish foods, prepare required amount of foods, advocate individual serving, and do not waste. Choose fresh and hygienic foods and appropriate cooking methods. Separate the cooked foods with raw foods when preparing them. If reheated, the cooked foods must be heated thoroughly. Learn to read food labels and choose the right foods. Eat at home as much as possible and enjoy the foods and family affection. Inherit the fine culture and advocate the civilized behavior of eating.

In order to make the Chinese Dietary Guidelines and balanced diet concept better understood and well spread, the Chinese Dietary Guidelines (2016) not only revises and released the Chinese Food Guide Pagoda (Figure 5.7) but also adds the Food Guide Plate (Figure 5.8) and the Food Guide Abacus (Figure 5.9).

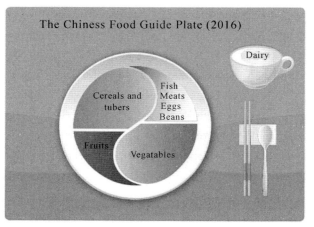

Figure 5.8　The Chinese Food Guide Plate

Source：Chinese Nutrition Society，2016.

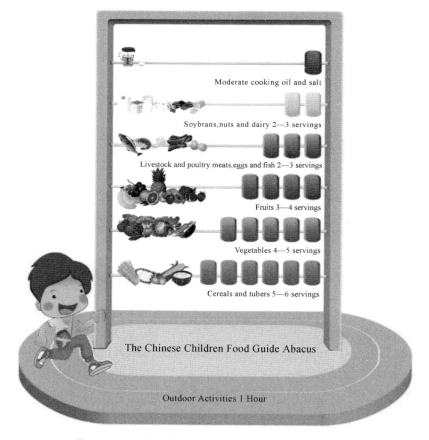

Figure 5.9　The Chinese Children Food Guide Abacus

Source：Chinese Nutrition Society，2016.

（3）The Dietary Guidelines for Indians

The first edition of Dietary Guidelines for Indians was published in 1998 and reprinted in 1999, 2003, 2005 and 2007. The second edition was released by National Institute of Nutrition（NIN）in 2011. In the Dietary Guideline for Indians, there are 15 dietary guidelines that provide a broad framework for appropriate action.

Guideline 1: Eat variety of foods to ensure a balanced diet.

Guideline 2: Provision of extra food and healthcare to pregnant and lactating women.

Guideline 3: Promote exclusive brestfeeding for six months and encourage breastfeeding till two years or more, if possible.

Guideline 4: Feed home based semi-solid foods to the infant after six months.

Guideline 5: Ensure adequate and appropriate diets for children and adolescents both in health and sickness.

Guideline 6: Eat plenty of vegetables and fuits.

Guideline 7: moderate use of edible oils and animal foods and very less use of ghee/butter/vanaspati.

Guideline 8: Avoid overeating to prevent overweight and obesity.

Guideline 9: Exercise regularly and be physically active to maintain ideal body weight.

Guideline 10: Restrict salt intake to minimum.

Guideline 11: Ensure the use of safe and clean foods.

Guideline 12: Adopt right pre-cooking processes and appropriate cooking methods.

Guideline 13: Drink plenty of water and take beverages in moderation.

Guideline 14: Minimize the use of processed foods rich in salt, sugar and fats.

Guideline 15: Include micronutrient rich foods in diets of elderly people to enable them to be fit and active.

An adequate diet, providing all nutrients, is needed throughout our lives. The nutrients must be obtained through a judicious choice and combination of a variety of foodstuffs from different food groups. The Figure 5.10 shows the Food Pyramid for Indians.

5.4.4   Food Label

5.4.4.1   Introduction of Food Label

With the development of society and improvement of living standards, food supplies have become more and more abundant, especially the prepackaged food. Now food supplies in supermarkets or farm product markets are really dazzling.

Food label (also called food labeling) refers to the words, graphics, symbols and all descriptions on the prepackaged food containers.

Food label is a description of food quality characteristics, safety characteristics and edible instructions. Food label includes food name, food ingredients, net quantity and specification, producer and/or distributor's name, address and contact method, production date and expiry date, storage condition, license number of food production, and standard

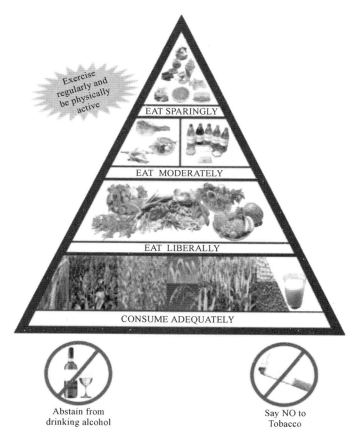

Figure 5. 10   The Food Pyramid for Indians
Source: National Institute of Nutrition, 2011.

code of product. Other information that should be labeled including irradiated food, genetically modified food, nutrition label, and quality grade. Several countries, such as the United States, Canada, Australia, Korea, China, and New Zealand, have mandatory food label.

Food label is a carrier of product information to consumers, and it is also one of the most important and direct means of communicating product information between buyers and sellers. It is one of the primary means by which consumers differentiate between individual foods and brands to make informed purchasing choices. It also makes it easier to compare similar foods to see which is healthier. Knowing how to read food label is especially important for someone with health condition, such as obesity, diabetes, high blood pressure or high cholesterol and need to follow a special diet. The more practice in reading food labels, the better will be in using them as a tool to plan healthy and balanced diet.

5. 4. 4. 2　Food Ingredients

Food ingredients (also called food ingredient list) refers to any substance that be used in the manufacture or processing of food, or exists (including in modified form) in the product, includes food additives. Food ingredients listing ingredients in a food by its common or usual name in descending order of predominance by weight. So, the ingredient that weighs the most is listed first, and the ingredient that weighs the least is listed last. Products containing ingredients consisting of several components must list the components in parentheses.

Food ingredients contain important nutrition information that can contribute to the consumer's assessment of a food's healthfulness. Use ingredient list can find out whether a food or beverage contains ingredients that are sources of nutrients you want to get less of, such as saturated fat (like shortening), trans fat (like partially hydrogenated oils), and added sugars (like syrups), and sources of nutrients you want to get more of, such as whole grains (like whole oats). In addition, some companies also list ingredients that often cause allergies, such as eggs, dairy, soy and nuts, this can help consumers avoid items causing problems. Food ingredient list is an important part of food label.

5. 4. 4. 3   Nutrition Label

Nutrition label refers to nutrition-and health-related information and description of food characteristics provided to consumers. It includes nutrition facts label, nutrition, and health claims.

Nutrition label may be either interpretive in nature, i. e. where colors or symbols are used to improve consumer understanding of the label information, or non-interpretive where quantitative nutrient data are provided without any interpretation.

Nutrition label intends to assist consumers in maintaining healthy dietary choices by providing important nutritional information at the point of purchase and it can be a cost-effective method of communicating nutrition information to consumers. It is also an important measure to ensure consumers' right to know, guide and promote healthy consumption. Improving people's diets is a public health priority and one tool the United States government has used to address this priority is by Nutrition Labeling and Education Act.

Nutrition label is one part of food label. Typically, food label studies focus on nutrition label. Nutrition facts label, nutrition claims and nutrition component function claims play important roles in conveying the products' diet and health information to consumers.

(1) Nutrition Facts label

Nutrition facts label (also called nutrition composition label) is usually represented by a tabular format which marked with the nutrients name and content, and percentage of daily value (%DV) in America or percentage of nutrient reference value (%NRV) in China.

The nutrition facts label is required on most prepackaged food in many countries, and most countries also release overall nutrition guides for general educational purposes. In some cases, the guides are based on different dietary targets for various nutrients than the labels on specific foods.

① The serving sizes are listed in standard measurements, such as cups or pieces. All of the nutrition information listed on the nutrition facts label is based on one serving of the food. Similar foods usually have similar serving sizes to make it easy for comparison.

② The calories listed show the amount of calories in one serving of the food. You can use this information to compare similar products and choose the one that is lower in calories. To achieve or maintain a healthy body weight, balance the number of calories you eat and drink with the number of calories you burn during physical activity and through your body's metabolic processes.

③ The nutrients contents are usually indicated in per servings of food in America or Canada, or in per 100 g (100 mL) or per servings of food in China. FDA suggests that the amounts of total fat, saturated fat, trans fat, cholesterol, sodium, total carbohydrate, dietary fiber, total sugars (includes added sugars), protein, vitamin D, calcium, iron and potassium that are in one serving must be listed. China suggests that list protein, fat, carbohydrate and sodium these four core nutrients must be listed. The nutrients content can enable you to compare foods to make healthy choices.

④ The Daily Value means the amount of a nutrient recommended per day for Americans 4 years of age and older or Nutrient Reference Value for Chinese. The Daily Value percent tells you how close you are to meeting your daily requirements for each nutrient, such as 5% DV or less is a little and 15% DV or more is a lot of a nutrient. It's based on a typical 2000 calorie diet. The DV can help you track whether you are getting enough or too much of all the nutrients you need in a day.

(2) Nutrition Claims

Consumers have long been interested in finding easier ways to identify healthful foods by looking at the labels when buying food. Claims are quick signals for consumers about what benefits a food or beverage they choose might have, and they can also encourage the food industry to reformulate products to improve their healthy qualities. Nutrition claims is one tool that can incentivize competition in the marketplace.

Nutrition claims means any claims which states, suggests or implies that a food has particular beneficial nutritional properties, such as energy level and protein content level. Nutrition claims include nutrient content claims and nutrient relative claims.

① Nutrient content claims: a claims describing the level of energy or nutrients content in food, such as "high", "low" or "no" and other terms.

② Nutrient relative claims: a claim after comparing the nutrients content or energy value with the same kind of food which consumers well known, such as "increased" or "decreased".

Most nutrition claims regulations apply only to those nutrients that have an established Daily Value. The requirements that govern the use of nutrient content claims help ensure that descriptive terms, such as high or low, are used consistently for all types of food products and are thus meaningful to consumers.

(3) Health Claims

Health claims are claims by manufacturers of food products that their food will reduce the risk of developing a disease or condition. For example, it is claimed by the manufacturers of oat cereals that oat bran can reduce cholesterol, which will lower the chances of developing serious heart conditions. Vague health claims include that the content of food is "healthy", "organic", "low fat", "non-GMO", "no sugar added", or "natural".

In some countries health claims also called nutrition component function claims. It refers to some nutrients that can maintain human body normal growth, development and normal physiological function, such as "calcium is a major component of teeth and bones and it can maintain bone density" and "protein contributes to tissue formation and growth".

Further, health claims are limited to claims about disease risk reduction, and cannot be claims about the diagnosis, cure, mitigation, or treatment of disease. Health claims are required to be reviewed and evaluated by FDA prior to use. An example of an authorized health claims: "Three grams of soluble fiber from oatmeal daily in a diet low in saturated fat and cholesterol may reduce the risk of heart disease. This cereal has 2 grams per serving. "

Health claims should be supported by scientific evidence and may be used on conventional foods and on dietary supplements to characterize a relationship between a substance and a disease or health-related condition, such as a healthy diet low in saturated and trans fats may reduce the risk of heart disease, (naming the food) is free of saturated and trans fats.

Reference to general, non-specific benefits of the nutrient or food for overall good health or health-related well-being may only be made if accompanied by a specific approved health claim.

① Calcium and osteoporosis: A food that claim to provide adequate in calcium to help reduce the risk for osteoporosis, a degenerative bone disease, must contain at least 200 mg calcium, no more phosphorus than calcium per serving, and calcium must be in a form that can be readily absorbed by the body.

② Fat and cancer: A food claiming that a low-fat diet may help to reduce the risk for developing some types of cancer should contain 3 g or less fat per serving or fish and game meats that are "extra-lean" (fewer than 5 g fat, fewer than 2 g saturated fat, and fewer than 95 mg cholesterol per serving).

③ Fiber-containing fruits, Vegetables and Grain Products and Risk of CHD: A food claiming to help reduce blood cholesterol levels and the risk for developing heart disease by providing fiber, must be or contain a fruit, vegetable or grain product, 3 g or less fat per serving, fewer than 20 mg cholesterol per serving, 1 g or less saturated fat per serving, and 15% or less calories from saturated fat, 0. 6 g or more dietary fiber per serving.

④ Folate or folic acid and neural birth defects: A food, claiming to reduce a woman's risk of having a child with a neural tube defect healthful diets with adequate content of folate, must meet or exceed the criteria for a good source: 40 mg folic acid per serving or at least 10% of Daily Value.

⑤ Omega 3-fatty acids: A food, claiming to provide omega 3-fatty acids must be low in both cholesterol and saturated fat based on the fact that there are supportive but not conclusive research findings showing that consumption of EPA and DHA omega-3 fatty acids may reduce the risk of coronary heart disease.

5.5 Nutrition and Disease

Nutrition plays an important role in the occurrence and development of some chronic diseases, such as cardiovascular and cerebrovascular diseases, diabetes mellitus, hyperlipidemia. In the following text, the role of nutrition in the occurrence, development, prevention and treatment of some nutrition-related chronic diseases are introduced.

5.5.1 Nutrition and Obesity

5.5.1.1 Definition of Obesity

Obesity is defined as having an excessive amount of body fat (or adipose tissue) that adversely affects health. It is characterized by excessive number and/or volume of adipocytes relative to other cell types. Another accepted definition is by reference to the body mass index (BMI). According to the WHO standards, adults with BMI between 25 kg/m^2 and 30 kg/m^2 are considered to be overweight. Those with BMI equal to or greater than 30 kg/m^2 are considered to be obese.

Being overweight doesnot necessarily mean obese. If a person's skeleton and muscle are particularly well developed, or there is severe edema, then weight can also be increased, so that the weight exceeds the standard weight, but this situation cannot be diagnosed as obesity.

5.5.1.2 Diagnosis of Obesity

There are many methods for obesity diagnosis. The commonly used methods can be divided into three categories: anthropometry, physiometry and chemometry.

Anthropometry includes height, weight, waist circumference, hip circumference, waist hip ratio, skin fold thickness and so on. Height and weight are the most commonly used anthropometric indicators. As the most commonly used anthropometry, BMI is a good index for the diagnosis of obesity. BMI is calculated as weight in kilogram divided by height in meter squared.

Physiometry measurement refers to measuring body composition according to physical principles, and then calculating body fat content. It includes bioelectrical impedance analysis, total body electrical conductivity, dual-energy X-ray, computerized tomography and magnetic resonance scanning.

Chemometry measurement is based on the theory of neutral fat which does not bind with water and electrolytes, so the tissue composition of the body can be calculated on the basis of fat-free components.

5.5.1.3   Epidemiology of Obesity

Obesity has now become an epidemic in developed and developing countries. The prevalence of obesity across the world continues to increase dramatically not only in adults, but especially among children and adolescents in recent decades.

A comprehensive analysis shows that about 2.2 billion people worldwide are overweight, accounting for one third of the world's total population, while about 712 million people are obese, accounting for 10% of the world's total population. Among the 20 most populous countries in the world, Egypt has the highest proportion of adult obesity (35%) and the United States has the highest proportion of child obesity (12.7%). Vietnam has the lowest proportion of adult obesity (1.6%) and Bangladesh has the lowest proportion of child obesity (1.2%). According to the Report on Nutrition and Chronic Diseases of Chinese Residents, the overweight and obesity rates of Chinese residents aged 18 and over in 2012 were 30.1% and 11.9% respectively according to Chinese standards. Males were higher than females, and cities were higher than rural areas.

Obesity itself is an independent disease, and it has now become an important public health problem worldwide. Obesity can lead to development of insulin resistance, and it is a potential risk factor for other diseases, such as type 2 diabetes, hypertension, cardiovascular disease, stroke, cancer, sleep apnea syndrome and other disorders. Obesity is also a significant risk factor for and contributor to increased morbidity and mortality. At present, obesity, as well as hypertension, diabetes mellitus and dyslipidemia are considered as the four most serious chronic diseases threatening human health and the leading nutritional disorders in the world.

5.5.1.4   Causes of Obesity

The balance between energy intake and expenditure determines a person's weight. Obesity is a chronic metabolic disease and the fundamental reason for obesity is that the body's energy intake is greater than the body's energy expenditure. If a person consumes more energy than he or she metabolizes, as a result, excessive energy is stored in the form of fat and the person gains weight (the body will store the excess energy as fat), and if a person consumes fewer energy than he or she metabolizes, he or she will lose weight. It is generally believed that obesity is caused by genetic and environmental factors, such as genetic susceptibility, lack of physical activity and overeating. A few cases are caused primarily by endocrine disorders, medications, or psychological factors. They interact in varying degrees to promote the development of obesity.

Genetic factors play a crucial role in determining an individual's predisposition to the weight gain and being obese. As knows a person is more likely to develop obesity if one or both parents are obese. Many studies have shown that there are a large number of different genes and their genetic re-arrangements that give rise to obesity. For example, one genetic cause of obesity is leptin deficiency. Leptin is secreted by white adipose tissues and it can inhibit food intake. Leptin conveys information to the hypothalamus regarding the amount of energy stored in adipose tissues and helps in the suppression of appetite and stimulates energy expenditure. If, for some reason, the body cannot produce enough leptin or leptin cannot signal the brain to eat less, this control is lost, and obesity occurs.

Physical activity levels have dramatically decreased in the past several decades. People spent more time on sedentary behaviors such as watching television, seeing mobile phone, surfing the internet, and playing video games. With a sedentary lifestyle, people can easily take in more calories every day than they burn off through exercise or normal daily activities. The myriad advances in technology developed over the past few decades which have made many tasks more efficient, but in the process human beings have ultimately decreased the number of energy expenditure.

Overeating leads to weight gain, especially if the diet is high in energy. It is well known that energy comes from fats, carbohydrates and proteins. Foods high in fat have high energy density. In recent years, increased dietary fat intake is an important reason for the increasing obesity rate in the world. The role of carbohydrates in weight gain is not clear, but carbohydrates increase blood glucose levels, which in turn stimulate insulin release by the pancreas, and insulin promotes the growth of fat tissue and can cause weight gain. Some scientists believe that simple carbohydrates contribute to weight gain because they are more rapidly absorbed into the bloodstream than complex carbohydrates and thus cause a more pronounced insulin release after meals than complex carbohydrates. This higher insulin release, some scientists believe, contributes to weight gain. Under the premise of controlling total energy intake, high protein diet can increase satiety and reduce energy intake, which is useful for obese people to lose weight. Overeating, especially eating fast food, skipping breakfast, eating most calories at night, consuming high-calorie drinks and eating oversized portions all contribute to weight gain.

Diseases such as hypothyroidism, polycystic ovary syndrome and Cushing's syndrome are also contributors to obesity. Other factors such as sleep debt, endocrine disruptors, mental disorders, depression and psychology also are factors that contribute to the obesity. Nowadays, some researchers believe that there is an interaction between intestinal microflora and obesity.

5.5.1.5　Prevention and Treatment of Obesity

The most important task for preventing obesity is to publicize the harm of obesity to human health, educate and guide residents to consume reasonable diet, correct unhealthy eating and living habits, take more part in outdoor activities and physical exercise to achieve and maintain an ideal and healthier weight.

The principle treatment of obesity is to achieve negative energy balance and promote fat decomposition. Treatment methods of obesity usually include:

① Controlling total energy intake. Energy supplied by diet must be less than energy consumed by the body, so the body can create a negative energy balance and promote the metabolism of excessive fat stored in the body for a long time until the body returns to normal level. On the basis of controlling total energy, macronutrients energy supply ratio should also be limited too. At present, it is generally accepted that diets for losing weight should be high in protein (energy supply ratio 20%—25%), low in fat (energy supply ratio 20%—30%), low in carbohydrate (energy supply ratio 45%—50%), and ensure supply of vitamins and minerals, increase intake of dietary fiber, supply some phytochemicals, distribute three meals reasonably and use reasonable cooking method;

② Increasing physical activity or exercise. Activity or exercise can not only increase energy expenditure and reduce fat, but also help maintain weight loss and prevent rebound, improve metabolic disorders, improve mood and healthy status, prevent many chronic diseases and increase compliance with dietary therapeutic. Whether or not dietary weight loss is carried out, physical activity and exercise should be an organic part of any weight loss plan. One of the best ways to lose body fat is through regular aerobic exercise, such as walking, cycling, stair climbing or swimming. It is recommended increase aerobic exercise more than 150 minutes per week to prevent further weight gain or to lose a modest amount of weight, or higher levels of physical activity as much as 200 to 300 minutes per week to get more significant weight loss;

③ Behavior change. A behavior modification program can help make lifestyle changes and keep weight lose off;

④ Prescription of weight-loss medications or weight-loss surgery.

5.5.2   Nutrition and Cardiovascular Diseases

5.5.2.1   Cardiovascular Diseases

Each heartbeat carries oxygen-rich blood to the body's tissues. The disfunctions of the heart and blood vessels are common in cardiovascular diseases, the disrupted blood supply hinders the ability of cells to perform their metabolic functions. People with cardiovascular disease may not be aware of that their weakness, fatigue, or shortness of breath are symptoms of a cardiovascular condition. However, when their condition takes a turn for the worse, the complications can be disabling and interfere with many aspects of daily life.

Cardiovascular disease (CVD) (also called heart disease) is a class of diseases that involve the heart, the blood vessels (arteries, capillaries, and veins) or both, the most common form of CVD, is caused by atherosclerosis in the coronary arteries that provide blood to the heart muscle. If atherosclerosis hinders blood flow in these arteries, which results in the deprivation of oxygen and nutrients leading to destroying heart tissue and causing a myocardial infarction (MI)—a heart attack. When the blood supply to brain tissue is blocked, a stroke happens. Both heart attack and stroke may result in disablement or even death.

Cardiovascular disease is the leading cause of deaths worldwide. In the United States, cardiovascular disease is responsible for approximately 36% of deaths. At the same time, cardiovascular deaths and disease have increased significantly in low-and middle-income countries. In addition, although most people assume that heart conditions are men's diseases, more women than men die each year from the various types of CVD.

5.5.2.2 Primary Hypertension

Hypertension is a clinical syndrome characterized by persistent elevation of systemic circulation arterial blood pressure. It is a common chronic systemic disease. Blood pressure was measured three times on different days without antihypertensive drugs, the systolic and/or diastolic blood pressures of systemic arteries were continuously elevated, and hypertension could be diagnosed if the systolic blood pressure $\geqslant$140 mmHg(18.7 kPa)and/or diastolic blood pressure$\geqslant$90 mmHg (12 kPa) (Table 5.20).

According to the *Report on Nutrition and Chronic Diseases of Chinese Residents* (2015 edition), in 2012, the prevalence of hypertension in adults aged 18 and over in China was 25.2%, with a preliminary estimate of 260 million people nationwide.

Table 5.20　Diagnosis and Grading of Hypertension

Category	SBP(mmHg)	DBP(mmHg)
Normal	<120 and	<80
Normal high value	120—139 and/or	80—89
Hypertension	$\geqslant$140 and/or	$\geqslant$90
Level 1 hypertension(Light)	145—159 and/or	90—99
Level 2 hypertension(Moderate)	160—179 and/or	100—109
Level 3 hypertension(Severe)	$\geqslant$180 and/or	$\geqslant$100
Simple systolic hypertension	$\geqslant$140 and	<90

(1) Etiology of Hypertension

The causes of most patients are unknown. Hypertension is the most common chronic disease and the most important risk factor of cardiovascular disease. It is a major complication of stroke, myocardial infarction, heart failure and chronic kidney disease. It not only causes high disability and mortality, but also seriously consumes medical and social resources and causes heavy burden to families and countries.

(2) Nutritional Treatment of Hypertension

According to the recommendations of the *Third Edition of the Guidelines for the Prevention and Treatment of Hypertension in China* (revised in 2010):

① Strict restriction of sodium salt intake: Sodium salt can significantly increase blood pressure and the risk of hypertension, while potassium salt can antagonize the effect of sodium salt on elevating blood pressure. The sodium salt intake of residents in China is significantly higher than the recommendation of WHO that the daily intake of sodium salt should be less than 6 g, while the intake of potassium salt is seriously inadequate. Therefore, all hypertensive patients should take various measures to reduce the intake of sodium salt as much as possible and increase the intake of potassium salt in food. Therefore, we should pay attention to: reduce cooking salt as much as possible, recommend the use of a quantifiable salt spoon; reduce the amount of sodium-containing condiments such as monosodium glutamate, soy sauce; consumet less or not all kinds of processed foods with high sodium content, such as salted vegetables, ham, sausages and all kinds of fried goods, increase the intake of vegetables and fruits, and use potassium-containing cooking salt for those with good kidney function.

② Weight control: Centralized obesity characterized by abdominal fat accumulation can further increase the risk of cardiovascular and metabolic diseases, such as hypertension. Appropriate weight loss and reduced body fat content can significantly reduce blood pressure. The most effective way to lose weight is to control energy intake and increase physical activity. In terms of diet, we should follow the principle of balanced diet, control the intake of high-calorie food (high-fat food, sugary drinks and alcoholic drinks), and properly control the consumption of staple food (carbohydrates). In terms of exercise, regular, moderate intensity aerobic exercise is an effective way to control body weight. The speed of weight loss varies from person to person, usually 0. 5—1 kg per week. For patients with severe obesity whose weight loss effect is not ideal by non-drug measures, they should use drugs to reduce weight under the guidance of doctors.

③ Quit smoking and limit alcohol: Smoking is an unhealthy behavior and one of the main risk factors for cardiovascular disease and cancer. Passive smoking also increases the risk of cardiovascular disease. Smoking can lead to vascular endothelial damage, significantly increasing the risk of atherosclerosis in patients with hypertension. Alcohol drinking should be controlled. The daily intake of alcohol should not exceed 25 g for men and 15 g for women. It is not advocated for patients with hypertension to drink alcohol. If they drink alcohol, they should have a small amount: the amount of liquor, wine (or rice wine) and beer should be less than 50 mL, 100 mL and 300 mL, respectively.

④ Reduce mental stress and maintain psychological balance: Long-term, excessive psychological reactions, especially negative psychological reactions, can significantly increase cardiovascular disease risk.

5. 5. 2. 3　Atherosclerosis

Atherosclerosis (AS) is a disease in which the inside of an artery narrows due to the build up of plaque. It is the main cause of coronary heart disease, peripheral vascular disease and cerebral infarction.

(1) Etiology of Atherosclerosis

There are many causes of atherosclerosis, which can be divided into internal causes (including genetic factors) and external causes (including environmental factors). The main external causes are hypertension, hyperlipidemia, smoking, obesity, too little exercise, psychological stress imbalance and diabetes, many of which are related to nutritional diet.

(2) Principles of Dietary Prevention and Treatment of Atherosclerosis

① Balanced diet: According to the current dietary problems, adjust the diet, food diversity, mainly grains, control the intake of white rice noodles, consume more coarse grains, coarse and fine mix, often consume dairy, legumes or their products, as well as appropriate amount of poultry, eggs, fish, lean meat, etc.

② Weight control: Losing weight and avoiding obesity in overweight people are the key strategies to prevent and treat cardiovascular diseases. Limit total caloric energy, fat intake accounts for less than 25% of total caloric energy, increase the intake of polyunsaturated fatty acids, reduce the intake of saturated fatty acids and trans fatty acids, P/S ratio is maintained at 1, appropriate intake of fish oil capsules, plant sterols can be selectd; control dietary cholesterol intake below 300 mg per day; appropriate supplementation of high-quality protein.

③ Restriction of sodium salt: Moderate restriction of sodium salt intake should not exceed 6g/d.

④ Consum more vegetables and fruits: It is best to be more than 400 g a day, take supplements of potassium, calcium, magnesium, vitamin C, vitamin E and B vitamins and ensure adequate dietary fiber every day.

⑤ Good lifestyle and eating habits: Small amount of meals, avoid overeating, quit smoking, limit alcohol, avoid strong tea, appropriate physical activity, reduce mental stress.

5.5.3　Nutrition and Diabetes Mellitus

Diabetes mellitus, an abnormality in glucose homeostasis, is a group of metabolic diseases in which a person has high blood sugar, either because the pancreas does not produce enough insulin, or because cells do not respond to the insulin that is produced. The incidence of diabetes mellitus is increasing rapidly in the world in the recent years. About 28% of persons with diabetes are unaware that they have it, because its damaging effects often appear before symptoms developing. It also leads to the development of other life-threatening diseases, including heart disease and chronic kidney failure.

5.5.3.1　Overview of Diabetes Mellitus

The term diabetes mellitus refers to metabolic disorders characterized by increased blood glucose concentrations and disordered insulin metabolism. As shown in Table 5.21, in type 1 diabetes, the abnormality is caused by complete or near-complete insulin deficiency, which is likely caused by autoimmune reactions that destroy the insulin-releasing β-cells of the pancreas. Type 2 diabetes is a relative insulin deficiency, a mismatch between insulin production and insulin requirements. There is no single cause for type 2 diabetes; rather, a number of primary genetic and environmental insults appear to be involved, and manifestations range from severe insulin resistance to limited insulin secretion (or some combination). Unlike type 1 diabetes, which is little influenced by genetic predisposition, type 2 diabetes has a strong genetic component (predisposition often accounts for greater than 90% of risk), though it does not result from a single gene modification. People with diabetes may be unable to produce sufficient insulin or use insulin effectively, or they may have both types of abnormalities.

Table 5. 21   Features of Type 1 and Type 2 Diabetes

Features	Type 1	Type 2
Age of onset	<30 years	>40 years
Prevalence in diabetic population	5%—10% of cases	90%—95% of cases
Associated conditions	Autoimmune diseases, viral infections, inherited factors	Obesity, aging, inherited factors
Major defect	Destruction of pancreatic beta cells; insulin deficiency	Insulin resistance; insulin deficiency (relative to needs)
Insulin secretion	Little or none	Varies; may be normal, increased, or decreased
Requirement for insulin therapy	Always	Sometimes

Normally, insulin secretions increase after food is ingested, and the insulin enables muscle and adipose cells to take up newly absorbed glucose from the blood. Insulin is also secreted between meals in smaller amounts to restrict the glucose raising actions of glucagon, a hormone that promotes glucose production in the liver (gluconeogenesis) and the breakdown of liver glycogen. In diabetes, on the one hand, decreased insulin secretion leads to insulin deficiency. Cells that are normally responsive to insulin may become resistant to its effects, or both. This situation leads to the decreased utilization of glucose in muscle and adipose cells and unrestrained gluconeogenesis in the liver, which leads to hyperglycemia, a marked elevation in blood glucose levels that can ultimately do harm to blood vessels, nerves, and tissues. A defect in insulin metabolism leads to the degradation of these nutrients, an increase in fatty acid and triglyceride levels in the blood, and muscle wasting due to insulin-mediated the synthesis of triglycerides and protein in body cells.

5.5.3.2   Medical Nutrition Therapy: Nutrient Recommendations

Medical nutrition therapy has a considerable influence on diabetes. The reasonable dietary choices can both lower blood glucose levels and slow the progression of diabetes complications. As always, the dietary plan must take personal preferences and lifestyle habits into account. Dietary plans need to be formulated to accommodate growth, lifestyle changes, aging, and any complications that develop. Although all members of the diabetes care team should understand the principles of dietary therapy, a registered dietitian is best suited to design and implement the medical nutrition therapy for diabetes patients. This section is about the nutrient recommendations for diabetes.

(1) Total Carbohydrate Intake

The amount of carbohydrate ingested has the greatest effect on blood glucose levels after meals, the more carbohydrate ingested, the greater the glycemic response. The carbohydrate recommendation is based in part on the individual metabolic needs (diabetes types or glucose tolerance degree) and individual preferences. In addition, the carbohydrate intake must be fairly consistent at meals and snacks to help reduce fluctuations in blood glucose levels between meals. Low-carbohydrate diets (less than 130 g per day), are not recommended.

(2) Carbohydrate Sources

Different carbohydrate-containing foods have different influences on blood glucose levels; for example, white rice consumption may cause blood glucose to rise more than would barley consumption. This glycemic effect of foods is affected by a number of factors including the amount of carbohydrate, type of sugar (glucose, fructose, sucrose, lactose), nature of the starch (amylose, amylopectin, resistant starch), the preparation method, the other foods included in a meal, and individual tolerances. The glycemic index (GI), a ranking of carbohydrate foods due to their average glycemic effect, has been compiled from the scientific literature; it is helpful for some individuals to make food choices. The GI is not a primary consideration when treating diabetes, however, because research investigating the possible benefits of low-GI diets on glycemic control have had confused results. In addition, there are considerable differences in individual responses to specific carbohydrate foods. Nonetheless, high-fiber, minimally processed foods, starchy foods, are among the foods frequently recommended for persons with diabetes.

(3) Fiber

Fiber recommendations for individuals with diabetes are similar to those for the general population. Therefore, people with diabetes are advised to consume fiber-rich foods such as legumes, whole-grain cereals, fruits, and vegetables in their diet. Although some studies have shown that very high intakes of fiber (50 g or more per day) may improve glycemic control, the benefits have mixed across studies, and for many individuals it is difficult to tolerated such large amounts of fiber.

(4) Sugar

It is a common misperception that people with diabetes need to avoid sugar and sugar-containing foods. In fact, table sugar (sucrose), made up of glucose and fructose, has a lower glycemic effect than that of starch. Because moderate consumption of sugar has not been shown to adversely affect glycemic level, sugar recommendations for people with diabetes are similar to those for the general population. Thus, sugars and sugary foods must be counted as part of the daily carbohydrate allowance.

Although it has a minimal effect on glycemic level, it is not advised fructose to be used as an added sweetener because excessive dietary fructose may adversely affect blood lipid levels. (Note that it is not necessary to avoid the naturally occurring fructose in fruits and vegetables.) It is found that sugar alcohols (such as sorbitol and maltitol) have lower glycemic effects than glucose, fructose, or sucrose, but their use has not been shown to significantly improve long-term glycemic control. Artificial sweeteners, also known as non-nutritive sweeter (such as aspartame, saccharin, and sucralose) contain no digestible carbohydrate and can be safely used in place of sugar.

(5) Dietary Fat

People with diabetes are at high risk of developing cardiovascular diseases. Therefore, saturated fat intake should be limited to less than 7% of total kcalories, trans fat intake should be minimized, and cholesterol intake should be limited to less than 200 mg daily.

(6) Protein

The protein intake in diabetes patients should be between 15% and 20% of energy intake, which is similar to the protein intake in the general population. Although small, short-term studies have indicated that diets with higher protein intakes may improve glycemic control, the long-term effects of such diets on diabetes management and complications are unknown. In addition, high protein intakes are discouraged because they may do harm to kidney function in some individuals.

(7) Micronutrients

Micronutrient recommendations for people with diabetes are similar to those for the general population. Vitamin and mineral supplementation is not recommended unless nutrient deficiencies develop; those at risk include the elderly, pregnant or lactating women, strict vegetarians, and individuals on kcalorie-restricted diets. Although some studies have suggested that supplemental chromium can improve glycemic control in type 2 diabetes, results remain unconsistent. At present, chromium supplementation is not recommended for type 2 diabetes patients.

5.5.4　Nutrition and Cancer

Cancer is a class of diseases characterized by out-of-control cell growth. There are over 100 different types of cancer, and each is classified by the type of cell that is initially affected. Cancer causes one in eight deaths worldwide and has overtaken cardiovascular disease (CVD) as the leading cause of death in many parts of the world. In 2018, the global cancer burden was estimated to have risen to 18.1 million new cases and 9.6 million deaths, and the top 3 most frequent cancers excluding non-melanoma skin cancer were lung cancer, prostate cancer and colorectum for males, and breast cancer, colorectum cancer and lung cancer for females.

5.5.4.1　How Cancer Develops

Some of human cells divide constantly to replace worn out or damaged cells in an orderly, regulated way. Billions of cells of your body are created each day, it is no wonder that it makes mistakes from time to time and creates abnormal cells. Usually your immune system recognizes these cells and repairs or eliminates them. Unfortunately, few abnormal cells escape from early surveillance mechanisms and finally develop malignant tumors.

The development of cancer, called carcinogenesis, often proceeds slowly and continues for several decades, because the process by which normal cells transform into invasive cancer cells and progress to cancer typically spans many years. The process of cancer is the result of a complex interaction involving diet, nutrition and physical activity, and other lifestyle and environmental factors, with host factors that are related both to inheritance and to prior experience, possibly through epigenetic change(Figure 5. 11). Such host factors influence susceptibility to cancer development, in particular related to the passage of time. This allows both opportunities to accumulate genetic damage, as well as impairment of function, for instance, DNA repair processes with ageing. The interaction between the host metabolic state and dietary, nutritional, physical activity and other environmental exposures over the whole life course is critical to protection from or susceptibility to cancer development. Once the tumors develop, they can disrupt the functioning of the normal tissue around it, and some tumor cells may metastasize, spreading to another tissue or organs in the body.

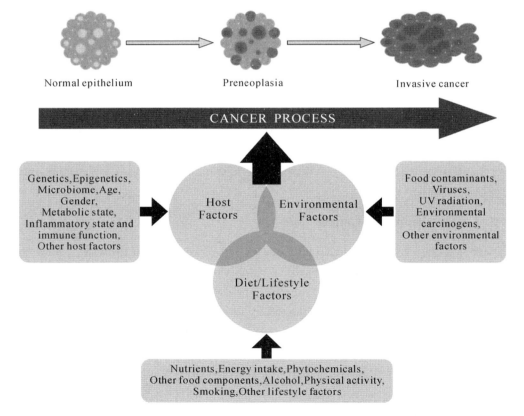

Figure 5. 11　Diet, Nutrition and Physical Activity, Other Environmental Exposures and Host Factors Interact to Affect the Cancer Process

Source: Diet, Nutrition, Physical Activity and Cancer: a Global Perspective. A Summary of the Third Expert Report, World Cancer Research Fund, 2018.

5. 5. 4. 2 Nutrition and Cancer Risk

(1) Body Fatness and Cancer

Like other environmental factors, cancer risk is strongly associated with diet and lifestyle. Certain food components may directly damage DNA or inhibit carcinogens formation in the body. In addition, nutrition-related disease obesity is a risk factor for a number of different cancers, including some relatively common cancers such as colon cancer and breast cancer. Obesity increases cancer risk, in part, by altering levels of hormones that affect cell proliferation, such as the sex hormones, insulin, and several kinds of growth factors. There is convincing evidence that greater body fatness is a cause of cancers of esophagus (adenocarcinoma), pancreas, liver, colorectum, breast (postmenopausal), endometrium and kidney. Greater body fatness is also probably a cause of cancers of the mouth, pharynx and larynx, stomach, gallbladder, ovary and prostate.

(2) Physical Activity and Cancer

Physical activity has a beneficial effect on cancer risk, likely through multiple mechanisms such as reductions in circulating oestrogen levels, insulin resistance and inflammation, which all have been related to cancer development at various anatomical sites when increased. Physical activity also contributes to the decrease of body fatness, in particular visceral fat, and therefore may have an additional indirect impact.

(3) Dietary Exposure and Cancer

Although studies in animals have suggested that fat-rich diets can promote tumor growth, evidence from population studies is confusing: high-fat diets often, but not always, is associated with high cancer rates. Within single populations, cancer rates do not reliably reflect fat intakes. In addition, the type of fat consumed may be important for tumorigenesis. Studies of colon and rectal cancers have shown that animal fats but not vegetable fat induce tumorigenesis.

Convincing evidences have indicated that consumption of alcoholic drinks is a risk factor for various forms of cancer including cancers of mouth, pharynx, larynx, liver, colorectum, breast, and oesophageal squamous cell carcinoma. Studies have suggested that higher ethanol consumption can induce oxidative stress through increased production of reactive oxygen species, which are genotoxic and carcinogenic. Alcohol may also act as a solvent for cellular penetration of dietary or environmental (e. g. tobacco) carcinogen, or interfere with retinoid and one-carbon metabolism and DNA repair mechanisms. In addition, acetaldehyde which is a toxic metabolite of ethanol oxidation, can be carcinogenic to some cell types such as colonocytes, owing to conversion of ethanol to acetaldehyde by colonic bacteria.

Food preparation methods are responsible for producing certain types of carcinogens. Some carcinogens are formed by cooking meat, poultry, and fish at high temperatures in these foods. For example, cooking meats at high temperatures results in the formation of heterocyclic amines (HCAs) and polycyclic aromatic hydrocarbons (PAHs), which have mutagenic potential through the formation of DNA adducts and have been linked to cancer development in experimental studies. In addition, carcinogens also accompany the smoke that adheres to food during grilling, and they are present in the charred surfaces of grilled foods. However, the cancer risk from eating such foods is unclear, because the biological actions of these carcinogens are influenced by other dietary components, including compounds in vegetables and other plant foods. In several population studies, consumption of well-cooked meats was associated with cancers of the stomach, colon, breast, and prostate.

A considerable number of human studies have shown a link between the consumption of fruits and vegetables and decreased incidences of certain cancers. Fruits and vegetables contain both nutrients and specific phytochemicals with antioxidant function, and these substances may prevent or reduce the oxidative reactions in cells which induce DNA damage. Phytochemicals may also help to prevent carcinogen production in the body and enhance immune functions that protect against cancer development. In addition, certain fruits and vegetables provide the B vitamin folate which plays crucial roles in DNA synthesis and repair. Thus, inadequate folate intakes may induce increased DNA damage.

Although research reports in the 1970s and 1980s suggested that a fiber-rich diet could prevent colon cancer, recent studies have cast doubt on the earlier analyses. The earlier studies based on the capability of colon cancer patients in recalling the foods which they had consumed during the preceding years, whereas more recent studies pay attention to more reliable-tracked the subjects' health behaviors and cancer out comes for extended periods (10 to 20 years). In addition, some studies that had shown fiber to be protective did not consider factors such as physical activity, smoking, or folate intake, all of which can affect cancer outcome. A fiber-rich diet may be protective against cancer, at least in part, through high levels of nutrients and phytochemicals.

5.5.4.3 Nutrition and Cancer Prevention Recommendations

The Third Expert Report of Diet, Nutrition, Physical Activity and Cancer released by World Cancer Research Fund made 10 cancer prevention recommendations in 2018. Each recommendation is intended to be one in a comprehensive package of behaviors that, when taken together, promote a healthy pattern of diet and physical activity conducive to the prevention of cancer.

(1) Be a Healthy Weight

Overweight and obesity, generally assessed by body mass index (BMI) and waist circumference, are now more prevalent than ever. Maintaining a healthy weight throughout life is one of the most important ways to protect against cancer and many other common non-communicable diseases. In order to prevent against cancer, it is necessary to keep your weight as low as you can within the healthy adult BMI range throughout life and avoid weight gain throughout adulthood.

(2) Be Physically Active

There is strong evidence that physical activity protects against cancers of the colon, breast and endometrium. Physical activity helps prevent excess weight gain and obesity; thus it may also indirectly contribute to a decreased risk of obesity-related cancers. It is recommended to be at least moderately physically active, and follow or exceed national guidelines, as well as limit sedentary habits.

(3) Eat a Diet Rich in Wholegrains, Vegetables, Fruit and Beans

It is recommended to consume a diet that provides at least 30 grams per day of fibre from food sources, include in most meals foods containing wholegrains, non-starchy vegetables, fruit and pulses (legumes) such as beans and lentils, eat a diet high in all types of plant foods including at least five portions or servings (at least 400 grams or 15 ounces in total) of a variety of non-starchy vegetables and fruit every day. Additionally, if you eat starchy roots and tubers as staple foods, eat non-starchy vegetables, fruit and pulses (legumes) regularly too if possible.

(4) Limit Consumption of "Fast Foods" and Other Processed Foods High in Fat, Starches or Sugars

There is strong evidence that diets containing greater amounts of "fast foods" and other processed foods high in fat, starches or sugars are cause of weight gain, overweight and obesity by increasing the risk of excess energy intake relative to expenditure. Great body fatness is a cause of many cancers. Furthermore, glycemic load probably causes endometrial cancer independently of its effect on body weight. Therefore, it is recommended to limit consumption of processed foods high in fat, starches or sugars, including "fast foods", many pre-prepared dishes, snacks, bakery foods, desserts, and confectionery such as candy.

(5) Limit Consumption of Red and Processed Meat

There is strong evidence that consumption of red meat and consumption of processed meat are both causes of colorectal cancer (red meat refers to all types of mammalian muscle meat, such as beef, veal, pork, lamb, mutton, horse and goat). Thus, it is necessary to limit consumption of red meat to no more than about three portions (about 350 to 500 grams cooked weight of red meat) per week, and consume very little, if any, processed meat.

(6) Limit Consumption of Sugar Sweetened Drinks

Regular consumption of sugar sweetened drinks is a cause of weight gain, overweight and obesity, because of the increase of the risk of excess energy intake relative to expenditure, whereas greater body fatness is a cause of many cancers. Therefore, it is recommended to drink mostly water and unsweetened drinks and not to consume sugar sweetened drinks.

(7) Limit Alcohol Consumption

Drinking alcohol is a cause of many cancers, including cancers of the mouth, pharynx, larynx, oesophagus (squamous cell carcinoma), liver, colorectum, stomach, kidney and breast. Therefore, for cancer prevention, it is best not to drink alcohol.

(8) Do Not Use Supplements for Cancer Prevention

There is strong evidence from randomized controlled trials that high-dose beta-carotene supplements may increase the risk of lung cancer in some people. There is no strong evidence that dietary supplements, apart from calcium for colorectal cancer, can reduce cancer risk. Therefore, high-dose dietary supplements are not recommended for cancer prevention, whereas it is best to meet nutritional needs through diet alone.

(9) For Mothers: Breastfeed Your Baby, If You Can

Lactation probably helps protect against breast cancer in the mother and promotes healthy growth in the infant, so breastfeeding is good for both mother and baby. This recommendation aligns with the advice of the World Health Organization, which recommends infants are exclusively breastfed for 6 months, and then up to 2 years of age or beyond alongside appropriate complementary foods.

(10) After a Cancer Diagnosis: Follow Our Recommendations, If You Can

All cancer survivors should receive nutritional care and guidance on physical activity from trained professionals. Unless otherwise advised, all cancer survivors are advised to follow these cancer prevention recommendations as far as possible after the acute stage of treatment.

5.5.5   Nutrition and Non-alcoholic Fatty Liver Disease

5.5.5.1   Non-alcoholic Fatty Liver Disease

Non-alcoholic fatty liver disease (NAFLD) refers to the hepatic manifestation of insulin resistance and the systemic complex known as metabolic syndrome characterized by hepatic steatosis in the absence of history of significant alcohol use or other known liver disease. NAFLD represent a spectrum of diseases ranging from simple hepatic steatosis to nonalcoholic steatohepatitis (NASH). NASH, a form of progression in NAFLD, can progress to fibrosis, hepatic cirrhosis and hepatocellular carcinoma (HCC). It is considered the most common chronic liver disease recently. If untreated, NASH can progress to hepatic cirrhosis and reduced liver function and increased risk of early mortality.

Currently, the "two hits hypothesis" and the disorder of bile acids (BAs) metabolism are widely recognized as the pathogenesis of NAFLD. The "two hits hypothesis" mainly involved the accumulation of fat in the liver and chronic inflammation and fibrosis of the liver. NAFLD/NASH is regarded as a hepatic manifestation of metabolic syndrome. Fat accumulation in the liver is closely related to metabolic disorders. Obesity and insulin resistance have been considered major drivers of lipid influx, which promote lipolysis of peripheral adipose tissue and increase the liver uptake of free fatty acids for de novo lipogenesis. Hyperinsulinemia and hyperglycemia can also inhibit the oxidation of fatty acids and accelerate lipogenesis. Once steatosis, as the first hit, have developed, chronic inflammation causing fibrosis may be precipitated by a variety of stimuli. Potential processes include oxidative stress and lipid peroxidation, mitochondrial dysfunction, adipocytokine/

cytokine imbalance, gut-derived bacterial endotoxins, hepatic stellate cell activation, and genetic factors. In addition to steatosis, a large amount of evidence indicated that the disruption of BAs homeostasis plays an important role in the pathogenesis of NAFLD/ NASH. BAs are amphipathic molecules synthesized from cholesterol in the liver and deliver into the intestinal lumen to aid in lipid emulsification and absorption of fat and fat-soluble vitamins. Besides, BAs act as ligands and bind to receptors such as liver nuclear receptors-farnesoid X (FXR), small heterodimer partner (SHP) and G-protein coupled membrane receptor (TGR5) to maintain the homeostasis of BAs, glucose and lipid. However, many studies have shown that patients with NAFLD/NASH have increased plasmatic and hepatic concentrations of BAs and have possessed a different mRNA and protein expression profile of hepatic nuclear receptors when compared with healthy person, suggesting that they can be associated with the progression of the disease.

5.5.5.2　Medical Nutrition Therapy: Nutrient Recommendation

Several studies have demonstrated that the reasonable dietary choices can both lower the weight and improve insulin resistance. As always, the dietary plan must take personal preferences and lifestyle habits into account.

(1) Total Carbohydrate Intake

A vast amount of data firmly demonstrated that high intake of carbohydrate, especially fructose, is associated with adverse progression of NAFLD. The nutrient recommendation is to restrict the intake of carbohydrate, a diet based on low-Glycemic Index products induce a significant higher weight loss and improve insulin resistance, and carbohydrate restriction could reduce glycemic load and serum triglycerides.

(2) Fiber

Fibers are mainly plant-derived carbohydrates which are generally resistant to human digestion. Intakes of dietary fiber is a protective factor against NAFLD, as it increases dietary fiber intake, blood LDL, fat accumulation in body, and resistance to insulin are decreased.

(3) Dietary fat

A large number of experimental data show that different types of dietary fat modulating hepatic triglyceride metabolism and accumulation in the liver, which plays an important role in the progression of NAFLD. Trans fatty acids (FAs) and saturated FAs have associated with insulin resistance and high cardiovascular risk. Excessive consumption of the trans FAs and saturated FAs up-regulated the lipogenic gene expression along with marked hepatic lipid accumulation in NAFLD, it can cause live steatosis, ALT elevations and insulin resistance and increase body weight and inflammatory mediators. Therefore, trans FAs and saturated FAs should be reduced in patients with NAFLD, especially in those with hypercholesterolemia. ω-3 PUFAs, EPA and DHA have anti-inflammatory activity in a variety of inflammatory diseases including diabetes and atherosclerosis. Studies have shown that ω-3 PUFAs can exert a beneficial effect on insulin resistance induced by high-fat diet by blocking the activation of NLRP-3 inflammatory body induced by metabolic stress. Furthermore, ω-3 PUFAs leads to the oxidation of fatty acid and decrease of fats by down-regulating sterol regulatory element binding protein 1c (SREBP-1c) and up-regulating peroxisome proliferator activated receptor a (PPAR-a). ω-3PUFAs supplementation effectively reduces fat synthesis and improves insulin resistance. Patients with NAFLD should be appropriately supplemented with fish oil, which is very convenient source of ω-3 PUFAs.

(4) Protein

Many studies have shown that moderately high protein content and a slightly lower glycemic index increase the completion rate of intervention and maintenance of weight loss, protein intake can improve NAFLD development, lack of protein and malnutrition lead to NAFLD development to NASH. Therefore, patients with NAFLD should receive a reasonable amount of protein supplement. At the same time, attention should be paid to the source of protein, with priority should be given to fish, poultry, and legumes derived protein.

5.6 Clinical Nutrition Therapy

Many chronic diseases including obesity, diabetes, hypertension, stroke, heart disease, gastrointestinal diseases, osteoporosis, and cancers are associated with nutrition status. Nutrition status means that the individual's nutritional needs are met at a physiological level. To reach the optimal nutritional status, nutrient intake should meet nutrient need (Figure 5.12). Nutrient intake includes food intake and nutrient absorption. Food intake is affected by many factors including disease condition, eating behavior, emotion, socioeconomic, etc. Nutrient absorption mainly depends on disease condition and physiologic stress. Nutrient need, also known as nutrient requirement, is influenced by psychologic stress, medications, trauma, infection, fever, age, gender, growth, body maintenance and well-being, etc.

Clinical nutrition therapy (CNT) or medical nutrition therapy (MNT) is a therapeutic approach to treating medical conditions and their associated symptoms *via* the use of a specifically tailored diet devised. The diet is based upon the patient's medical record, physical examination, functional examination and dietary history. Clinical nutrition therapy focuses on maintaining or improving the nutrition status by avoiding or treatment of malnutrition. Malnutrition contains over-nutrition and under-nutrition. Under-nutrition is very common in hospitals. Nutrition status of patients in hospitals is influenced by illness conditions and the related treatments (Figure 5.13). Some studies showed that among the 40% of the patients, who were undernourished at admission; about 75% lost further weight during hospitalization. In China, the hospitalized patient malnutrition rate was about 15%—60%. Under-nutrition patients have prolonged hospital stays and higher mortality. The

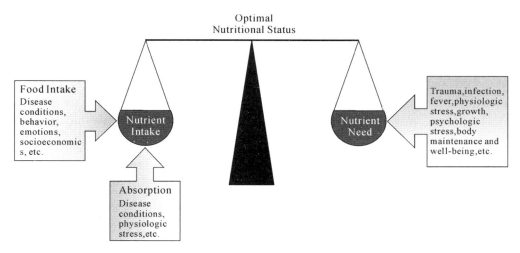

Figure 5. 12　A Balance Between Nutrient Intake and Nutrient Need

Source：MAHAN L K, RAYMOND J L. Krause's Food & the Nutrition Care Process[M]. 14th ed. Elsevier, 2017.

benefits of an appropriate nutrition intervention can improve both short-term and long-term outcomes of many diseases. In spite of it may be not obvious or immediate, the nutritional assessment and essential nutrition support are important for patients in hospital.

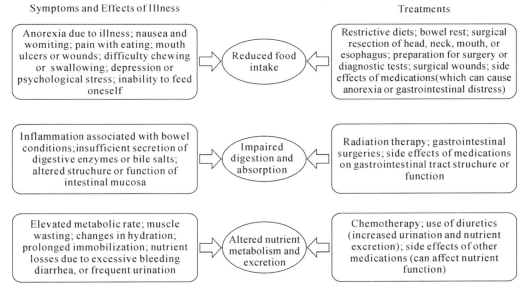

Figure 5. 13　Ways in Which Illness Can Affect Nutrition Status

Source：ROLFES S R, PINNA K, WHITNEY E. Understanding Normal and Clinical Nutrition[M]. 8th ed. Cengage Learning, 2008.

5.6.1　Nutrition Assessment

Screening and assessment of nutritional status is the most basic work in nutrition care process. The significance of assessment of nutritional status is that it provides the personalizing information to prevent or manage an individual's disease, or promote an individual's health. In terms of health promotion, regular assessment of nutritional status can detect inadequate nutrition in the early stage, allowing interventions to implement by improving dietary intake and lifestyle before developing a more serious deficiency status. In terms of management of an individual's disease, assessment of nutritional status can identify nutritional problems which need to be improved to manage the disease via nutrition intervention.

5.6.1.1　Nutrition Screening

Nutrition screening, conducted by any qualified health care professional, identifies patients or clients who might have nutrition problem. The common screening criteria include current body weight, history of weight loss, and poor dietary intake. Sometimes, additional information is collected in a nutrition screening, such as severity of disease, history of nutrition risk, use of modified diet, current nutrition support, presence of wounds, the life stage, etc. Based on nutrition screening, patients who are potential at nutritional risk, who are already at nutritional risk, and who need further assessment can be identified.

(1) Nutrition Screening Data Collection

① Dietary intake: For hospitalized patients in facilities that serve meals, food intakes can be directly observed and analyzed. This method can also reveal a person's food preferences, changes in appetite, and any problems with a prescribed diet.

② Anthropometry: Anthropometric measurements can reveal problems related to both over-nutrition and protein-energy malnutrition. Body weight and height (length) are the most widely used anthropometric measurements and help to evaluate growth in children and nutrition status in adults. Other index includes body composition test, upper-arm skin-fold, and upper-arm circumference, waist, hip circumference, and calculation of the corresponding indicators, such as waist-to-hip ratio, waist height ratio, body mass index (BMI), etc.

Basic anthropometric measurements include:

Height: Height(length) measurement (Figure 5.14 and Figure 5.15) is usually applied to normal nutritional status evaluation.

Body Weight: Body weight is one of the most convenient and useful indicators of nutritional status. Ideal Body weight: Ideal body weight is a very useful tool to check the appropriate weight for an individual. It is very essential to maintain ideal body weight to prevent any health risks. Broca formula (adult): Ideal weight(kg) = Height(c)m − 105; Children above 2 years old Ideal weight(kg)=Age×2+8.

BMI is the most common tool used for assessing the significance of your body weight in

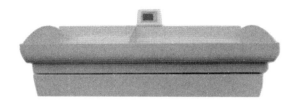

Figure 5. 14   Baby Body Length and Weight Measurement Bed

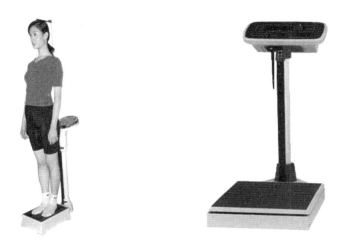

Figure 5. 15   Adult Height and Weight Measurement Instrument

relation to your health. The BMI must be interpreted with caution in the young (Table 5. 22), the elderly, and in athletes. In short, a simple snapshot of BMI cannot be interpreted in terms of the future risks of developing nutrition-associated complications (NACs) unless the direction of loss and the interplay of factors causing the loss are evaluated.

Table 5. 22   The BMI Value for 7 to 18 Years Old Male and Female of Overweight
and Obesity Children in China

Age	Overweight for Boy	Obesity for Boy	Overweight for Girl	Obesity for Girl
7—	17. 4	19. 2	17. 2	18. 9
8—	18. 1	20. 3	18. 1	19. 9
9—	18. 9	21. 4	19. 0	21. 0
10—	19. 6	22. 5	20. 0	22. 1
11—	20. 3	23. 6	21. 1	23. 3
12—	21. 0	24. 7	21. 9	24. 5
13—	21. 9	25. 7	22. 6	25. 6
14—	22. 6	26. 4	23. 0	26. 3

(to be continued)

continued

Age	Overweight for Boy	Obesity for Boy	Overweight for Girl	Obesity for Girl
15—	23. 1	26. 9	23. 4	26. 9
16—	23. 5	27. 4	23. 7	27. 4
17—	23. 8	27. 8	23. 8	27. 7
18—	24. 0	28. 0	24. 0	28. 0

Source: Group of China Obesity Take Force, Body Mass Index Reference Norm for Screening Overweight and Obesity in Chinese Children and Adolescents [J]. China Epidemiology, 2004, 25(2):97-102.

Skinfold thickness: Skinfold thickness is a good indicator of body fat or calorie reserves, since approximately 50% of adipose tissue is located in the subcutaneous area. It often includes triceps, biceps, under the shoulder blade angle (figure 5. 16). The normal value is 12. 5 mm for men and 16. 5 mm for female in America, 8. 3 mm for men and 15. 3 mm for female in Japan and China.

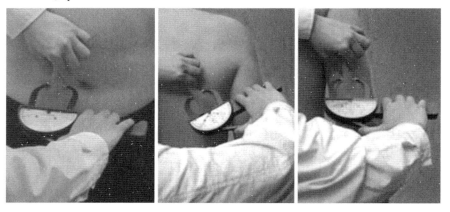

Figure 5. 16   Measurement of the Abdomen, Under the Shoulder Blade and Triceps Skinfold
Thickness

Other indexes: Circumference, includes upper arm circumference, chest circumference, waist circumference, hip circumference, etc. often used to evaluation of regional muscle and fat distribution.

③ Clinical examination: Clinical examination (physical examination) is a non-specific method useful in severe malnutrition, for example, Marasmus or Kwashiorkor, when obvious signs are present. However, it only detects about 25% of moderate cases of malnutrition. It confirms the presence of under or over-nutrition. While under-nutrition is often recognized, malnutrition may require a higher index of suspicion than over-nutrition. Their interpretations are listed in Table 5. 23 according to different anatomic sites and organ systems.

Table 5. 23   Clinical Signs of Nutrient Deficiencies

Body System	Acceptable	Signs of Malnutrition	Other Possible Causes
Hair	Shiny, firm in scalp	Dull, brittle, dry, loose; falls out (PEM*); corkscrew hair (copper)	Excessive hair bleaching; hair loss from aging, chemotherapy, or radiation therapy
Eyes	Bright, clear pink membranes; adjust easily to light	Pale membranes (iron); spots, dryness, night blindness (vitamin A); redness at corners of eyes (B vitamins)	Anemia, unrelated to nutrition; eye disorders; allergies
Lips	Smooth	Dry, cracked, or with sores in the corner of the lips (B vitamins)	Sunburn, windburn, excessive salivation from ill-fitting dentures or other disorders
Mouth and gums	Red tongue without swelling, normal sense of taste; teeth without caries; gums without bleeding, swelling, or pain	Smooth or magenta tongue (B vitamins), decreased taste sensations (zinc); swollen, bleeding gums (vitamin C)	Medications, periodontal disease (poor oral hygiene)
Skin	Smooth, firm, good color	Poor wound healing (PEM, vitamin C, zinc); dry, rough, lack of fat under skin (essential fatty acids, PEM, B vitamins); bruising, bleeding under skin (vitamin C and K)	Poor skin care, diabetes mellitus, aging, medications
Nails	Smooth, firm, pink	Ridged (PEM); spoon shaped, pale (iron)	
Other	—	Dementia, peripheral neuropathy (B vitamins); swollen glands at front of neck (PEM, iodine); bowed legs (vitamin D)	Disorders of aging(dementia), diabetes mellitus (peripheral neuropathy)

* PEM: Protein-Energy Malnutrition

Source: ROLFES S R, PINNA K, WHITEY E. Understanding Normal and Clinical Nutrition[M]. 8th ed. Cengage Learning, 2008.

④ Laboratory biochemical examination: Biochemical tests are useful in the detection of early or mild to moderate malnutrition. Serum, urine, fetal and immune skin tests is the most common check specimen. While there is no single irrefutable measure of nutritional status, proficiency in detecting malnutrition in its early stages is essential for effective treatment and prevention of adverse clinical outcomes.

Plasma protein: Plasma proteins as indicators of protein depletion and deficiency are the role of the acute-phase response in their regulation. Albumin, pre-albumin (PA), transferring (TF), and retinol binding protein (RBP) are all negative acute-phase reactants.

In children with Kwashiorkor, one week of treatment induces a doubling of PA and RBP with no change in albumin. TF is sensitive to iron status (increasing in response to a deficiency), and RBP will change in response to alterations in vitamin A status. Plasma albumin of less than 30g/L is often used as an index of malnutrition but it may be unreliable.

Urinary creatinine excretion: Index reflects total body muscle mass and parallels its changes closely. With calorie deprivation, muscle is catabolized as fuel and creatinine excretion falls. Patients on diuretics such as those with cardiac and liver failure and those with renal disease are especially likely to have low excretions of creatinine.

(2) Nutrition Screening Tool

There are several nutrition screening tools. Nutritional risk screening in 2002 (NRS 2002), which was developed by European scholars in 2002, is mainly used for medical-surgical hospitalized patients. The screening criteria for NRS 2002 include BMI, weight loss, dietary intake, and severity of disease. This screening should be done within 24 hours for a hospitalized patient by a nurse or a dietitian in 10 to 15 minutes.

Malnutrition Universal Screening Tool (MUST), developed by the British Association for Parenteral and Enteral Nutrition (BAPEN), is a screening tool that contains five steps to identify adults, who are malnourished. MUST includes three data collections: BMI, weight loss percentage (unplanned weight loss in 3—6 months), and acute disease effect (likely to be no nutritional intake for more than 5 days).

Malnutrition Screening Tool (MST) is a simple, easy to use, and two questions screening tool. It gives a score from 0 to 5 to show the level of malnutrition risk. If a score is 2 or more, it indicates the risk of malnutrition (Table 5.24).

Table 5. 24　Malnutrition Screening Tool (MST)

Malnutrition Screening Tool	
1. Have you/the patient lost weight recently without trying?	
No	0
Unsure	2
Yes, how much(kg)?	
1—5	1
6—10	2
5—11	3
>15	4
Unsure	2
2. Have you/the patient been eating poorly because of a decreased appetite?	
No	0
Yes	1
Total Score:	

Source: Ferguson M et al. Development of a Valid and Reliable Malnutrition Screening Tool from Adult Acute Hospital Patients[J]. Nutrition, 1999, 15: 458.

Mini Nutritional Assessment (MNA) is a nutrition screening tool for 65 or more than 65 years old patient population in clinics, long term care facilities and hospitals. The data collected by MNA includes the decrease of food intake, weight loss, mobility, any psychological stress or acute disease, has dementia or not, and BMI or calf circumference.

5.6.1.2   Nutrition Assessment

Nutrition assessment is a process that a registered dietitian makes a comprehensive evaluation for an individual's nutrition status by using all the collected data including dietary intake, anthropometric measurements, laboratory biochemical examination, clinic examination, as well as health, dietary, supplement, medication, family and social histories. Nutrition assessment is the first step of nutrition care process.

(1) Health and Family Histories

The information such as family history of diseases, current and past health conditions, allergies, past or recent surgeries, and so on should be considered in a nutrition assessment, because they may be nutrition related problems. For example, an overweight client or patient with dyslipidemia and the family history of heart attack may need a more urgent nutrition intervention than those without the health problem and family history. Although dyslipidemia is hereditable somehow, nutrition intervention can meliorate the condition and prevent the cardiovascular disease or prolong the onset of cardiovascular disease. Wasting diseases, trauma, recent major surgery, gastrointestinal tract disease, and the end stage of cancer may lead to nutrition deficiency. Therefore, before malnutrition happens, a dietitian should identify the risk in a nutrition assessment, carry out a nutrition intervention in time, and then improve the patient's medical and health condition.

(2) Nutrition and Dietary Histories

Inadequate dietary intake leads to nutrition deficiency due to vomiting, anorexia, anosmia, ageusia, dysphagia, chewing problems, medication intakes, inability to eat (some patients with dementia or stroke), etc. Therefore, in a nutrition assessment, a dietitian usually records the mouth-gastro-intestinal symptoms (as above) at the beginning. The purpose of collection of dietary histories is to identify a person's eating habits and to estimate the average daily nutrient intake and to determine the patient who is at high risk of having or developing a nutritional problem. The commonly dietary survey methods have been described in public health section and each method has advantages and disadvantages. Obtaining the patients' food intake data is a challenge for an assessor's skill and training. The nutrient intake can be estimated using dietary analysis software or tables of food composition, and nutrition intake levels can be compared with RNI or AI values. Another option is to compare the food guideline such as Chinese dietary guideline:

How to get an accurate diet history? Step 1, estimation of portion sizes. The methods of estimate portion sizes include using food models, showing patients with household measures such as the serving size, or using the common household items or parts of body. Step 2, evaluation of nutrient intake. Methods to calculate nutrient intake include diet analysis software, food database, and exchange lists. Step 3, determination of intake adequacy. The common way to identify if the patient's intake is adequate or not is to compare with standards such as Dietary Reference Intakes (DRIs) and estimate energy expenditure. Previous assessment data can be used as a reference. Nutrition requirements may be altered for specific diseases or medical conditions, for example, protein requirements should be increased for patients with wound healing or trauma; Potassium and magnesium intake should be reduced for patients with end stage chronic kidney disease; Potassium needs may be increased while on loop diuretics.

(3) Supplement and Medication Histories

Food and drug, food and supplement, drug and supplement may interact with each other. For example, many drugs interact with grapefruit. Intake of antihyperlipidemic drugs such as atorvastatin, lovastatin, and simvastatin should avoid grapefruit. Since vitamin K increases blood clotting, patients who are taking anticoagulant drug (e. g. warfarin) should maintain consistent vitamin K intake. Therefore, dietitian need to inform patients which foods are rich in vitamin K, and patients should not consume them too much at a time. In a word, the interaction between drug, supplement, and food can influence drug effectiveness and nutrition status. Therefore, dietitian must to know the supplement and medication history of a patient or client in a nutrition assessment.

(4) Subjective and Objective Data

① Subjective data: Subjective data is information provided by the patient, family members or. It typically obtained through interviews with patient, family members or caregivers. Examples of subjective data includes dietary intake, weight history, gastrointestinal symptoms, lifestyle habits, and previous nutrition care or interventions.

② Objective data: Objective data obtained from verifiable source, commonly found in medical record. Examples of objective data includes anthropometrics, laboratory or biochemical tests, nutrition-focused physical exam, and client medical history.

(5) Anthropometric Assessment

The anthropometric data is used for assessment of growth, estimation of body composition, screening for nutrition risk, and identifying goals for nutrition intervention and monitoring changes after intervention implemented. In addition to collect data of weight, height, and the growth (infants, children, and adolescences), factors affecting body weight also need to be considered, such as edema, ascites, diuretic therapy, amputation, and intravenous fluids.

① Evaluation of body weight: The formula to calculate % Ideal Body Weight (IBW) is: % IBW=[Current Body Weight (CBW)/IBW] * 100. 90.5%—109% is within normal level; 80% — 90% is mild deficit/malnutrition/wasting; 70%—79% is moderate deficit/malnutrition/wasting; < 70% is severe deficit/malnutrition/wasting. Another way to evaluate body weight is to use percentage of Usual Body Weight (% UBW). The formula to calculate % UBW is: % UBW = (CBW)/UBW * 100. When interpret % UBW, 85%—

95% is mild deficit/malnutrition; 75%—84% is moderate deficit/malnutrition; <75% is severe mild deficit/malnutrition.

② Assessment of body weight change: The percentage of weight change is used for assessing weight change. The formula for weight change is: % weight change＝(UBW－CBW)/ UBW *100. The assessment of weight change is showed in the Table 5.25.

Table 5.25　The Assessment of Weight Change

Time Frame	Significant Weight Loss	Severe Weight Loss
1 week	1%—2% UBW	>2% UBW
1 month	5% UBW	>5% UBW
3 months	7.5% UBW	>7.5% UBW
6 months	10% UBW	>10% UBW

③ Adjusted body weight: Adjusted Body Weight (ABW) is mainly used for calculating energy requirement for obesity. The formula is: ABW＝[(CBW－IBW) * 0.25]＋IBW. Although there is very little research in establishing this formula, it is frequently used in weight management.

④ Adjustments for Amputations: For patients with amputations, there are three formulas as below.

● Estimated pre-amputation body weight＝CBW/(100%－% amputation)×100;

● Estimated post-amputation body weight＝(100%－% amputation)/100%×pre-amputation weight;

● Estimated IBW (post-amputation)＝(100%－% amputation)/100%×IBW for original height.

The percentages of amputation (% amputation) are listed in Table 5.26.

Table 5.26　The Percentage of Amputations

Parts of Amputation	Percentage
Entire arm	5%
Forearm and hand(below the elbow)	2.3%
Hand	0.7%
Entire leg	16%
Below the knee amputation	5.9%
Foot	1.5%

⑤ Adjustment for spinal cord injuries.

● IBW for paraplegics: subtract 5%—10% from IBW (90%—95% of IBW);

● IBW for Quadriplegics: 10%—15% from IBW (85%—90% of IBW).

⑥ Assessment of growth (pediatrics): WHO Growth Charts are commonly used for assessing growth for infants and children. The assessment of pediatric weight/height/head circumference is listed in the Table 5. 27.

Table 5. 27　The Assessment of Pediatric Weight/Height/Head Circumference

Growth Chart Percentile	Indication
BMI-for-age>95th%	Obese
Weight-for-length>95th%	Overweight
BMI-for-age and weight-for-length 85th—95th%	At risk for overweight
BMI-for-age and weight-for-length <5th%	Under weight
Length-for-age <5th%	Short stature
Head circumference <5th or >95th %	Development problem Possible Protein-Energy Malnutrition (PEM)

(6) Biochemical/Laboratory Data

Biochemical/laboratory data is very important because it is very useful when reviewed in conjunction with other assessment data. When reviewing laboratory values for nutrition assessment, dietitians should keep in mind that they need to know factors affecting blood chemistries and to monitor lab results over time.

① Assessment of protein status: There is a correlation between Protein-Energy Malnutrition (PEM) and poor lab outcomes. No single test alone sensitive or specific enough to identify PEM. When under metabolic stress, protein metabolism is altered. When assessing protein status, both somatic protein and visceral protein should be reviewed. Somatic protein status is a measure of the protein in skeletal muscle. Visceral protein status is a non-muscular protein status, including organs and visceral proteins, and proteins found in blood.

There are several lab values can be used for assessment of visceral protein status. Creactive protein (CRP), synthesized by liver, is used to assess degree of stress or inflammation. CRP is increased with infection, stress, surgery, trauma, and heart disease. Albumin, also synthesized by liver, maintains oncotic pressure transport protein. It is a prognostic indicator for morbidity, mortality, loss of consciousness, and severity of illness. Prealbumin, primarily synthesized in liver, serves as a transport protein for thyroxine carrier protein for retinol-binding protein. It is increased with corticosteroid use and renal failure while decreased with malnutrition, infection, and inflammation stress. Transferrin, synthesized in liver, is an iron-binding transport protein. It is increased with iron deficiency anemia and dehydration while decreased with infection, inflammation, liver disease, and starvation. Retinol-binding protein, synthesized in liver, transports molecule for vitamin A. It is increased with dehydration and renal disease while decreased with overhydration, liver disease, vitamin A deficiency, and stress.

To assess somatic protein status, Creatinine-Height Index (CHI) is the direct measurement. The formula of calculation of CHI is: CHI = (actual 24 hours urinary creatinine/expected 24 hours urinary creatinine) * 100. 80% — 100% CHI means well nourish; 60%—80% CHI is mild depletion of protein; 40% — 59% means moderate depletion of protein; less than 40% CHI means severe depletion of protein. CHI can be increased with catabolic or emotional stress, exercise, and trauma. CHI can be decreased with protein-free diet, elderly age, compromised renal function, and muscle atrophy.

② Basic metabolic panel and comprehensive metabolic panel: Basic Metabolic Panel (BMP) includes the following lab values: sodium (Na^+), Potassium (K^+), Chloride (Cl^-), Carbon dioxide (CO_2), Glucose, Blood Urea Nitrogen (BUN), and Creatinine (Cr). The fishbone-typical method of charting labs is as showed in Figure 5.17. Na^+ and K^+ indicate fluid balance and acid-base balance. K^+ also play an important role in neurotransmission and muscular contraction. BUN, the end-product of protein metabolism, is primarily used to assess kidney function. It is increased with renal failure, dehydration, and gastrointestinal bleeding while decreased with acute malnutrition, inadequate protein intake, and overhydration. Creatinine, end-product of skeleton muscle metabolism, is also primarily used to evaluate kidney function. Enhanced creatinine may indicate renal failure. Lower creatinine can used as a marker of lower muscle mass and malnutrition. Blood glucose is increased with diabetes, trauma, stress, and corticosteroid use while decreased with insulin overdose, end-stage liver disease, and starvation.

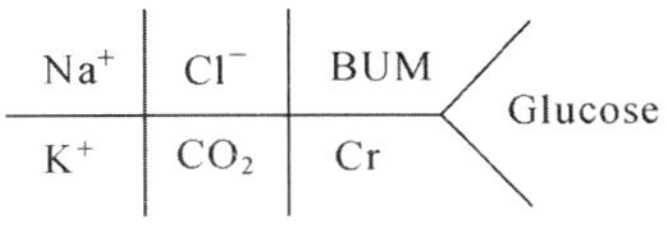

$$
\begin{array}{c|c|c}
Na^+ & Cl^- & BUM \\
\hline
K^+ & CO_2 & Cr
\end{array} \Big\rangle \text{Glucose}
$$

Figure 5.17   Fishbone Chart of Basic Metabolic Panel (BMP)

In addition to the lab values from the BMP, comprehensive metabolic panel also include calcium, phosphorus, magnesium, albumin, total protein, and liver function tests.

③ Hematologic assays to assess iron status and types of anemia: There are two types of anemia, microcytic anemia and macrocytic anemia. Iron deficiency anemia, Anemia of Chronic Disease (AOCD), acute blood loss, and thalasessemia belong to microcytic anemia, which characterized by abnormal red blood cells. Anemia due to vitamin B12 or folate deficiency is macrocytic anemia, which decreases ability to synthesize new blood cells. The differential diagnosis of anemia showed in Table 5.28.

Table 5.28   The Differential Diagnosis of Anemia

Type of Anemia	Hbg	Hct	MCV	Serum Iron	Ferritin	TIBC
Iron deficiency or chronic blood loss	↓	↓	↓	↓	↓	↑
AOCD	↓	↓	Normal or ↓	↓	Normal or ↑	↓

(to be continued)

continued

Type of Anemia	Hbg	Hct	MCV	Serum Iron	Ferritin	TIBC
Vitamin B12 Deficienc	↓	↓	↑	↑	Normal	Normal or ↓
Folate Deficiency	↓	↓	↑	↑	Normal	Normal or ↓
Acute Boold Loss	↓	↓	Normal			↑
Inflammation /Infection/ Stress					↑	↓

Note: Hemoglobin (Hgb), Hematocrit (Hct), Mean Corpuscular Volume (MCV), Total Iron Binding Capacity (TIBC)

(7) Nutrient Need Estimation

① Estimation of energy needs: The components of total energy expenditure include basal metabolic rate (BMR), physical activity (PA), and thermic effect of food (TEF). Because the measurement of BMR is difficult, resting metabolic rate (RMR) is used to replace BMR. Energy needs are estimated via predictive equations. Data commonly used for calculating energy needs contains age, sex, height, and dosing weight. Dosing weight could be CBW, IBW, or adjusted BW. The factors can affect dosing weight including edema, ascites, etc.

- Predictive energy equation for RMR: (weight in kilogram, height in centimeter)

Harris-Benedict equation for RMR

Men: RMR=66. 5+13. 8×weight+5. 0×height−6. 8×age

Women: RMR=655. 1+9. 6×weight+1. 8×height−4. 7×age

Mifflin-St Jeor equation for RMR

Men: RMR=10×weight+6. 25×height−5×age+5

Women: RMR=10×weight+6. 25×height−5×age−161

- Total energy expenditure (TEE):

TEE=RMR * activity factor (AF) or RMR * injury/stress factor (IF)

Some clinicians use both an AF and an IF, but they may overestimate energy needs. Selection of appropriate AF or IF shows in the Table 5. 29.

Table 5. 29 Activity Factors and Injury Factors for Energy Calculation

Activity Factoes(AF)	Injury/Stress Factors(IF)
Resting/bedfast:1. 0—1. 4	Medical:1. 1—1. 2
For hospitalized patient confined to bed:1. 1—1. 2	Surgery:1. 1=1. 4
For hospitalized patient out of bed:1. 2—1. 3	Cancer:1. 1—1. 4
Sedentary/light activity:1. 4—1. 6	Infection:1. 0—1. 4
Moderate activity:1. 6—1. 8	Sepsis:1. 3—1. 4
Highly active:2. 0	Skeletal or blunt trauma:1. 2—1. 4

(to be continued)

continued

Activity Factoes(AF)	Injury/Stress Factors(IF)
	Head injury:1. 5
	Critical illness/major surgery/trauma 　Mechanical ventilation:1. 2—1. 4 　Off ventilator, 2—3 weeks:1. 6—1. 8
	Burns 　≤20％ Body surface area:1. 2—1. 5 　20％—40％ Body surface area:1. 6—1. 8 　＞40％ Body surface area:1. 8—2. 0

- Estimated needs in the critically ill patient:

Ireton-Jones equation (1992) for TEE

Non-ventilated patients:

$$TEE = 629 - 11 * age + 25 * weight (kg) - 609 * (O)$$

O means obese, 0 if not obese, 1 if obese (＞30％ above IBW)

Ventilated patients:

$$TEE = 1925 - 10 * age + 5 * weight (kg) + 281 * (S) + 292 * (T) + 851 * (B)$$

S=1 if male, 0 if female

T=1 if trauma, 0 if no trauma

B=1 if burns, 0 if no burns

- Estimating energy needs using kcal/kg (Table 5. 30):

$$TEE = kcal * IBW (kg)$$

Table 5. 30　Estimating Energy Needs Using Kcal/kg

Non-Stressed Patiens Multiply IBW in kg by:(kcal/kg)					Stressed Patients Multiply IBW in kg by:(kcal/kg)	
Weight Status	1	2	3	4	Health Status	Normal
Overweight	20	25	30	35	Basal energy needs	25—30
Normal weight	25	30	35	40	Ambulatory(wt. maintenance)	30—35
Underweight	30	35	40	45	Malnutrition with mild stress	40
1. Sedentary: confined to chair or bedrest. 2. Light: Mostly seated or standing, with arm movements. 3. Moderate: frequent movements involving arms and legs, walking briskly. 4. Marked: Walking uphill, activities requiring intermittent but frequent spurts of enegy.					Severe injuries/sepsis	50—60
					Extensive burns	80

Source: ESVELT B, DEHOOG S. The Role of the Clinical Dietitian and Modified Diets, Clinical Nutrition[J]. Philadelphia, WB Saunders, 1984,1:156-170.

Since the TEE estimated by the equations above is higher than the actual TEE for Chinese population, therefore, the TEE of Chinese should be 95% of TEE calculated by all the equations listed above. All the predictive equations are estimations, health practitioner should use their clinical judgment to determine actual factor to use. Calculations just give estimates of kcal needs. Monitoring weight to determine if adjustments are needed is very important.

② Estimation of protein requirement: For healthy adults, DRI of protein is 0.8 g/kg body weight. For population with plant-based dietary pattern, the recommendation of protein is 1.16 g/kg body weight. For obese population, IBW is used to estimate protein needs.

Protein factures depending on diagnosis or conditions: such as renal disease: stage 1—2: 0.8 g/kg, GFR<25 mL/min predialysis: 0.6—0.75 g/kg; hemodialysis: 1.2 g/kg; peritoneal dialysis: 1.2—1.3 g/kg; cancer: 1—1.5 g/kg, depending on degree of weight loss and therapy; cancer cachexia: 1.5—2.5 g/kg; inflammatory bowel disease: 1—1.5 g/kg; hepatitis: 1—1.5 g/kg; cirrhosis: 1—1.2 g/kg; encephalopathy, acute: 0.6—0.8 g/kg; stroke: 1—1.25 g/kg; pulmonary disease: 1.2—1.5 g/kg; pressure ulcers or wounds: 1.25—1.5 g/kg; underweight (BMI<18.5): 1.25—2 g/kg.

③ Estimation of fluid needs: There are two common methods for adults. One is using 1 mL fluid per 1 kcal of estimated energy needs. Another one is that the fluid needs are calculated based on body weight. Young adult (16—30 years old): 35—40 mL/kg; Adult: 30—35 mL/kg; Adult (55—65 years old): 30 mL/kg; Adult (>65 years old): 25 mL/kg.

5.6.1.3　Comprehensive Nutrition Evaluation

The goals of nutritional assessment are to define accurately the nutritional status of an individual patient, to identify clinically relevant malnutrition, and to use assessment tools to monitor changes in nutritional status during nutritional support. Comprehensive nutrition evaluation with Subjective Global Assessment (SGA) is usually used (Table 5.31). According to all of these parameters' ratings, SGA results in a 3-level classification: normal nourished, moderate malnourished (or at risk of malnutrition), and severe malnourished (or poor nutrition status).

Table 5.31　The Content and Assessment Standards of SGA

Index	A Grade	B Grade	C Grade
1. Weight change in past two weeks week	no change increased	decrease <5%	decrease >5%
2. Dietary intake change	no change	decrease	noteating/low, calorie
3. Gastrointestinal symptoms that persisted for >2 weeks	none / diminished	mild nausea, vomiting	Severe nausea vomiting
4. Activities ability to change	none / loss	able to ambulate	bedridden

(**to be continued**)

continued

Index	A Grade	B Grade	C Grade
5. Stress response	none / low stress	moderate stress	high stress
6. Muscle wasting	none	mild wasting	severe wasting
7. Triceps skinfold thickness	normal	slightly reduced	severe reduction
8. Ankle edema	none	slightly edema	severe edema

Above 8, it is at least five belong to Class C or B grade that can be individually defined as heavy or moderate malnutrition.

Source: JIAO G Y, JIANG Z. Clinical Nutrition[M]. 3th ed. Beijing: People's Health Publishing House, 2011: 154-155.

Another tool for comprehensive nutrition evaluation is the Mini Nutrition Assessment (MNA) Long Form which can be found on the website of Nestle Healthcare Nutrition. It includes screening and assessment. In screening part, there are six questions for scores including food intake, weight change, mobility, any psychological stress or acute disease, neuropsychological problems, and BMI. In assessment part, several questions would be asked, such as lives independently, medication intake, pressure sores or skin ulcers, meal consumption, protein intake, fruits or vegetable intake, fluid intake, mode of feeding, self view of nutritional status, health status, mil-arm circumference, and calf circumference. The scores are recorded and calculated. The malnutrition indicator score will be the sum of the total screening score and the total assessment score.

5.6.2　Enteral Nutrition Support

There are two alternate modes of feeding to provide nutritional support for patients with special needs. We first examine ways of feeding when the gastrointestinal tract can still be uesd—enteral nutrition (EN). Then, we will review the alternative of nutrient feeding directly into the vein when the gastrointestinal tract can not be uesed—parenteral nutrition (PN).

In hospitalized patients, especially those with hypermetabolic illness or injury, protein-energy malnutrition is a serious concern. Often a highly personalized aggressive nutritional program provided by the skilled hospital nutritional support team is lifesaving. Many patients who require nutritional support over an extended time can continue this therapy at home with continuous follow-up care and monitoring and reduced costs.

Clinical nutrition therapy (CNT), in fact, is a nutrition care process namely: nutrition assessment, nutrition diagnosis, nutrition intervention, nutrition monitoring and evaluation. Nutrition intervention, that is nutrition support method, is an important part of modern medicine. It includes enteral nutrition (EN) and parenteral nutrition (PN).

EN: Nutrients formulated are delivered to the gastrointestinal (GI) tract to meet a patient's nutritional needs. Enteral nutrition includes oral diets or supplements, but more often refers to the use of tube feedings, which supply nutrients directly to the stomach or intestine via a thin, flexible tube.

PN: Provides nutrients intravenously to patients who do not have adequate gastrointestinal functional. Enteral nutrition support is usually preferred, partly to avoid the expense and complications associated with intravenous feedings and partly to preserve health GI function.

Nutrition support make patients who cannot and should not, or will not eat achieve and maintain good nutritional status, decrease length of stay, fatality and disability of disease, malnutrition and increase quality of life. For different inpatients, their nutrition conditions are also different. Therefore, we have to choose optimum EN or PN mode for inpatient including condition, chance, route, formular, etc. (Figure 5. 18).

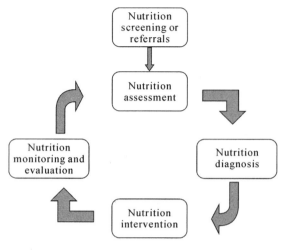

Figure 5. 18　The Nutrition Care Process
Source: ROLFES S R, PINNA K, WHITNEY E. Understanding Normal and Clinical Nutrition [M]. 8th ed. London: Cengage Learning, 2008.

5. 6. 2. 1　Classification of Enteral Nutrition

(1) Oral Feeding

Most of the oral nutrition supplements (ONS) are supply in the form of drink and nutritionally complete. These "drinks" can be shipped during the day between meals and have beneficial effects on nutritional status and outcome. The way suits for upper gastrointestinal tract swallowing function well and no obstruction in patients. In addition, the oral intake also fixes hospital regular meals (normal diet, soft diet, semi-liquid and liquid diets), the treatment of dietary (adjusted the nutrients diet) and test meal (such as OGTT for DM), etc.

(2) Tube Feeding

Nutrients are moved into the intestinal through nutrition tube (Figure 5. 19). Enter tube feeding (ETF) suits for insufficient nutritional by oral, or upper gastrointestinal tract swallowing function deficiency and obstruction in patients, and tube feeding more than 4 weeks.

Feeding route: Tube feeding route depends on the medical condition, expected duration of tube feeding, and potential complications of a particular rout.

Nasogastric tube feeding (NG), fixing burn, short bowel syndrome, etc., prepared for short-term.

Nasointenstinal (NI) tube (nasoduodenal tube, nasojejunal tube), suitable for infant, the aged, pancreatitis, etc., prepared for longer-term.

Stomy feeding, including gastrostomy, jejunostomy, fixing coma, intestinal fistula, etc., prepared for longer-term.

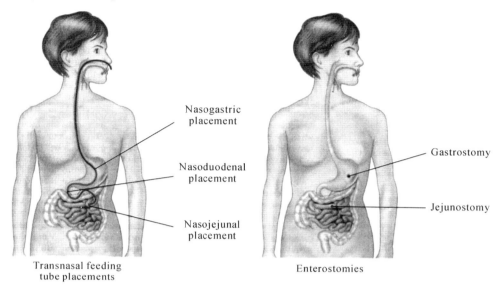

Figure 5.19   Tube Feeding Routes

Source: ROLFES S R, PINNA K, WHITNEY E. Understanding Normal and Clinical Nutrition[M]. 8th ed. London: Cengage Learning, 2008.

Enteral nutrition infusion system: Enteral nutrition was transferred by the pathway including infusion pump, enteral feeding tube and infusion system (Figure 5.20 and Figure 5.21). The delivery of intermittent and continuous feedings can be controlled with an infusion pump.

Tube feeding delivery techniques may be classified as bolus feeding (delivery of about 250 to 400 milliliters in less than 20 minutes), intermittent feeding (delivery of about 250 to 400 milliliters over 20—40 minutes) and continuous feeding (slow delivery of formula at a constant rate over an 8-to- 24 hour period) according to patient condition.

5.6.2.2   Types of Enteral Nutrition Formular

Enteral nutrition is flow regime by the way of oral or tube feeding. According to nutrition sources, enteral formulas are categorized four types:

Stand formulas (polymeric formulas): Stand formulas contain most intact proteins and polysaccharides. Intact proteins (protein that has not been hydrolyzed) or hydrolyzed protein (semi-elemental diet) as nitrogen source and polysaccharides are suitable for oral or tube feeding, such as homogenized diet (made by self or commodity), mixed milk, intact protein-based on-elemental diet (milk formula, lactose-free formula, dietary fiber formula).

Elemental formulas: Elemental formulas also called hydrolyzed, chemically defined diet (CDD) or monomer formulas, are low molecular which require minimal digestive effort and easily absorbed without leaving much residue. Carbohydrates are present as

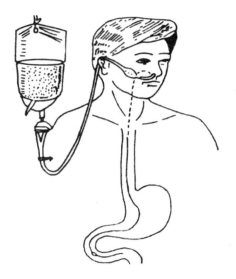

Figure 5. 20　Nasogastric Tube

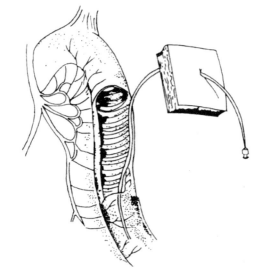

Figure 5. 21　Jejunum Colostomy

oligosaccharides, sucrose and glucose. Proteins are present in form of short chain peptides and fat is usually present in the form of medium chain triglycerides (MCT) along with small amounts of essential fatty acids. As these have been partially or fully predigested, they are easily absorbed for patients who cannot eat ordinary foods.

Modular formulas (nutrient module): Modular formulas are single macronutrients used for people with unique nutrient combination to treat their illnesses. They exist as glucose polymers, protein powders, and fat emulsions.

Special formulas: Special formulas also called disease-special nutrients formulas, are designed to meet the specific nutrient needs of patients with particular illnesses. Products have been developed for individuals with liver, kidney, lung disease, and glucose intolerance.

5. 6. 2. 3　Complications Associated with Enteral Tube Feeding

Complications associated with ETF may be primary of mechanical, gastrointestinal and metabolic nature. Complications associated with the procedures of enterostomy tube are infrequent include reaction to anesthesia, perforation of adjacent organs, bleeding, and infection. Special precautions should be taken when feeding into the small bowel due to the lack of gastric volume or acidity.

Mechanical complications may be caused by tube clogging. It is important to check tube for displacements or kinks, change tube if necessary, flushing the tube with water when medication is administered.

Gastrointestinal complications: may be caused by nausea or vomiting, constipation, diarrhea. Please administer enteral formulas at room temperature, decrease rate of infusion, volume, concentration of formulas, etc.

Metabolic complications may be caused by dehydration, serum electrolyte and mineral disturbances. Please monitor fluid balance with special interest in kidney function, serum values of electrolytes, urea, and creatinine.

5.6.2.4   Monitoring Enteral Tube Feeding

Monitoring the nutritional support given is essential to maintain metabolic stability and promote recovery (Table 5.32). Clinical, anthropometric, and biochemical parameters should be monitored before the start and throughout the period of feeding.

Residual volume in stomach should be monitored every 2 to 4 hours, and feeding should be halted if the residual volume exceeds 1.5 times the hourly rate. Residual volume greater than 200 mL for a nasogastric tube or greater than 100 mL for a gastrostomy tube is a cause for concern, but residual volumes are not reliable if tube diameter is less than 10 French.

Table 5.32   Suggested Monitoring Protocol for Enteral Nutrition

Tolerance	Nausea; Vomiting; Diarrhea; Constipation; Abdominal distension
Nutrition and metabolic	Body weight; Serum Na＋, K＋, osmolality; Acid base balance; Blood glucose, urea, nitrogen; Serum Mg＋＋, Ca＋＋, PO$_4$＋＋; Urine examination; Liver function tests
Mechanical	Confirm tube patency and location before each use; Irrigate feeding tube for intermittent feeds; Crushed medication administration

(1) Monitoring the Tube-Fed Patient

The nutritional support team carefully monitors all patients who are being nourished by tube-feeding. The nursing staff administering the formula to the patient should check for gastric residuals or gastric emptying rate, noting any signs of abdominal distention or bloating, and monitors usual vital signs—temperature, pulse, and respiration. Attending nurses also should monitor the formula flow rate and record the intake and output of formula and fluid. The nutritional support clinical dietitian should monitor tolerance for the formula, state of hydration, and nutritional status response following laboratory test panels commonly included in nutritional support assessment protocols. Also to be monitored are any other special test results related to the patient's disease status or metabolic complications, such as insulin-dependent diabetes mellitus (IDDM), traumatic injury, or sepsis.

(2) Formula Tolerance

Gastrointestinal signs such as vomiting, abdominal distention or bloating, and stool frequency and consistency are to be noted (see To Probe Further above). If these occur, the feeding many need to be adjusted to a less concentrated formula that feeds the patient more slowly with continuous rather than intermittent bolus feeding until tolerance improves and symptoms subside.

Daily urine tests for glucose and acetone for the first week or so. according to protocol, reflect carbohydrate tolerance. If test results continue to be negative in the nondiabetic, these tests may be discontinued. Blood glucose monitoring may be used instead of urine testing. Patients who are diabetic or those who are severely stressed with sepsis may have difficulty metabolizing carbohydrate. Rather than reducing the formula carbohydrate needed for energy, sometimes insulin is given.

(3) Hydration Status

Daily weights, compared with a baseline weight before starting the formula, help indicate hydration status. Daily separate input and output measures and records of formula and water are essential. Sudden weight changes indicate hydration imbalance and need to be investigated. Signs of dehydration include weight loss; poor skin turgor; dry mucous membranes; low blood pressure from decreased blood volume; and increased levels of serum protein, blood cells, and hematocrit. Signs of overhydration include weight gain, edema, jugular vein distention, and elevated blood pressure. Regular protocol monitoring includes serum tests for glucose, potassium, sodium, chloride, albumin, complete blood cell counts, and blood urea nitrogen along with periodic tests for urine specific gravity. Dehydration indicators include elevated blood levels of sodium, chloride, glucose, and urea and elevated levels of hematocrit and urine specific gravity. Severe dehydration is critical and life-threatening. It can be prevented by careful monitoring and supplying the patient's daily fluid requirements with needed water given through the tube. If it does occur, the feeding is to be stopped and intravenous rehydration with a 5% glucose solution usually follows.

(4) Nutritional Response

In addition to body weights and selected laboratory values described previously, usual protocol of enteral nutrition support programs includes the following basic monitoring assessments of patient response.

① Kcalorie calculation: Daily during the first week then weekly thereafter, compute the kcalories in the amount of formula actually taken in by the patient and compare with kcalories in the amount of formula ordered.

② Nitrogen balance study: Using laboratory tests of urinary urea nitrogen and urine creatinine for initial baseline assessment, take measurements daily for the first week and weekly thereafter, together with calculations of dietary(formula) nitrogen intake.

③ Energy expenditure: Estimate energy expenditure initially and repeat the estimate when a change in patient situation occurs.

④ Serum albumin: With a 21-day half-life, serum albumin is a basic indicator of general body protein status to be measured every 2 weks. Serum prealbumin, with a rapid 2-day half-life, thus reflecting current status, is increasingly being used also.

⑤ Serum iron and transferrin or total iron-binding capacity: Measure these basic indicators of iron status and nutritional anemia risk every 2 weeks.

⑥ Serum magnesium: Measure serum mangnesium, an indicator of the degree of malnutrition, every week, or more frequently in severe malnutrition.

5. 6. 3   Parenteral Nutrition Support

When a patient intestinal function is inadequate, enteral formulas cannot meet nutrient needs, PN is a lifesaving option for critically ill persons. Parenteral nutrition (intravenous nutrition), delivers nutrients by intravenous. It should be administered to patients whose gastrointestinal tract is not functioning and who may become malnutrition after long-term intravenous feeding. Unfortunately, the procedure is costly and associated with a number of potentially dangers complications. Parenteral nutrition support according to input ways can be classified:

Partial parenteral nutrition (PPN): Deliver partial or total nutrients via peripheral veins. PPN is used most often in patients who require short periods nutrition support (7 to 10 days) and do not have high nutrients as hypertonic solutions (protein, energy) irritate small veins with a low blood flow, causing phlebitis or thrombosis of the vein.

Total parenteral nutrition (TPN): Provide partially or all of the nutrition a patient requires *via* central veins. With a large blood flow, nutrient concentrations are high solution for longer periods (above 4 weeks). The most commonly used central vein is subclavian vein.

5. 6. 3. 1   Indications and Contraindications for Parenteral Nutrition

(1) Indications for Parenteral Nutrition

Patients who are unable to meet nutrition needs through oral diet or enteral nutrition. Patients with the following conditions are often considered parenteral nutrition: ① severe nutritional risk or protein-energy malnutrition; ② gastrointestinal dysfunction; ③ intestinal obstruction, digestive tract fistula, short bowel syndrome; ④ inflammatory bowel disease; ⑤ acute hemorrhage necrotic pancreatitis, AHNP.

When deciding to initiate PN, a dietitian should use critical thinking involving in considering all aspects of patient and weigh the risk and the benefit of PN. Usually length of time for gastrointestinal tract inaccessible and nutrition status are to be considered.

(2) Contraindications for Parenteral Nutrition

Except patient consuming oral diet and functioning gastrointestinal tract, there are several contraindications for PN: ① water, electrolyte turbulences, acid-base imbalance; ②shock, organ failure; ③terminally ill (almost die); ④risk outweigh potential benefit; ⑤ expect PN to last less than 14 days

5. 6. 3. 2   Parenteral Nutrients

Parenteral solutions are composed of small molecules of nutrients that best suited to meet patient requirement. Because nutrients are provided intravenously, they must be given in forms that are safe to be injected directly into the bloodstream. The basic requirements: sterile, non-toxic pyrogen, the pH and osmotic pressure is appropriate, intermiscibility and good stability, easy to use, and safe.

Amino acids: Parenteral solutions contain all of the essential and non-essential amino acids, concentration range from 3.5% to 15% are used for TPN. Disease-specific amino acids solutions are available for patients with liver failure, kidney failure and metabolic stress. Amino acids provide 4 kcal per gram calories. Recommended protein delivery is 0.8—2.0 g/kg/day.

Calculation of amino acids content of PN solution: for example: calculate gram and energy of amino acids in 700 mL of 8.5% amino acids; 700 mL×8.5%=59.5 g; 59.5 g×4 kcal/g=238 kcal.

Carbohydrate: Dextrose is the main source of energy in patients. 5%, 10%, 25% and 50% injection often be used in clinical. Dextrose provides 3.4 kcal per gram calories. Excess dextrose leads to excessive CO_2 production. Inadequate dextrose administration cannot provide enough energy for the brain and nerve system.

Calculation of dextrose content of PN solution: for example: how many mL of 50% dextrose needed to provide 595 kcal from dextrose? 595 kcal/3.4 kcal/g=175 g; 175 g/50%=350 mL.

In practice of PN, glucose infusion rate (GIR), which stated in mg/kg/min, is also an important monitoring parameter for safety. Time (min) refers to total number of minutes PN delivered. The maximum rate of glucose infusion is 4 to 7 mg/kg/min.

Calculation of GIR: For example, calculate the GIR for 420 g dextrose delivered over 24 hours for 70 kg patient (mg/kg/min). First step: convert gram of dextrose to mg, 420 g×1,000=420,000 mg.

Second step: convert hours to minutes, 24 h×60=1440 min.

Third step: GIR=420,000/70/1440=4.2 mg/kg/min.

Lipids: Lipid emulsions supply essential fatty acids and are a significant source of energy. The emulsions usually contain triglycerides, phospholipids and glycerol. Lipids delivery usually presents as intravenous fat emulsion (IVFE). Varying concentrations available include 10%, 20%, and 30% IVFE. Fat emulsions provide about 10 kcal per gram calories.

Calculation of dextrose content of PN solution: For example, how many kcal in 350 mL of 20% lipid emulsion? 20 g×10 kcal/g=200 kcal; 200 kcal×350 mL/100 mL=700 kcal.

Fluids and electrolytes: such as 10% sodium chloride, potassium chloride and calcium gluconate, respectively, 25% magnesium sulfate.

Vitamins and trace minerals: Commercial multivitamin and trace mineral preparations are routinely added to parenteral solutions including zinc, copper and selenium, except Fe.

5.6.3.3　Infusion Way and Formulation for Parenteral Nutrition

(1) Infusion System for Parenteral Nutrition

① Parenteral nutrition catheter, mainly central vein catheter made by polyurethane, silicon rubber including single-lumen central venous catheter, dual-lumen central venous catheter, and triple-lumen central venous catheter (Figure 5.22).

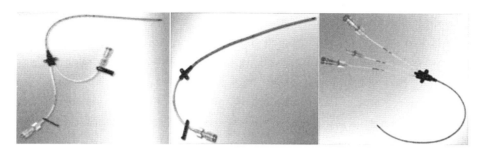

Figure 5. 22   Parenteral Nutrition Catheter

② Infusion pump: It can show the speed and volume of transfusion with security alarm device (Figure 5. 23).

③ In-line terminal filter: It can filter bacteria and particles except pyrogen.

④ Bags include mono-chamber TPN bag and dual-chamber TPN bag.

⑤ Mixer device: It concludes automixer, multitask operating system (MOS) controlled by computer.

(2) Formulation for Parenteral Nutrition

① Bottles of the infusion: each nutrient composition single bottle infusion, respectively.

② 2-to-1: A parenteral solution that contains dextrose, amino acids, and electrolyte solution mixed, with y-shaped pipe or tee connection *in vitro* with fat emulsion, then infusion at the same time.

③ Total nutrient admixture (TNA) or all-in-one (AIO): All the parenteral nutrition components are mixed and then infused in a container under aseptic conditions.

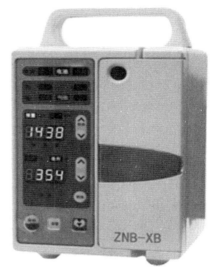

Figure 5. 23   Parenteral Nutrition
Infusion Pump

5. 6. 3. 4   Parenteral Nutrition Complications

Parenteral nutrition is a complex treatment that requires skills from a variety of disciplines. because It is not only costly but also poses a number of potentially dangerous complications. There are several complications as follow.

(1) Infection

Infection is the primary complication related to PN. It is mainly associated with catheter-related infections (septicemia), or enteric bacterial translocation (bacteremia). The reasons of infection include contamination during insertion, long-term catheter placement, formula contamination, and catheter entrance site infection.

(2) Metabolic Complications

If patients are severely malnourished due to severe illness, once too much nutrition supplement is consumed or nutrition support is given, electrolyte disturbances, hypomagnesemia, hypophosphatemia, and hypopotassemia, which can be fatal, may occur within the first few days. These electrolyte or metabolic disturbances appeared after refeeding is called refeeding syndrome. It is an acute laboratory alteration associated with infusion of glucose, lipid, amino acids and electrolytes. Except electrolyte disturbances, hypomagnesemia, hypophosphatemia, and hypopotassemia, other metabolic complications include essential fatty acid deficiency, hyperglycemia, intestinal mucosa barrier hypofunction, hyperlipidemia, hyperammonemia, trace element deficiency, uremia, etc.

(3) Technical Complications

Technical complications are associated with operations and intubation, catheter indwelling and infusion technology such as air embolism and pneumothorax. The complications contain air embolism, arteriovenous fistula, catheter fragment embolism, central vein thrombophlebitis, cardiac perforation, endocarditis, hydromediastinum, pneumothorax or tension pneumothorax, subclavian hematoma, subcutaneous emphysema, etc.

(4) Gastrointestinal Complications

Since disuse of gastrointestinal tract or excess glucose/lipid delivery, there are several gastrointestinal complications such as cholestasis, gastrointestinal villous atrophy, and hepatic abnormalities.

5.6.3.5　Parenteral Nutrition Monitoring

Patients receiving parenteral nutrition should be carefully monitored. Intense monitoring should be conducted for first few days, thereafter the monitoring frequency can be decreased after patient reaches goal feeding and stabilizes. The frequency of parenteral nutrition monitoring is showed in Table 5.33. Monitoring includes:

(1) PN effect observation: weight fluctuations, plasma proteins, water intake and output, etc.

(2) Catheter monitoring: observation of the catheter position to prevent potential infection.

(3) Laboratory detection: such as the patient metabolic status (energy consumption, respiratory quotient, blood gas analysis, plasma osmotic pressure), hepatic and renal function, serum biochemical parameter and nutrients, especially serum glucose, the tolerance to lipids.

(4) Nutrition assessment, especially anthropometric measurements should be performed frequently. The most important thing is to decide when it is appropriate to initiate enteral nutrition or oral nutrition.

Table 5. 33　Parenteral nutrition monitoring

Parenteral Nutrition Monitoring		
What should be monitored	Frequency	
	Initial Period	Later Period
Food intake and output	Daily	Daily
Weight	Daily	Weekly
Catheter site	Daily	Daily
Temperature	Daily	Daily
Serum glucose	Daily	Every 3 weeks
Serum triglycerides	Weekly	Weekly
Serum electrolytesDaily	Every 1—2 weeks	
Liver function enzymes	Every 3 weeks	Weekly
Hemoglobin, hematocrit	Weekly	Weekly
Platelets	Weekly	Weekly
Blood urea nitrogen	Every 3 weeks	Weekly

5. 6. 4　Food for Special Medical Purpose (FSMP)

Foods for special medical purposes refer food formulations used to manage the diets of people with specific chronic diseases or conditions under medical or physician supervision. These special foods are intended for people whose nutritional requirements cannot be met by normal foods. Our knowledge base in the area of nutrition and health-related diseases has grown much larger over the past 50 years. Among the available therapeutic tools, specific therapeutic dietary ingredients and food-based formulations play a key role in preventing or mitigating disease and other health-related conditions except for drug therapy. Clinical patients are prone to be suffering from malnutrition, and malnutrition is one of the important factors that cause clinical treatment complications and delay in recovery. Therefore, clinical nutrition support with special medical use formula as an important component plays a key role in the clinical treatment process.

5. 6. 4. 1　History of FSMP

In USA, FSMP is called as medical foods. Medical foods have been widely recognized as having an important role in enteral nutrition since the 1970s. Prior to 1972, medical foods using under a physicians' care were classified as drugs. As defined by the Orphan Drug Act (1988 Amendment) (USA) medical foods is a kind of foods which is formulated to be consumed or administered orally under the supervision of a physician, and which is intended for the dietary management of specific disease or condition for which distinctive nutritional requirements, based on recognized scientific principles, and are established by medical evaluation. Furthermore, medical foods in the US are classified into the following categories: nutritionally complete formulas, nutritionally incomplete formulas, formulas for metabolic (genetic) disorders in patients over 12 months of age, and oral rehydration products. The criteria that clarified the statutory definition of medical foods can be found in the FDA's regulations. At present, the management of medical foods is relatively loose in the United States, medical foods do not require pre-approval from the FDA for marketing.

The Codex Alimentarius Commission (CAC) is a body charged by the Food and Agriculture Organization (FAO) of the United Nations and the World Health Organization (WHO) with developing an international food code (food standards, guidelines and recommendations) under the FAO/WHO Joint Food Standards Programme. The CAC defined medical foods as for special medical purposes (FSMPs) and identified a specific target population for their use in 1991. Moreover, in order to meet the special nutritional needs of infants with particular disorders, diseases or other medical conditions, the CAC formulated the "Standard for infant formula and formulas for special medical purposes intended for infants, CODEX STAN 72—1981, Amended 2007" (CAC, 1981), which stipulates those medical foods that can be administered to infants under the age of 12 months. According to the Codex Standards, FSMP is a category of foods for special dietary uses which are specially processed or formulated and presented for the dietary management of patients, may be used only under medical supervision. They are intended for the exclusive or partial feeding of patients with limited or impaired capacity to take, digest, absorb or metabolize ordinary foodstuffs or certain nutrients contained therein, or who have other special medically-determined nutrient requirements, whose dietary management cannot be achieved only by modification of the normal diet, by other foods for special dietary uses, or by a combination of the two.

In EU, FSMP is defined as "food specially processed or formulated and intended for the dietary management of patients, including infants, to be used under medical supervision; it is intended for the exclusive or partial feeding of patients with a limited, impaired or disturbed capacity to take, digest, absorb, metabolize or excrete ordinary food or certain nutrients contained therein, or metabolites, or with other medically-determined nutrient requirements, whose dietary management cannot be achieved by modification of the normal diet alone. " The category of FSMPs includes nutritionally complete foods, nutritionally complete foods with a nutrient-adapted formulation, and nutritionally incomplete foods.

In Australia and New Zealand, the Food Standards Australia and New Zealand (FSANZ) established two standards for FSMPs: "Food for special medical purposes, Standard 2.9.5" (FSANZ, 2012) and "Infant Formula Products, Standard 2.9.1" (FSANZ, 2012). However, there is no specific product classification in Australia and New Zealand. In Japan, medical foods are referred to as "Foods for Sick", which need a Ministry of Health seal of approval before being allowed on the market. Additionally, many other countries (Canada, Singapore, Vietnam, Republic of Korea, etc.) have formulated their standards for medical foods based on the CAC's standard, usually including some further refinements.

In China, under General Principles of Food for Special Medical Purpose (GB 29922—2013), FSMP refer the formula foods specially processed and prepared in order to meet special needs for nutrient or diet of those suffering from food intake restriction, disorder of digestive absorption, disorder of metabolic or certain diseases. Such foods must be used alone or together with other foods under the guidance of doctor or clinical nutritionist. Food for special medical purposes means food specially processed or formulated and intended for the dietary management of patients, including infants, to be used under medical supervision; it is intended for the exclusive or partial feeding of patients with a limited, impaired or disturbed capacity to take, digest, absorb, metabolize or excrete ordinary food or certain nutrients contained therein, or metabolites, or with other medically-determined nutrient requirements, whose dietary management cannot be achieved by modification of the normal diet alone. These products are to be used under the guidance of doctors or clinical dietitians. They can only be sold from or by a medical practitioner or dietitian; a medical practice, pharmacy or certain other institutions; or appropriate distributors. This is helpful to manage the possible risk of inappropriate use and to help consumers seek professional health advice.

The development of FSMP in China is mainly divided into the following 4 stages:

(1) Initial Stage (1970—2000)

With the development of clinical nutrition at this stage, the clinical effects and social value of FSMP has been recognized gradually. For instance, the clinical application of FSMP has been reported in Beijing in 1974. In the 1980s—1990s of the 20th century, the unique position of nutrition disciplines in the health care system clearly manifested.

(2) Emphasis Stage (2002—2009)

In 2002, the Chinese Medical Association made the classification of FSMP, various government agencies began to gradually clarify their health insurance policies. In 2006, the China Nutrition Improvement Action Plan clearly stated the importance of correct nutrient consumption for health. At this stage, the requirement for the technology and function of FSMP increased in China, the progress during this stage established a scientific basis to adjust and improve FSMP.

(3) Improvement Stage (2009—2015)

In 2014, the "food" status of FSMP was claimed in the new food safety law. In 2015, CFDA issued the "Administrative Measurement for the Registration of Formula Foods for Special Medical Uses (Trial)". It ensured the basic need for the quality and safety of formula FSMP, and made registration conditions, production Enterprise capabilities, clinical trials and so on clear.

(4) Standardization Stage (2016—)

Under the comprehensive system, FSMP officially enters standard product registration, production and promotion. FSMP industry has stepped into initial stage of development.

5. 6. 4. 2　Classification of FSMP

In China, two categories in which FSMP can be classified: FSMP for infants 0—12 months of age and the FSMP for people over one year old.

(1) FSMP for Infants (0—12 months of ageas)

FSMP for infants contain following six classes: ① lactose-free formula food or low lactose formula food; ② partially hydrolyzed milk protein formula food; ③ extensively hydrolyzed milk protein formula or amino acid-based formula food; ④ formula food for premature infants or low birth weight infants; ⑤ breast milk nutrition food; ⑥ formula food for disorder of amino acid metabolism.

(2) FSMP for People over One Year Old

① Full nutritional formula food: The formula foods of special medical purpose that may be used as single nutrition source to meet the nutritional requirements of the target group. These products contain all the necessary nutrients at appropriate levels so that they may be used as the sole source of nutrition for a patient when taken in a sufficient quantity. This quantity will depend for example on the age, body weight and medical condition of the patient as recommended by a health care professional. They may be used as a sole source of nutrition to replace the total diet, either orally or via an enteral tube. They may also be used for partial feeding of the patient, depending on nutritional needs and in accordance with the recommendations of the health care professional. Full nutritional formula food is divided into two classes: applicable to 1—10 years crowds or applicable to crowds older than 10 years.

② Specific full nutritional formula food: The formula foods of special medical purpose that may be used as single nutrition source to meet the nutritional requirements of the target group with certain disease or medical state. These products are aimed at taking into account the specific nutritional needs associated with a disease or range of diseases, disorders or medical conditions. These products may constitute the sole source of nourishment for the persons for whom it is intended. There are 13 categories of specific full nutritional formula food below:

- Full nutritional formula food for diabetes;
- Full nutritional formula food for disease of respiratory system;
- Full nutritional formula food for nephrophathy;
- Full nutritional formula food for tumour;
- Full nutritional formula food for hepatopathy;
- Full nutritional formula food for muscle attenuation syndrome;
- Full nutritional formula food for trauma, infection, operation and other stringent state;
- Full nutritional formula food for inflammatory bowel disease;
- Full nutritional formula food for food protein allergy;

- Full nutritional formula food for intractable epilepsy;
- Absorbing barrier of gastrointestinal tract and pancreatitis;
- Full nutritional formula food for metabolic disorder of fatty acid;
- Full nutritional formula food for obesity and lose fat operation.

③ Non-full nutritional formula food: The formula foods of special medical purpose may meet the partial nutritional requirements of the target group, not applicable to be regarded as single nutrition source. These products either do not contain all the essential nutrients or contain them in quantities or balance specific for a disease, disorder or medical condition, which means the products are not suitable to be used as the sole source of nourishment. They are used for partial feeding by the patient in addition to normal foods, an adapted diet, other FSMP products or parenteral nutrition. There are 5 categories of non-full nutritional formula food: nutrient module, electrolyte formula, thickening module, fat (fatty acid) module and carbohydrate module. Nutrient module includes protein (amino acids) module, liquid formula and formula for the disorder of amino acid metabolism.

5.6.4.3 The Differences between FSMP and General Food, Health Food, or Drug

FSMPs are different to therapeutic goods which are used to treat or cure a medical condition. Meanwhile, FSMPs also differ in a number of ways from other foods. In accordance with Food Safety Law in China, food can be divided into two categories: general food and special food. Under the category of special food, there are health food, infant formula food and FSMP. Among them, infant formula food is easy to be distinguished from other foods because of its obvious characteristics. However, general food, health food, as well as FSMP are often confused by the public. The differences of these three types of food forms are summarized in 4 aspects, and added the drug to make a comparison, to help the public distinguish these product categories correctly.

In China, the differences of usage, formula, registration and label claim of FSMP with general food, health food or drug are listed in Table 5.34 to Table 5.37.

Table 5.34 The Differences Between FSMP and General Food, Health Food or Drug in Usage

Category	Main Usage
General food	Provide energy and nutrients to human body, to maintain the normal metabolism.
Health food	With the purpose of adjusting body function. These products focus on the health function, such as "assisting blood sugar reduction", "supplying vitamins & minerals".
FSMP	As a nutritional supplement, provide nutrition supports for patients. These products focus on the nutrition support, rather than health function.
Drug	Used to prevent or treat disease.

Table 5. 35　The Differences Between FSMP and General Food, Health Food or Drug in Formula

Category	Formula
General food	Contain proper nutrients, and are harmless to human body.
Health food	Contain functional components, and will not cause any acute, subacute or chronic harm to human body. General food ingredients, approved new food raw materials, substances which are both used as food and drug in China, etc., are all allowed to use in health food.
FSMP	Rich in nutrients (e. g. protein, fat, carbohydrate, vitamins, minerals, etc.), can meet the special dietary need for people under different disease condition. The product formula shall comply with GB 25592/GB 29922. Except for the nutrients and optional components stipulated in above standards, it is forbidden to add neither other bioactive substances nor drugs.
Drug	Contain bioactive components, and are allowed to have side effects.

Table 5. 36　The Differences Between FSMP and General Food, Health Food or Drug in Registration

Category	Requirements	Regulations
General food	No product registration or filing requirements before marketing	—
Health food	Product registration or filing	Administrative Measures on Health Food Registration and Filing
FSMP	Product registration	Administrative Measures on FSMP Registration
Drug	Product registration	Administrative Measures on Drug Registration

Table 5. 37　The Differences Between FSMP and General Food, Health Food or Drug in Label Claim

Category	Label Claim
General food	1. When the nutrient content reaches the requirements of GB 28050, it is allowed to make content claim or function claim of that nutrient on the label, and the expression shall be indicated in accordance with GB 28050. 2. It is forbidden to claim health function or disease prevention/treatment.
Health food	1. Indicate the approved health function on the label, such as "assisting blood sugar reduction" and "supplying vitamin C". 2. It is forbidden to claim disease prevention or treatment.
FSMP	1. Indicate the formula characteristic, and specify the suitable crowds in accordance with the product category. 2. It is forbidden to claim health function or disease prevention/treatment.
Drug	Claim the indications of the drug.

5. 6. 5　Diet-drug Interactions

A medical drug (or medicine) is a chemical used for the prevention and treatment of symptoms, or cure of diseases. Pharmacology is the study of drugs, their properties and effects. Pharmacotherapy is how to use drugs to treat disease or/and maintain health. Nutrition intervention and pharmacotherapy are sometimes integrated and coordinated. Specific nutrients from diet or nutrition status may influence the actions of specific drugs. Drugs can also interact with nutrients. Therefore, understanding the basic principles of pharmacology is very important for professionals in nutrition intervention.

5.6.5.1　Pharmacokinetics

How does a drug work in the body? A drug usually binds to a specific receptor on the cell membrane to trigger or alter specific enzymatic reactions. This process is the initiation of drug action in the body. The alteration of enzymatic reactions can be stimulation or inhibition of them, which changes the physiological function of the cells. Because drugs need to bind to the receptors for their actions, drugs are designed to match the shapes of the specific receptors.

After administration of drugs, the process of the drugs in the body is called pharmacokinetics. Pharmacokinetics is the study of drug absorption, distribution, metabolism, and excretion. At any phase of pharmacokinetics, drugs may interact with nutrients; drugs may result in altered nutrition status; or nutrients or health/condition interact with drugs.

(1) Absorption

The absorption of a drug means a drug moves from the site of administration to circulatory or lymph system. The mechanisms of absorption for drugs are similar to the absorption of nutrients, including passive diffusion, facilitated diffusion, and active transport. Drugs should be dissolved and thus absorbed by gastrointestinal tract. Thereby, dissolution must occur before absorption. Excipients are those substances added to the drugs that may influence dissolution. Several factors in gastrointestinal tract influence the absorptions of drugs such as the portion, the pH, and the surface area of the gastrointestinal tract. The chemical properties of the drug also affect the absorption. Fat-soluble drugs can cross the cell membrane easily.

(2) Distribution

The distribution of a drug means the delivery of drug to the target site. It is affected by the binding of the drug to proteins in blood, the circulation, and the binding of the drug to tissue surfaces. The more drugs that are combined to the target sites, the less drug is freed in the blood.

(3) Metabolism

The metabolism of a drug means the inactivation (biotransformation) of the drug for excretion. This process is predominately done in liver, a little in gastrointestinal tract. Cytochrome P-450 isoenzymes (CP450) are the family enzyme system responsible for drug metabolism. Most of CP450 are found in liver. Some are found in gastrointestinal tract. Some substances including inducers and inhibitors may interact with CP450 enzymes to alter drug levels and effects. Inducers stimulate CP450, increase drug metabolism, and decrease drug effect. In contrast, inhibitors reduce the action of CP450, decrease drug metabolism, and enhance drug effect.

(4) Excretion

The excretion of a drug means the elimination of drug from body. Most of drugs are excreted by urine or bile. Some of drugs are excreted by lungs, bowel, or breast milk. The nephrons in kidney are responsible for urinary excretion of drugs. They filter drugs out from the blood and concentrate into urine. Drugs can also be reabsorbed in nephrons.

5. 6. 5. 2　Diet-drug Interactions

Drug-nutrient interaction involves kinetic changes to a drug caused by a nutrient or the alteration of nutritional status caused by a drug. Food-drug interaction involves the interactions that affect the way a drug may impact nutritional status or the way food may affect drug efficacy. The interactions can happen in dissolution, absorption, metabolism, and excretion of drugs. Health professionals should be very familiar with the interactions and have the sensibility of the potential interactions in clinic patient care.

(1) Effect of Food/Nutrients on Drug Kinetics

① Alter drug dissolution: Dissolution of drug must occur before drug absorbed. The nutrition-related factors affected drug dissolution includes gastric pH, gastric empty rate, and any diseases or conditions changed gastrointestinal tract function. Most of drugs prefer to dissolve in acidic solution, for example, the gastric acid. People with achlorhydria, a condition of reducing gastric acids, experience a less therapeutic effectiveness of drug due to decreased dissolution of the drug. The time of drug dissolution is affected by gastric emptying rate. Medications such as metoclopramide can affect gastric emptying time. Gastrointestinal tract conditions such as vomiting and diarrhea also decrease the dissolution of drugs.

② Alter drug absorption: Drug absorption can be influenced by the presence of food, alcohol, or dietary supplements by several ways. The effects of drugs for the therapeutic purpose depend on the absorption of drugs. Increasing absorption can enhance the drug action, while decreasing absorption can reduce the drug effect. The effect of food/nutrients on medication absorption can be summarized as three ways. The first, the presence of food may decrease the rate or the extent of drug absorption. For example, anti-osteoporosis drug alendronate cannot be absorbed when ingested with a meal or up to 2 hours after a meal. The second, chelate complexes that are formed with certain drugs and the mineral cations such as Ca, Mg, Fe, and Zn from foods decreases drug absorption. For example, ingestion of ciprofloxacin and dairy products together can form an insoluble chelate complex, thus absorption of ciprofloxacin is decreased. The third, the presence of food may increase the absorption of some drugs. A high fat diet increases the dissolution and the absorption of lipid-based drugs.

③ Alter drug distribution: Drug distribution is influenced by the circulation, which affected by age, disease status, etc. For example, drug distribution is enhanced for patient with vasodilation. Body composition and albumin level also affect drug distribution. Low albumin level causes the decrease of drug binding sites and increases unbounded drug, which enhances the drug effects. For example, warfarin (an anticoagulant drug that prevents stroke and heart attack) can induce bleeding in hypoalbuminemia patients.

④ Alter drug metabolism: Diet may alter the metabolism of some drugs. Food/nutrients serve as an inhibitor or inducer for the drug metabolic enzyme system. Drug effectiveness and the side effects can be altered by food/nutrients. For example, grapefruit reduces the metabolism of some drugs by inhibiting the activity of cytochrome P450 3A4 isoenzymes. Serum drug levels increase and cause toxicity. The herb product St. John's wort/hypericum, which is used for the treatment of depression, induces cytochrome P450 3A4 isoenzymes. St. John's wort/hypericum increases the metabolism of some drugs and cause therapeutic failure for those drugs.

⑤ Alter drug urinary excretion: Dietary intake, acid-base balance, and hydration status can change the urinary condition and thereby alter the drug reabsorption and excretion. For example, lithium, which is a drug to treat with manic-depressive psychosis, are reabsorbed at the same sites with sodium in the kidney. High sodium intake increases sodium and lithium execration.

(2) Effect of Drugs on Food/Nutrients

① Alter nutrient absorption

Drug can change the absorption of nutrients. Drug may damage mucosal surface, and thereby may reduce nutrient absorption. Drug may alter gastric acidity. For example, antiulcer drugs such as a proton pump inhibitor are used for a long time that may decrease the absorption of iron, thiamin, and vitamin B12, since an acid environment increases the absorption of those nutrients. Ingestion of some drugs with foods may reduce the absorption of nutrients, drugs, or both. For example, Antibiotics such as tetracycline chelate with calcium, magnesium, iron, and zinc from foods.

② Alter nutrient metabolism: Drug can alter the metabolism of nutrients. Drug may increase the metabolism of nutrients leading to increase the requirements for the nutrients or increase the risk of deficiency for the nutrients. The drugs of anticonvulsants such as phenobarbital and phenytoin enhance the metabolism of folic acid, vitamin D and K. Long term use may result in deficiencies of the nutrients. Drug may interrupt the action of vitamin. For example, antituberculosis drug isoniazid inhibits vitamin B6 to convert to the active form.

③ Alter nutrient excretion: Drug can alter the excretion of nutrients. Drug may increase or decrease the urinary excretion of nutrients. For example, loop diuretics such as furosemide increase the excretion of many minerals such as sodium, potassium, calcium, magnesium. Thiazide diuretics increase reabsorption of calcium and decrease the excretion of calcium.

(3) Effects of Drugs on Nutritional Status

① Appetite changes: Drugs may suppress or increase appetite. Amphetamines, which treat with the disease of attention deficit hyperactivity disorder for children, may suppress appetite and lead to malnutrition in children. Many chemotherapy drugs can also cause loss of appetite. Most antipsychotic drugs stimulate appetite and increase body weight.

② Gastrointestinal changes: Drug may present in the saliva. The antibiotic clarithromycin enters into the saliva and cause a bitter taste. Drug may change oral bacteria. For example, antibiotics tetracycline may lead to oral yeast overgrowth. Drug may also cause abnormal sense of taste, dry mouth, and increase stomatitis and glossitis. Furthermore, drug induced dry mouth or throat or mucositis result in dysphagia. Drug may alter stomach mucosa leading to nausea, vomiting, bleeding, and ulceration. Drug can change intestinal bacteria, and some drugs cause constipation.

③ Systemic metabolic changes: Drug may exacerbates glucose intolerance. For example, corticosteroid impair glucose or insulin tolerance and cause new onset diabetes. Drug may also result in dyslipidemia such as increasing triglycerides and cholesterol. Antipsychotic risperidone increases the level of triglycerides.

④ Renal or urinary effects: Drug can cause urinary retention, urinary frequency or acute renal failure. Oxybutynin, which is a bladder control agent and used for reducing frequent urination, can lead to urinary retention. Calcitonin treated with osteoporosis can enhance urinary frequency. Several drugs can result in acute renal failure.

5.6.5.3 Specific Drugs and Their Effects on Diet/Nutritional Status

(1) Coumadin (Warfarin)

Coumadin, which is an anticoagulant, reduces the formation of blood clots. Coumadin used to treat or prevent blood clots in veins or arteries reduces the risk of stroke and heart attack. Vitamin K enhances blood clotting. If increasing vitamin K intake for patients treated with Coumadin, the effect of Coumadin on reducing blood clots is decreased. If patients treated with Coumadin decrease vitamin K intake, the effect of Coumadin on reducing blood clots is enhanced, which may cause bleeding. Therefore, the recommendation of vitamin K intake for patients treated with Coumadin is that vitamin K intake should be consistent from day to day. Vitamin K presents abundantly in dark green, leafy vegetables such as cooked spinach and other greens. Soybeans, green peas, and black-eyed peas are also rich in vitamin K.

(2) Monoamine Oxidase Inhibitors (MAOIs)

Monoamine oxidase (MAO) is responsible for inactivating the neurotransmitters such as dopamine, norepinephrine, and serotonin in the brain. Low levels of these three neurotransmitters are associated with depression and anxiety. Monoamine oxidase inhibitors (MAOIs) are drugs that block this inactivation, and thereby increases the activated levels of these three neurotransmitters. MAO is also responsible for breaking down another amine called tyramine. Therefore, MAOIs inhibits MAO, resulting in the increase of neurotransmitters and tyramine. Increasing tyramine level in the blood can cause sudden increase of blood pressure and may cause stroke. Tyramine presents in nature foods such as any overripe fruits, chicken and beef livers, broad-beans, tofu, eggplant, and in processed food such as fermented foods, cheeses, smoked or pickled meat, poultry, or fish, soy sauce, yogurt. For patients treated with MAOIs should limit tyramine in their diet and consume foods which are fresh or properly stored.

(3) Grapefruit

Grapefruit contains a high amount of furanocoumarin, which inhibits cytochrome P450 3A4 isoenzymes in the intestinal cells. In large amounts, furanocoumarin can inhibit hepatic cytochrome P450 3A4 isoenzymes. The body uses cytochrome P450 3A4 isoenzymes to break down certain drugs so that they can be excreted from the body. Thereby, grapefruit can result in the increase of drug effect and the risk of toxicities. The effect of grapefruit on drug metabolism can keep up to 24—72 hours after consumption. Numerous drugs are subjected to such metabolic interactions, such as statin which is used to treat hyperlipidemia, cyclosporines that are immunosuppressants, antihistamines, anti-infective agents, antiarrhythmic, calcium channel blockers, and benzodiazepines.

(4) Alcohol and Medications

Alcohol can interacts with many medications. Alcohol can have central nerve system effects such as sedation and depressed respiration. when consumes with drugs including narcotics or antidepressants. Alcohol can cause hepatotoxicity when intakes with acetaminophen medications. Alcohol may cause gastrointestinal bleeding when consumes with aspirin or nonsteroidal anti-inflammatory drugs (NSAIDS). Alcohol can either decrease or increase drug effect. Alcohol reduces warfarin effects on blood clots. Alcohol can also enhance insulin effects for people with diabetes. Some drugs alters alcohol metabolism in the body. For example, cephalosporins can inactivate hepatic aldehyde dehydrogenase and thereby increase the level of acetaldehyde in the blood when intake with alcohol. The severe symptom is acetaldehyde toxicity including headache, dizziness, nausea, vomiting, and physical discomfort.

5.7　Foodborne Illness

The relationship between food and health includes two aspects, including nutrition and food safety problems. Toxic substances (including pathogenic microorganisms) in food may cause health hazards when they enter the human body.

5.7.1　Overview of Foodborne Illness

5.7.1.1　Definition and Characteristics

Foodborne disease/illness is any disease resulting from the consumption of contaminated food or beverages which may contain pathogenic bacteria, parasites, viruses or certain chemicals. Natural toxins contained in editable plants and animals can also cause foodborne illness. Foodborne illness is one of the most widely distributed and common diseases worldwide. Cases of foodborne illness occur daily in all countries, from the most developed to the least developed countries. It is an important global public health problem.

The term of "foodborne illness" is gradually developed from "food poisoning". Both terms are often used interchangeably by consumers. However, the definition of "foodborne disease" has wider scope than that of "food poisoning". Foodborne illness also includes allergic reactions and other conditions where food acts as a carrier of the allergen. In 1984, "foodborne illness" as an official professional terminology term was used to replace the "food poisoning" by the WHO.

The most common symptoms of foodborne diseases can be ranged from an upset stomach to more serious symptoms, including nausea, diarrhea, fever, vomiting, abdominal cramps, and dehydration. The victims may experience different type and severity of symptoms by the type of pathogen in food, amount of contaminated food consumed, and the individual's health status.

5.7.1.2　Factors Contribute to the Foodborne Illness

Foodborne illnesses are mainly caused by contaminated food and the food with nature toxins. Biological, chemical, and physical factors are contributed to contaminated food. With more than 200 known diseases being transmitted through food, pathogens are the most significant cause.

(1) Biological hazards

Biological hazards include parasites and microorganisms such as bacteria, viruses, and prones. Bacteria and viruses are the most common causes of foodborne illness, and in every food safety program, controlling these biological hazards is a primary goal.

Bacteria are one-celled microorganisms with a cell wall but no nucleus. They exist in a variety of shapes, types and properties. Some pathogenic bacteria are capable of spore formation and thus, highly heat-resistant (e. g. *Clostridium botulinum*, *C. perfringens*, *Bacillus subtilis*, *B. cereus*). Others are capable of producing heat-resistant toxins (e. g., *Staphylococcus aureus*). Most pathogens are mesophilic with optimal growth temperature range from 20 to 45℃ (68 to 113°F). However, certain foodborne pathogens (termed psychrotrophs) are capable of growth under refrigerated conditions or temperatures less than 10℃ (50°F). The most well documented psychrotrophic foodborne pathogens are *Listeria monocytogenes*, and *Yersinia enterocolitica*. *Listeria monocytogenes*, for example, will grow (albeit slowly) at temperatures just above freezing (approximately 33—34°F). Certain strains or serotypes of *Bacillus cereus*, *Clostridium botulinum*, *Salmonella* spp., *E. coli* O157 : H7, and *Staphylococcus aureus* may also grow slowly under refrigeration conditions.

Viruses are particulate in nature and multiply only in other living cells. Thus, they are incapable of survival for long periods outside the host. While greater than 100 types of enteric viruses have been shown to cause foodborne illness, the most common foodborne

virus pathogens are Norwalk virus, Noroviruses (formerly known as Norwalk-like viruses),
Rotavirus, Astrovirus, and Hepatitis A.

Parasitic Protozoa are one-celled microorganisms without a rigid cell wall, but with an
organized nucleus. They are larger than bacteria. Like viruses, they do not multiple in
foods, only in hosts. The transmissible form of these organisms is termed a cyst. Protozoa
that have been associated with food and water-borne infections include *Entamoeba
histolytica*, *Toxoplasma gondii*, *Giardia lamblia*, *Cryptosporidium parvum* and
Cyclospora cayatenensis.

Multi-cellular Parasites are animals that live at the expense of the host. They may occur
in foods in the form of eggs, larvae, or other immature forms. Trichinosis has been an
important reportable pathogen associated with undercooked pork. Other parasites of concern
include flatworms or nematodes (associated with fish), cestodes or tapeworms (usually
associated with beef, pork, or fish) and trematodes or flukes.

(2) Chemical Hazards

Chemicals may present in food naturally or added improperly or intentionally during
agricultural producers, food processors or consumers. Naturally occurring chemicals are
toxins and food allergens that produced by biological organisms. Chemical contaminants
from human include agricultural chemicals such as pesticides, fertilizers, food additives,
metals, and chemical residues.

(3) Physical Hazards

Foreign material such as stones pieces of glass, staples, wood, and bone fragments
from animals can result in physical hazards. Theses can entry food from food-processing,
poor food-handling, and in retail food establishments. It can harm human if the people
swallow the food with pieces of glass. Glasses are often used as packing material for foods,
which must be avoiding breakage container to prevent slivers of glass get into food.

5.7.1.3　Classification of Foodborne Illness

Foodborne illness may be classified as infection, intoxication, or toxin-mediated
infection. Foodborne infections are caused by eating biological hazards along with food.
Intoxications are caused by consuming food that contains a toxic chemical. Some toxins are
produced by microbes. Food intoxications may also be caused by consume poisonous plants,
fish or food contain chemicals such as pesticides or cleaning agents. Toxin-mediated
infection is caused by eating foods are contaminated by harmful microorganisms that produce
toxins inside the human body. The different between toxin-mediated infection and
intoxication is toxin of toxin-mediated is produced inside the human body.

5.7.2　Microbial Foodborne Illness

Microbes or their toxic by-products most typically cause foodborne illness. Of all the
foodborne complaints reported, bacterial causes are at the top of the list followed by viral,
parasitic, and fungal contamination.

5.7.2.1　Factors to Microbial Foodborne Illness

Generally, there are three key factors contribute to microbial foodborne illness. They are ① contamination-pathogens must be present in the food; ② growth—in some cases they must also have the opportunity to multiply in the food in order to produce an infectious dose or sufficient toxin to cause illness; ③ survival—when present at a dangerous level they must be able to survive in the food during its storage and processing. Pathogens can get into food through many ways (Figure 5.24).

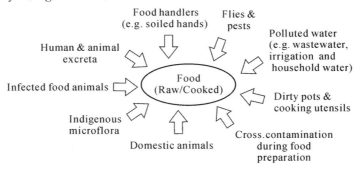

Figure 5.24　Sources of Microbial Contamination

5.7.2.2　Microorganism Growth Condition—FAT TOM

FAT TOM is a mnemonic device that describes the six favorable conditions required for the growth of foodborne pathogens. It is an acronym for food, acidity, time, temperature, oxygen and moisture. Each of the six conditions that foster the growth foodborne pathogens are defined in the following Table 5.38.

Table 5.38　FAT TOM for Conditions of Microorganism Growth

Food	Some foods promote microorganism growth more than others. Protein-rich foods such as meat, milk, eggs and fish are most susceptible.
Acidity	Foodborne pathogens require a slightly acidic pH level of 4.6—7.5, while they thrive in conditions with a pH of 6.6—7.5. The Food and Drug Administration (FDA) regulations for acid/acidified foods require that food be brought to a pH of 4.5 or below.
Time	Food should be removed from "the danger zone" (see below) within two hours, either by cooling or heating. While most guidelines cite two hours, a few indicate that four hours is still safe.
Temperature	Foodborne pathogens grow best in temperatures between 41 ℉ (5℃) to 135 ℉ (57℃), a range referred to as the temperature danger zone (TDZ). They thrive in temperatures that are between 70 ℉ (21℃) to 120 ℉ (49℃).
Oxygen	The presence of oxygen can be both helpful and harmful to the growths of pathogens. Aerobic oxygen need oxygen to grow, whereas anaerobic pathogens do not.
Moisture	Water activity (Wa) is a measure of the water available for use and is measured on a scale of 0 to 1.0. Foodborne pathogens grow best in foods that have a Wa between 0.86 and 1.0.

5. 7. 2. 3   Bacteria Pathogens

Harmful bacteria are common cause of foodborne illness. According the pathogenesis, the mechanism of bacteria foodborne illness can be cataloged as pathogen bacterial infection and intoxication. The difference between infection and intoxication is briefly described in Table 5. 39.

Table 5. 39   Comparison of Infection and Intoxication

	Infection	Intoxication
Pathogens	Bacteria	Bacterial toxins
Incubation	Longer (>4 h)	Shorter (1—2 h)
Fever	Yes	No
Antibiotics	Use	Do not use

(1) Mechanism of Bacterial pathogenesis

① Infection: Infection occurs when living bacteria are ingested with food in numbers sufficient for some to survive the acidity of the stomach, one of the body's principal protective barriers. These survivors then pass into the small intestine where they multiply and produce symptoms. Infections can be invasive or non-invasive. In non-invasive infections, the organism attaches itself to the gut surface or epithelium to prevent itself from being washed out by the rapid flow of material through the gut. It then multiplies, colonizing the surface. Invasive pathogens are not confined to the intestinal lumen but can penetrate the cells lining the gut. In some cases their penetration is limited to the immediate vicinity of the gut. Some pathogens invade the mucosa of the large intestine rather than the small intestine, producing inflammation, superficial abscesses and ulcers, and the passage of dysenteric stools containing blood, pus and large amounts of mucus. In other cases, microbial invasion is not restricted to the gut's immediate locality and the organism spreads further through the body, producing symptoms other than diarrhea at sites remote from the gut itself, as for example in brucellosis, listeriosis, typhoid and paratyphoid fevers.

② Intoxication: With foodborne intoxications, the bacteria grow in the food producing a toxin. When the food is eaten, it is the toxin, rather than the microorganisms, that causes symptoms. Since the toxin is ingested with the food there is no direct person-to-person spread, as can occur with some enteric infections, and the incubation period (the time between consumption of the food and the appearance of symptoms) tends to be shorter, generally of the order of one or two hours or even less in some cases. This is because the toxin begins to act as soon as it reaches the site of action, whereas with infections the microorganism need time to multiply in the body.

(2) Common Bacterial Pathogens

The most common bacterial foodborne pathogens are *Salmonella*, Campylobacter jejuni, Escherichia coli O157 : H7 and Clostridium perfringens.

① *Salmonella*: According WHO ranking, *Salmonella* has caused the most common foodborne illness worldwide. In the past few years, large outbreaks of illness caused by *Salmonella*-contaminated eggs and peanut products have made the headlines in the USA. They are microscopic living creatures that pass from the feces of people or animals to other people or other animals. *Salmonella* are typically motile, non-spore-forming, Gram-negative, rod-shaped bacteria. Currently, there are approximately 2,400 types (serovars) of *Salmonella*. *Salmonella typhimurium* has been the species that accounts for most foodborne illnesses related to this bacterium. Another species, *Salmonella enteritidis*, has been associated with foodborne diseases resulting from consumption of contaminated undercooked eggs. *Salmonella Heidelberg* has caused outbreaks associated with raw produce. *Salmonella* DT104, a specific serotype, is resistant to a wide range of antibiotics.

Associated Food: Salmonella is widespread in the environment and is associated with all animal species, including mammals, birds, reptiles, and amphibians. It has been found in water, soil, insects, animal feces, raw meats, poultry, seafood, and on factory and kitchen surfaces. While these are common sources, *Salmonella* has been isolated from numerous other food sources as well. A variety of food has caused salmonellosis outbreaks, including meat, poultry, eggs, milk and dairy products, fish and shrimp, and cream-filled desserts and topping.

Symptoms: Acute symptoms of salmonellosis may include nausea, vomiting, abdominal cramps, diarrhea, fever, and headache. Typically, symptoms develop 12—72 hours after ingestion of contaminated food. Most persons infected usually recover without treatment after four to seven days. As with many foodborne pathogens, young children, the elderly, and the immunocompromised are the most likely targets of *Salmonella* infections. Depending on host factors, such as the age and health of the host, the infective dose has been estimated to be less than a thousand cells for many of the strains, and as low as 15—20 cells for some strains.

Prevention: *Salmonella* bacteria can survive for weeks outside a living body, and they are not destroyed by freezing. Ultraviolet radiation and heat accelerate their demise; they perish after being heated to 55℃ (131°F) for 90 min, or to 60℃ (140°F) for 12 min. To protect against *Salmonella* infection, heating food for at least ten minutes at 75℃ (167°F) is recommended, so the centre of the food reaches this temperature.

To control *Salmonella* foodborne illness, several ways may be taken:

● Thoroughly cook all poultry, poultry products, eggs, ground meat products and fish.

● Use only pasteurized milk.

● Thoroughly wash hands before and handling raw meat, poultry and egg products.

● Use clean utensils and surfaces to prepare foods.

● Wash utensils, cutting boards and surfaces thoroughly with hot soapy water and rinse before preparing foods.

② *Campylobacter*: Bacteria of the genus *campylobacter* are Gram-negative rods that are spirally curved and motile. Because these organisms are microaerophilic, they require only a low level of oxygen to survive. With respect to growth temperatures, bacteria in the genus *Campylobacter* are generally mesophilic, with a growth range from about 25℃ to 45℃ and optimal growth at 37℃ or 42℃ for the thermophilic species. These organisms are normally found in wild birds, poultry, pigs, cattle, domesticated animals, unpasteurized milk, and contaminated water. They are transmitted to humans by fecal-oral routes and by ingestion of contaminated water and ice, but most commonly by consuming raw or undercooked meat.

Associated Food: Most cases of *Campylobacter* infections are associated with eating raw or undercooked poultry. Other common sources of *Campylobacter* include cattle, pigs, sheep, ostriches, shellfish, dogs, cats, unpasteurized milk, contaminated water and ice. Fruits and vegetables can also be a source of infection when washed with contaminated water or when prepared on the cutting board that was used for raw poultry meat and then unwashed.

Symptoms: The symptoms associated with this disease are usually flu-like: fever, nausea, abdominal cramping, vomiting, enteritis, diarrhea, and malaise. Symptoms begin within 2—5 days after ingestion of the bacteria, and the illness typically lasts 7—10 days. Because most people normally recover from this infection on their own, treatment is not usually necessary. However, antibiotics such as azithromycin and erythromycin are effective against campylobacter, and can be prescribed for patients with severe diarrhea. Recurrence of this disease can occur up to three months after pathogen ingestion.

Prevention: Several ways to prevent campylobacteriosis

- Thoroughly cook meat, poultry and fish.
- Proper sanitation of food contact surfaces and utensils.
- Proper hand washing after handling raw meat, poultry and seafood .
- Use pasteurized milk.
- Use a safe water supply.

③ *Vibrio parahaemolyticus*: *Vibrio parahaemolyticus* is a naturally occurring bacterium that inhabits coastal brackish marine waters throughout the world and is commonly found in the seacoastal area of South China. This organism requires salt to survive and appears in higher concentrations during the warmer summer months. If ingested in sufficient numbers, this bacterium can cause illness such as gastroenteritis. Illnesses linked with this organism have been associated with the consumption of raw or improperly cooked seafood. Foodborne infections caused by *V. parahaemolyticus* are fairly common in Asia. Outbreaks tend to be concentrated along coastal regions during the summer and early fall when higher water temperatures favor higher levels of bacteria. Since the infection is categorized as a short-term illness with no long-term complications, many cases are not reported, and/or many of those infected simply assume it was the flu or a short bout of food poisoning. When patients go to the doctor, many laboratories do not have the proper selective media or equipment to screen for *V. parahaemolyticus.*

Associated Food: *Vibrio parahaemolyticus* is a naturally occurring estuarine organism that can be taken up and concentrated by mollusks, such as clams and oysters, as they feed. Outbreaks of illness related to *V. parahaemolyticus* typically occur by ingesting raw or undercooked seafood and shellfish (especially oysters), or through cross-contamination of cookware or utensils. The bacteria proliferate rapidly when contact surfaces are not cleaned properly or the seafood is not kept out of the temperature "danger zone".

Symptoms: The most common symptoms of consuming *Vibrio parahaemolyticus* is watery diarrhea, nausea, vomiting, abdominal cramping, headache, fever and chills. Incubation time usually occur after 15 hours, but can begin as early as 4 hours and as late as 36 hours after exposure and continue for up to 3 days. It is categorized as a short illness, and after recovery there are no prolonged effects. However, in rare instances those who are either immunocompromised or particularly sensitive to its toxin may experience more severe effects. An open wound or abrasion on the skin that is exposed to seawater, fish, or shellfish can also harbor *V. parahaemolyticus*, causing skin or soft tissue infections. As the vast majority of cases of *V. parahaemolyticus* food infection are self-limiting, treatment is not typically necessary. In severe cases, fluid and electrolyte replacement is indicated.

Prevention: Seafood and shellfish are considered Potentially Hazardous Foods because foodborne pathogens increase in number if temperature abuse occurs. In other words, most foods in this category should be kept at either above 57℃ (135℉) (after cooking) or below 5℃ (41℉) (storage), with temperatures in the middle being considered part of the "danger zone." As a rule of thumb, foods should spend no more than 4 hours in the "danger zone" temperature range. Shellfish are an exception and may be transported and received at 7℃ (45℉). Once a product is frozen, it is important to maintain a proper freezer temperature to avoid product thawing. Labeling properly stored foods is also helpful to ensure that others handling the food in the future will know exactly how long a food product has been stored. To prevent *V. parahaemolyticus* contamination, seafood including oysters must be thoroughly cooked; use proper hand washing techniques and practice good personal hygiene; keep proper sanitation of food contact surfaces and utensils; and use a safe water supply.

④ *E. coli* O157 : H7: *Escherichia coli E. coli* is a bacterium from the family *Enterobacteriaceae* usually found in the digestive system of healthy humans and animals and transmitted through fecal contamination. There are hundreds of known *E. coli* strains, with *E. coli* O157 : H7 being the most recognized. *E. coli* are found everywhere in the environment but mostly occupy animal surfaces and digestive systems, making it important to thoroughly wash anything that comes into contact with these surfaces. *E. coli* O157 : H7 are Gram-negative rods that have been variously described as verotoxigenic *E. coli* (VTEC) or shiga-like toxin producing *E. coli* (SLTEC). Most recently, the designation has been simplified to shiga-toxin producing *E. coli* (STEC) in recognition of the similarities of the toxins produced by *E. coli* O157 : H7 and *Shigella dysenteriae*. These potent toxins are the cause of severe damage to the intestinal lining of those infected. The toxins produced by *E. coli* O157 : H7 are responsible for the symptoms associated with infection such as hemorrhagic colitis, hemolytic uremic syndrome (HUS), and even death. The organism can survive at low temperatures and under acidic conditions, making it difficult to eradicate in nature. The organism has a low infective dose and can be transmitted from person to person, as well as in food products.

Associated Food: Sources of *E. coli* O157 : H7 infections include undercooked or raw hamburgers, sheep, pigs, goats, poultry, game meat, alfalfa sprouts, unpasteurized fruit juices, dry-cured salami, lettuce, cheese curds, unpasteurized or raw milk, contaminated water and ice, and person-to-person transmission. Fruits and vegetables can cause infection from contact with contaminated water. The most common source of infection, however, is caused by consuming undercooked or raw meats. Because there appears to be a low infective dose for this organism (10—100 cells), adequate sanitation and/or proper processing of foods is critically important.

Symptoms: The acute disease associated with this organism is named hemorrhagic colitis. The symptoms characteristic to this disease are watery and/or bloody diarrhea, fever, nausea, severe abdominal cramping, and vomiting. Because most people recover from this infection on their own, treatment is usually not necessary. Symptoms can appear within hours or up to several days after ingestion of the bacteria, and the illness usually lasts 5—10 days. Some individuals may develop HUS. In the very young, this disorder can cause renal failure, hemolytic anemia, or even permanent loss of kidney function. In the elderly, these symptoms may occur, as well as thrombotic thrombocytopenic purpura (TTP) (HUS with additional neurological dysfunction and/or fever).

⑤ *Clostridium botulinum*: *Clostridium botulinum* (*C. botulinum*) is the bacterium that causes botulism. These Gram-positive organisms are characterized by their slightly curved, motile, and anaerobic rods that produce heat-resistant spores. The spores, which are very resistant to a number of environmental stresses such as heat and high acid, can become activated in a low acid (pH greater than 4.6), anaerobic, high moisture environment with temperatures ranging from 3℃ to 43℃ (38℉ to 110℉). Spores allow the bacteria to survive in adverse environmental conditions and germinate once conditions become more favorable. *C. botulinum* is ubiquitous in nature, often found in soil and water. Although the bacteria and spores in themselves do not cause disease, the production of botulinum toxin is what leads to botulism, a serious paralytic condition that can lead to death. There are seven strains of *C. botulinum* based on differences in antigenicity among the toxins, each characterized by its ability to produce a protein neurotoxin, enterotoxin, or haemotoxin. Types A, B, E, and F cause botulism in humans, while types C and D cause botulism in animals and birds. Type G was identified in 1970 but has not been determined as a cause of botulism in humans or animals.

Associated Food: Foodborne botulism results from the ingestion of pre-formed toxin in food. Botulinum toxin can be found in foods that have not been properly handled or canned and is often present in canned vegetables, meat, and seafood products. Infant botulism occurs when infants ingest *C. botulinum* spores that germinate and produce toxin in the intestine. Honey is a common dietary source of *C. botulinum* spores and, therefore, infants less than one year of age should not consume honey.

Symptoms: Botulinum toxin is a neurotoxin, thus it affects the nervous system and is characterized by descending, flaccid paralysis that can cause respiratory failure. Foodborne botulism produces symptoms beginning in 6 to 36 hours, though some can even start after two weeks. Symptoms include double and blurred vision, slurred speech, difficulty swallowing, dry mouth, diarrhea, nausea, and muscle weakness that descends through the body. Recovery occurs with prompt administration of antitoxin and respiratory intensive care. Deaths that occur within the first two weeks of botulism are often the result of pulmonary or systematic infection and failure to recognize the disease. Often the symptoms of foodborne botulism are mistaken for symptoms associated with stroke, chemical intoxication, myasthenia gravis, and Guillain-Barre syndrome. Tests such as brain scans, spinal tap exams, nerve conduction exams, electromyography (EMG), and a tensilon exam can distinguish the above diseases from botulism.

Treatments: In infant botulism, infants may appear lethargic, constipated, have poor feeding patterns, and have a weak cry. Infants can be treated with antibiotics to kill *C. botulinum* in the body and antitoxin to neutralize the toxin. Infant botulism is less fatal than foodborne botulism, with $<2\%$ mortality rate.

Prevention: During the canning process, foods undergo a hot fill process and oxygen is removed, leaving the food in an anaerobic environment. Certain foods, such as meat, are able to bind oxygen to create an anaerobic environment that allows *C. botulinum* to grow. Home canning processes for low acid foods are extremely risky because the time and temperature food are heated are often inadequate. On a commercial scale, improperly handled food products have also contributed to outbreaks. The preventive method can be: (ⅰ) Proper preservation methods for canning low acid foods (vegetables, meat, poultry). (ⅱ) Acidification of foods below pH 4.6. (ⅲ) Reduction of water activity to 0.85 or below. (ⅳ) Avoid the use of honey with infants. (ⅴ) Do not temperature abuse vacuum packaged food or MAP (modified atmosphere packaged) food.

⑥ *Staphylococcus*: *Staphylococcus aureus* is part of the natural microflora of humans. The bacteria grow to higher numbers in pimples, sores and when someone has a cold. The bacteria grow best at our body temperature. *S. aureus* can multiply rapidly in food held at room temperature and the toxin can be produced by the microorganism growing in the food. This toxin is called an enterotoxin because it causes gastroenteritis or inflammation of the lining of the intestinal tract. Thorough cooking destroys the *Staphylococcus aureus* bacteria, but the toxin is very resistant to heat, refrigeration, and freezing. When *Staphylococcus* bacteria get into warm food and multiply, they produce a toxin or poison that causes illness. The toxin is not detectable by taste or smell. While the bacteria itself can be killed by temperatures of 120 F, its toxin is heat resistant; therefore, it is important to keep the staph organism from growing. *Staphylococcus* bacteria are found on the skin and in the nose and throat of most people; people with colds and sinus infections are often carriers. Infected wounds, pimples, boils and acne are generally rich sources. *Staphylococcus* also is widespread in untreated water, raw milk and sewage.

Associated Food: Foods commonly involved in staphylococcal intoxication include protein foods such as ham, processed meats, tuna, chicken, sandwich fillings, cream fillings, potato and meat salads, custards, milk products and creamed potatoes. Foods that are handled frequently during preparation are prime targets for staphylococci contamination.

Symptoms: Symptoms include abdominal cramps, vomiting, severe diarrhea and exhaustion. These usually appear within one to eight hours after eating staph-infected food and last one or two days. The illness seldom is fatal.

Prevention: Keep food clean to prevent its contamination, keep it either hot (above 140 °F) or cold (below 40 °F) during serving time, and as quickly as possible refrigerate or freeze leftovers and foods to be served later.

⑦ *Listeria*: This bacterium is quite special because it can survive for long periods under adverse conditions, and its ability to grow at refrigeration temperatures, *Listeria* has since become recognized as an important foodborne pathogen. *L. monocytogenes* is frequently carried by humans and animals. The organism can grow in the pH range of 4.4 to 9.6. It is salt tolerant and relatively resistant to drying, but easily destroyed by heat. (It grows between 32 °F and 113 °F).

Symptoms and Associated Food: Listeriosis primarily affects newborn infants, pregnant women, the elderly and those with compromised immune systems. In a healthy non-pregnant person, listeriosis may occur as a mild illness with fever, headaches, nausea and vomiting. The incubation period is a few days to several weeks. Recent cases have involved raw milk, soft cheeses made with raw milk, and raw or refrigerated ready-to-eat meat, poultry or fish products.

Prevention: Preventive measures for listeriosis include maintaining good sanitation, turning over refrigerated ready-to-eat foods quickly, pasteurizing milk, avoiding post-pasteurization contamination, and cooking foods thoroughly.

(3) Mycotoxins

Mycotoxin is a toxic secondary metabolite produced by organisms of the fungi kingdom, commonly known as molds. One mold species may produce many different mycotoxins, and the same mycotoxin may be produced by several species. Some molds have the ability to produce toxic metabolites, known as mycotoxins, which can produce a range of disorders from gastroenteritis to cancer. More than 300 mycotoxins have been identified but only a relatively small number have been shown to occur in foods and feeds at levels sufficient to cause concern.

Aflatoxins are a type of mycotoxin produced by *Aspergillus* species of fungi, such as *A. flavus* and *A. parasiticus*. The umbrella term aflatoxin refers to four different types of mycotoxins produced, which are B_1, B_2, G_1, and G_2. Aflatoxin B_1, the most toxic, is a potent carcinogen and has been directly correlated to adverse health effects, such as liver cancer, in many animal species. Aflatoxins are largely associated with commodities produced in the tropics and subtropics, such as cotton, peanuts, spices, pistachios and maize. Mycotoxins can also present in milk, meat and their products as a result of animals consuming mycotoxin-contaminated feed.

Other mycotoxins have a range of other health effects including kidney damage, gastrointestinal disturbances, reproductive disorders or suppression of the immune system. For most mycotoxins, a tolerable daily intake (TDI) has been established, which estimates the quantity of mycotoxin which someone can be exposed to daily over a lifetime without it posing a significant risk to health.

5.7.3　Chemical Contamination

Chemical hazards in foods can arise from a number of different sources (Figure 5.25). Food can be contaminated by many points from harvest to the consumer. Sources of food contamination commonly are air, water, soil, ingredients, animals, food handlers, and packaging materials. Therefore, some fresh fruits or vegetables can be contaminated when they are washed or irrigated by contaminated water. Water can be contaminated by animal manure, human sewage or pesticide residue. Meat and poultry carcasses can become contaminated during processing, such as slaughter with small amounts of fecal material in the intestines of the animal.

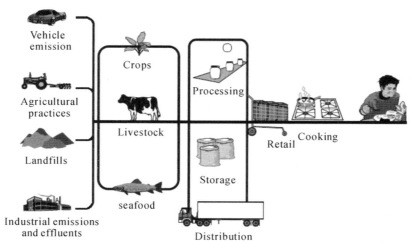

Figure 5.25　Diagram of Chemical Hazards from Different Sources

5.7.3.1　Industrial and Environmental Contamination

Modern industry produces huge numbers of chemical products and by-products. These can contaminate the environment and food chains, ultimately contaminating the human food supply itself. Most attention in this area has focused on heavy metals such as mercury, cadmium and lead, and organics such as polychlorinated biphenyls (PCBs). All of the above mentioned are now widespread in the environment though their concentrations are usually low, except in cases of industrial accidents and environmental disasters.

5.7.3.2　Agricultural Contamination

Foods can also carry residues of pesticides and veterinary drugs. Organochlorine pesticides were identified in the early 1970s as a particular problem since they persist in the environment, accumulate in the fatty tissues and increase in concentration as they pass up the food chain. Contamination is particularly associated with foods such as milk, animal fats, fish and eggs. As a result of concerns over their potential carcinogenicity and harm to the environment, the use of organochlorine pesticides has been restricted in many countries and residue levels in foods have shown a decline over recent years. They do however remain important in many developing countries. Residue levels in foods from developing countries are generally higher, but data are not available from many countries.

Organochlorine pesticides have increasingly been replaced by organophosphorus compounds. These do not persist in the environment or animal tissues for long periods and survey data have shown that they are seldom present in foods. However, they pose a serious health risk when ingested at high concentrations.

There are four causes of pesticides contamination:

(1) Contamination During Transport or Storage

Typical cases involved powders such as sugar or flour which were transported or stored with a pesticide or in a place previously contaminated with pesticide.

(2) Ingestion of Seed Dressed for Sowing

Mainly associated with organic mercury fungicides, such outbreaks occurred particularly during times of food shortage when treated seeds were distributed after farmers had already sown their own grain. Local people were unable to read the warning label on the bags or mistakenly believed that washing off the dye also removed the pesticide.

(3) Mistaken Use in Food Preparation

This occurs when pesticides are mistaken for food materials such as sugar, salt and flour.

(4) Misuse in Agriculture

Pesticides have been found in food or water due to misuse near harvesting time, misuse of containers, contamination of ground water and use of excessively high doses in agriculture.

Residues of veterinary drugs such as antibiotics can also find their way into milk or meat. In many cases the long-term effects of these on human health are not known but they can, for example, provoke strong allergic reactions in sensitive people. They can also encourage the spread of antibiotic resistance in bacteria, making treatment of human infection more difficult, and for this reason it has been recommended that antibiotics used in human medicine should not be used in animals. Antibiotic residues in milk that is used to produce fermented products can interfere with the fermentation process by inhibiting the desirable lactic acid bacteria. Normally this is just a technical problem resulting in economic loss but, when it occurs, pathogens present in the milk may grow and pose a health hazard later. For these reasons many countries have regulations prohibiting the sale of milk from cows being treated for mastitis and milk is routinely tested for the presence of antibiotic residues.

A few hormonal agents are used for growth promotion in farm animals (e. g. bovine somatotropin hormone, or BST). Minute residues of these drugs do not pose a risk for consumers, although there are different opinions on the acceptability of these drugs and monitoring is necessary to ensure that permitted limits are not exceeded.

5.7.3.3　Food Processing Contamination

Chemical contaminants can sometimes be introduced as a result of food processing and storage. Drinking water can be contaminated from lead used in water storage tanks and piping and this has on occasion caused cases of lead poisoning in children. Lead-based solder used in certain types of can is the major source of lead in canned foods, and processors in many countries have now adopted non-soldered cans as a simple remedy for this problem. Lead can also leach into foods stored in inadequately glazed earthenware pots. When pots are glazed at temperatures below 1,200℃, much of the lead in the glaze will remain soluble and if the pots are used to store acidic foods such as pickles or fruit juices then the product can become contaminated. Apple juice that caused a fatal case of lead poisoning contained 1,300 mg/L lead after three days storage in such a jar.

Chemicals have been deliberately added to foods since the earliest times. Before the advent of accurate analytical methods this was largely uncontrolled and open to abuse, but nowadays their use is subject to much closer regulation. Food additives can serve a number of purposes, such as preservative, antioxidant, acidity regulator, emulsifier, colour, flavour or processing aid. The health implication of additives is constantly under review by national regulators and international bodies such as JECFA who recommend ADI levels on the basis of data from toxicological studies. Additives such as some food colorings have occasionally been banned as a result of such studies. Where additives are allowed, permitted levels of use are prescribed for specified foods. Occasional problems may arise, however, with unscrupulous or ill-informed food processors that use non-permitted additives such as boric acid or excessive levels of permitted ones.

Nitrates and nitrites occur naturally in the Nitrates and nitrites occur naturally in the environment and are also deliberately added to some processed foods as a preservative and color fixative. They are, for example, particularly important for controlling the growth of *Clostridium botulinum* in cured meats. Under suitable conditions, the presence of nitrate/nitrite can lead to the formation of nitrosamines which are known to cause cancer in mammals. Studies have shown that food preparation techniques such as malting grain, smoking, drying and broiling of meat and fish and the frying of cured promote the formation of nitrosamines.

To reduce exposure to these compounds, good manufacturing practices are recommended which include addition to foods of the minimum amounts of nitrates/nitrites necessary to achieve their functional purpose and the use of nitrosation inhibitors such as ascorbate.

5.7.4   Natural Toxicants in Food

As opposed to man-made chemicals such as pesticides, veterinary drugs or environmental pollutants that get into our food supply, toxins can be present due to their natural occurrence in food. Natural toxins found inherently in foods of plant and animal origins can be harmful when consumed in sufficient quantities.

Toxic compounds are produced by a variety of plants and animals. Natural toxins may be present serving specific function in the plant and animal or evolved as chemical defense against predators, insects or microorganisms. These chemicals have diverse chemical structures and are vastly different in nature and toxicity.

5.7.4.1   Natural Toxins Present in Food of Plant Origin

Of over 300,000 different plant species in the world, at least 2,000 species are considered to be poisonous. Cases of poisoning are often reported when wild species of mushrooms, berries or other plants are ingested. Globally, only hundreds of plant species are commonly eaten, yet many of them can become toxic to the body if they are taken in excess or if they are not properly treated before consumption. Depending on the species, the edible parts of plants vary, which may include foliage, buds, stems, roots, fruits and tubers, and so are their poisonous parts.

Plants from the same genera may exhibit similar or vastly different toxicities. The amount and the distribution of the toxins present in a plant vary according to the species as well as the geographical conditions where it is grown.

In general, plant organs that are important for survival and reproduction, such as flowers and seeds, will concentrate defense compounds. These compounds may be more rapidly synthesized or stored at certain stages of critical growth, i. e. in buds, young tissue or seedlings as in the case of potato sprouts.

Common examples of natural toxins in food plants include glycoalkaloids in potatoes, cyanide-generating compounds in bitter apricot seeds and bamboo shoots, enzyme inhibitors and lectins in soya beans, green beans and other legumes.

5.7.4.2   Natural Toxins Present in Food of Animal Origin

Natural toxin of animal origin may be a product of metabolism or a chemical that is passed along the food chain. While poisoning after eating terrestrial animals is relatively uncommon, poisoning due to marine toxins occurs in many parts of the world. Marine toxins produced by toxic microalgae are accumulated in shellfish, crustacean and finfish following their consumption. Tetrodotoxin, a potent marine neurotoxin, is thought to be produced by certain bacteria. It is found in over 90 species of puffer fish and may cause lethality after ingested even a small amount. Seafood poisoning commonly reported in coral reef fish is due to the presence of ciguatoxin that may be found in more than 300 species of fish. Histamine produced by bacterial spoilage of scombroid fish causes another kind of seafood poisoning.

There are approximately 1,200 species of poisonous and venomous animals in the world. While most of them are not used as food, care must be taken to avoid the poisonous glands or tissue containing the toxins when these animals are used as food. Glands of some animals that are not considered poisonous or venomous when ingested can also cause food poisoning such as gall-bladder of grass carp which contains the cyprinol related chemicals.

5.7.5　Principles of Prevention of Foodborne Illness

Since foodborne illness is a significant public health challenge in the world, preventing foodborne illness is an essential point to insure food safety and quality. HACCP (Hazard analysis and critical control points) systems currently are used for controlling food safety hazards and prevent food contamination. HACCP is referred as the prevention of hazards rather than finished product inspection. The HACCP system can be used at all stages of a food chain, from food production and preparation processes including packaging, distribution, etc. There are seven principles of HACCP:

Principle 1: Conduct a hazard analysis. Plans determine the food safety hazards and identify the preventive measures the plan can apply to control these hazards. A food safety hazard is any biological, chemical, or physical property that may cause a food to be unsafe for human consumption.

Principle 2: Identify critical control points. A critical control point (CCP) is a point, step, or procedure in a food manufacturing process at which control can be applied and, as a result, a food safety hazard can be prevented, eliminated, or reduced to an acceptable level.

Principle 3: Establish critical limits for each critical control point. A critical limit is the maximum or minimum value to which a physical, biological, or chemical hazard must be controlled at a critical control point to prevent, eliminate, or reduce to an acceptable level.

Principle 4: Establish critical control point monitoring requirements. Monitoring activities are necessary to ensure that the process is under control at each critical control point. In the United States, the FSIS is requiring that each monitoring procedure and its frequency be listed in the HACCP plan.

Principle 5: Establish corrective actions. These are actions to be taken when monitoring indicates a deviation from an established critical limit. The final rule requires a plant's HACCP plan to identify the corrective actions to be taken if a critical limit is not met.

Corrective actions are intended to ensure that no product injurious to health or otherwise adulterated as a result of the deviation enters commerce.

Principle 6: Establish procedures for ensuring the HACCP system is working as intended. Validation ensures that the plants do what they were designed to do; that is, they are successful in ensuring the production of a safe product. Plants will be required to validate their own HACCP plans. FSIS will not approve HACCP plans in advance, but will review them for conformance with the final rule.

Verification ensures the HACCP plan is adequate, that is, working as intended. Verification procedures may include such activities as review of HACCP plans, CCP records, critical limits and microbial sampling and analysis. FSIS is requiring that the HACCP plan include verification tasks to be performed by plant personnel. Verification tasks would also be performed by FSIS inspectors. Both FSIS and industry will undertake microbial testing as one of several verification activities.

Verification also includes 'validation'—the process of finding evidence for the accuracy of the HACCP system (e. g. scientific evidence for critical limitations).

Principle 7: Establish record keeping procedures. The HACCP regulation requires that all plants maintain certain documents, including its hazard analysis and written HACCP plan, and records documenting the monitoring of critical control points, critical limits, verification activities, and the handling of processing deviations.

(Sun Guiju, Pang Daohua, Qiu Lianglin, He Canxia, Tang Chunlan, Feng Dan, Zou Zuquan, Yang Danting, Ding Yusong, Ye Yang, Zha Longying, Zhang Xiaohong, Wang Lijun, Yang Yan, Li Yonghua, Wang Shaokang, Guo Xin, Yuan Zhiqiong, Feng Qing)

Exercises

Chapter 6   Social, Psychological, and Behavioral Factors and Health

6.1   Social Factors and Health

Social factors have a broad impact on health and play an important role in the occurrence, prognosis, and prevention of diseases. Social factors include elements such as environment, population, and the level of civilization (politics, economy, culture, etc.). With the development of social economy and the advancement of medical science and technology, people's understanding of health and disease is deepening and developing. The study of the relationship between social factors and health is the most basic research field in preventive medicine.

6.1.1   Social Economy and Health

Social economy includes a country's economic development level, as well as its residents' clothing, food, housing, transportation, and social security. Therefore, social economy and population health are closely related. Economic development provides a material basis for public health, while the population's health plays a critical role in developing productivity and economic prosperity. In general, countries with a high gross national product (GNP) per capita have a high level of science and technology, good working conditions and nutrition, rich material and cultural life, and complete medical and health care and public facilities, which are beneficial to improve residents' health conditions and overall level of health.

6.1.1.1   Economic Development Level and Health

Statistical data shows a very close relationship between a country or region's level of economic development and the health of its residents. This is generally reflected in the following aspect: As a country's economic level improves, the health of its residents also gradually improves. Countries at different economic levels show significant differences in health levels. Usually, the indicators reflecting the level of economic development and residents' health status are used to analyze the impact of economic factors on health. Economic development indicators mainly consist of GNP, GNP per capita, health expenditure per capita, and so forth. Health indicators include natality, mortality, infant mortality, average life expectancy, etc. Social and economic factors not only affect residents' health status directly, but also indirectly through health services. Different levels of social and economic development are important factors for the difference in resident's health level in different countries. Therefore, a country or society with economic development and abundant materials can provide adequate food nutrition, good living and working conditions and medical services, which support residents' health.

6.1.1.2   Socioeconomic Status and Health

Socioeconomic status refers to the position of an individual or group in a class society. Studies suggest that socioeconomic status is the most decisive factor affecting an individual's health and life expectancy. In addition, a stable and sustained relationship exists between people's socioeconomic status and their health. Sociologists often use social and economic status as a means to predict people's behavior, using education, income, and occupation as the three most common indicators to measure social and economic status. In health research, education reflects a person's ability to proactively access social, psychological, and economic resources; occupation reflects a person's social status, rights and responsibilities, level of physical activity, and health risks; income reflects a person's ability to consume, housing conditions, nutrition, and access to health care resources. Education, income, and occupation are inextricably linked to socioeconomic status, and inequalities in these factors affect health services and health outcomes related to race and gender. For example, people with low incomes and less education (usually women and certain ethnic minorities) have higher mortality rates than those with more education and wealth, and the gap continues to grow. Information from the World Health Organization (WHO) confirmed that health status, health behavior, the accessibility and use of health service, and social economic status change among different racial or ethnic groups, genders, education, and income.

6.1.1.3   Impact of Economic Development on Health

Economic development affects health in three primary ways: providing people with necessary nutrition conditions, ensuring the investment of basic medical care costs, and providing a better environment for people's work and life. Economic development has promoted the improvement of national health in many ways. Socioeconomic development has provided people with sufficient food, good labor and living conditions. The improvement of social economic level and the accumulation of social wealth are conducive to promoting the development of social security, legal systems, science, education, culture and health, and increasing the opportunities for people to improve their quality of life. Economic development is conducive to increasing health investment, promoting the development of health services, and encouraging residents' use of health services.

Despite its positive impacts, economic development has also brought some new health problems, mainly in the following aspects: ① Emergence of modern social diseases—modern social diseases refer to a series of diseases related to social modernization and the development of material civilization, such as venereal diseases, suicide, drug abuse, alcoholism, teenage pregnancy, and mental disorders. The increasing abundance of material possessions, the popularity of electronic equipment, chemicals and other items, has caused "civilization diseases" such as air-conditioning syndrome, computer syndrome and Internet addiction, and the number of people with bodily dysfunctions has increased year by year. ② Increase of negative social events—with the development of economy, traffic accidents soar; the data shows that 1.2 million people die on the road every year all over the world. In 2011, 210,821 road traffic accidents occurred in China, resulting in 62,387 deaths and 237,421 injuries, with direct economic losses exceeding 1 billion renminbi. At the same time, social conflicts such as unbalanced economic development and the widening gap between rich and poor have increased violence and crimes. ③ Increase of psychological stress factors—one of the characteristics of modern society is its fast pace, which carries with it a demand for high efficiency of work. The fast pace of modern life complicates interpersonal relationships and increases stress events, which tends to exacerbate people's psychological tension and cause psychosomatic diseases and mental diseases. ④ Aggravation of environmental pollution—industrial production and residents' daily lives discharge a large number of pollutants that will cause environmental pollution upon entering the water, atmosphere and soil, where they destroy the ecological balance and normal living conditions, and have direct, indirect, or potentially harmful effects on human health. ⑤ Increase of social floating population—economic development will inevitably lead to the increase of population flow. A large number of rural surplus laborers flooding into the city will bring many health problems, such as increased risk of infectious disease transmission, which is not conducive to implementing health care policies.

The essence of social economy development is the improvement of social productivity. People are the most important factor in productivity. The improvement of population health will certainly promote social and economic development, mainly in the following aspects: ① Improvement of population health status promotes economic development. Improved health, longer life expectancy, and longer working life, can create more wealth. At the same time, improving the health level also means improving the intelligence level. In today's highly developed science and economy, increased intelligence level is a prominent factor for improving productivity and developing social economy. ② Reduced resource consumption. Improved population health means fewer illnesses and injuries, which can conserve many social services, especially health resources.

6.1.2　Social Culture and Health

Among the social factors that affect human health, culture plays a significant role. In its sixth report, WHO noted that "Once people's living standards exceed their minimum needs, and the use of means of livelihood is conditionally determined, cultural factors would play an increasingly important role in health."

6.1.2.1　Connotation and Characteristics of Culture

In a broad sense, culture refers to the totality of both social wealth and spiritual wealth. A more narrow definition casts culture as ideology, including ethics, religious belief, philosophy, art, customs, education, science, technology, and knowledge. Generally speaking, culture can be divided into three types: intelligent culture, normative culture, and ideological culture. Intelligent culture mainly affects people's health by influencing their living environment and lifestyle, normative culture affects people's health by dominating their behaviors, and ideological culture affects people's health mainly by influencing people's psychological processes and spiritual life. Different cultural types have overlapping effects on people's health.

Culture displays the following basic characteristics:

(1) Co-existence

Culture is a set of shared concepts, values, and codes of conduct that make an individual's capacity for behavior acceptable to the collective. Culture and society are closely related; culture cannot exist without society, and society cannot exist without culture. Cultural inconsistencies exist within the same society.

(2) Inheritance

A society's core culture comes from historical tradition, which has a clear internal structure and rules. Each historical era contains unique characteristics by which this era may be identified. Culture has both positive and negative influences on later generations.

(3) Complexity

No cultural phenomenon exists in isolation, but rather culture contains various forms and elements. Different cultures can penetrate into each other through human activities and are formed by the combination of various cultural elements.

(4) Differences

Human beings live in a certain cultural pattern, which inevitably reflects the differences among regions, nations, and countries. Human production activities will be engraved with the brand of cultural characteristics, or even directly expressed as the meaning of culture.

6.1.2.2　Education and Health

Education belongs to a normative culture and is a significant means of human socialization. Education level is an important index to reflect the cultural level and quality of a country and a nation. Many studies have shown that education has a greater impact on health than improvements in income, employment, and living conditions. A strong correlation exists between education and health status; the more educated the individual, the less likely he or she is to contract diseases. In addition, education level also has a significant impact on the health of the next generation. The infant mortality rate of illiterate women is 2.5 times that of women with more than 10 years of education. In the United States, research indicates that mothers with more than 16 years of education are about 50% less likely to have children of low birth weight than mothers with less than 9 years of education.

The main ways that education affects health are as follows: ① Education affects people's choice of lifestyle. People with a higher education tend to choose a healthy lifestyle.

② Education affects people's use of health services. People with a high education level better understand the importance of preventive health care and make more reasonable use of health services. ③ Education affects people's health by influencing their employment opportunities, income, and other factors.

6.1.2.3　Custom and Health

Custom is a behavior pattern or norm observed by generations of families and kindred in a specific social and cultural area. A habit is a pattern of action that has been reinforced by repetition or repeated practice and becomes necessary. Custom refers to a stylized way of action in a group of people's lives, which is passed down from generation to generation and is closely connected with their daily activities. Because different ethnic groups have different physical characteristics and living habits, the distribution of diseases among different ethnic groups is partly determined by physical characteristics, but living habits also have a great influence on health. For example, the western way of eating separately is much more hygienic than sharing dishes around a table. Although sharing food can enhance communication and close feelings to a certain extent, it facilitates the spread of disease. For example, many bacteria, viruses, and other pathogenic microorganisms are present in sputum, and sputum can survive for a long time and become a source of infectious diseases.

6.1.2.4　Religion and Health

Religion is the subjective reflection of the natural and social forces that dominate people's daily life. It is the summation of the belief and code of conduct with the worship and will of a god or gods as the core. Buddhism, Islam, and Christianity are the three major world religions in modern society.

Religion and its relationship with mental health is a complex problem. Many studies have found that religion may help to improve mental health. A 2002—2005 survey to study the causal relationship between religious activities and health in China showed that participation in religious activities significantly improved the health and reduced the mortality of the elderly, and helped to form social capital of the old when they participated in religious activities. But there are also contradictory conclusions, such as the 1978 mass suicide of 909 members of the Peoples Temple, led by American Jim Jones. The effect of religious belief on health is two-sided, but the mechanism is still unclear.

6.1.3　Health Service and Health

Health services are comprehensive public welfare actions taken by the state and society in the prevention and treatment of diseases, protection, and improvement of residents' health. Health services are required for promoting the all-round development of human beings and providing a basic condition for economic and social development. Health services are one of the four major factors that affect people's health. They can reduce the occurrence of diseases through preventive health care and health education, rehabilitate patients and restore the labor force through medical treatment, and effectively improve social productivity.

6. 1. 3. 1 Health Resource and Health

Economic globalization is the main development trend of today's society. With increasing urbanization, people's living standards have been greatly improved. Therefore, people's demand for medical and health services is also growing correspondingly. The investment and allocation of health resources have a great influence on population health. Studies demonstrate that increased health resources, including health care providers can, on the whole, significantly improve health outcomes. In China, from 2005 to 2014, the number of health technicians per thousand people increased from 3. 41 to 5. 56, an increase of 62. 83%. The number of hospital beds per thousand people increased from 2. 56 to 4. 83, an increase of 88. 32%. The substantial increase of health resources resulted in a decline of population mortality and further improved national health. Studies also show that increasing financial and human resources have a significant positive impact on public health. However, in China, economic and health development among various regions is unbalanced; in particular, the central and western regions lag behind the southeast regions in terms of health resources and economic strength. Different health resources accumulated throughout a region's past will lead to different levels and understanding of health in residents of underdeveloped versus developed areas. The unequal distribution of health resources cannot guarantee the health of the majority of people, which is not conducive to the improvement of a group's health level.

6. 1. 3. 2 Health Care Systems and Health

The health care system refers to the comprehensive policies and measures adopted by a country or a region to solve the problem of residents' prevention and treatment of diseases, including basic elements such as the collection, distribution, and payment of health expenses, as well as the way health services are supplemented and managed. Forms of health care vary in different countries around the world, but they can be classified as the following five main models.

(1) The Universal Government-funded Health Care Model

Universal government-funded health care (also known as single-payer health care) is available to all citizens regardless of their income or employment status. Some countries may provide health care to non-citizen residents, while some may require them to buy private insurance. Under this system, health service planning, health resource allocation, medical and health equipment and facilities belong to the state. In this model, the coverage of health services is wide, which can guarantee the fairness of people's health to a certain extent. Canada, Australia, Bhutan, Botswana, Brazil, Brunei, Cuba, Denmark, Finland, Greece, Iceland, Italy, Kuwait, New Zealand, North Korea, Norway, Oman, South Africa, Spain, Sweden, and United Kingdom follow this model, though some differences may exist among them.

(2) The Universal Public Insurance Health Care Model

Usually, countries following this health care model provide workers with social insurance. The government withholds part of their wage, which is divided between the employee and the employer. People who don't have a legal contract of employment and/or can't register as unemployed may be eligible to pay a certain amount of money for health insurance. This model may help to solve the problem of medical services being unattainable due to economics, and it also reduces the occurrence of excessive medical treatment, corruption, and other phenomena because the supply and the demand share medical expenses. Therefore, this model can remedy market failure to a certain extent and improve the efficiency of medical services, but it requires the government to be responsible for the price and quality of medical services. China, Japan, France, Colombia Hungary, Poland, Romania, Russia, Slovakia, and South Korea follow this model.

(3) The Universal Public-private Insurance Health Care Model

In this system, some people receive health care via primary private insurance, while others, who are ineligible for private insurance, receive insurance from the government. Chile, Germany, Mexico, and Peru follow this health care model.

(4) The Universal Private Health Insurance Model

In this system people receive health care via private insurance, usually subsidized by the government for low-income citizens. Netherlands and Switzerland follow this model.

(5) The Non-universal Insurance Health Care Model

In this system some citizens have private health care insurance, some are eligible for subsidized public health care, and some are not insured at all. India, Jordan, Paraguay, and United States follow this model.

6.2　Psychological Factors and Health

With the development of social policy, economy, and culture, psychological factors have a greater influence on health. Social psychological factors are very complex; various factors in the social environment will inevitably affect people's psychological activities, resulting in emotional changes and impacts to health. In 2013, relevant statistics from China Mental Health Association showed the incidence of depression in China was about 3%—5%. In 2017, the prevalence of anxiety disorders in China was about 4.98%. Currently, more than 26 million people suffer from depression, but the consultation rate of depression in China is less than 10%. Students, unemployed residents, and laid-off workers are the most commonly afflicted group, with depression being most notable among college students.

6.2.1　Psychological Factors and Health

Psychological factors refer to the psychological process of movement and change, including people's feelings, perceptions, and emotions. Psychological phenomenon is the manifestation of psychological processes and personality. Psychological processes consist of the cognitive process, emotional process, and volitional process. Personality includes tendencies and psychological characteristics. The pathogenesis of psychological factors is believed to be caused by psychosocial factors stimulating the central nervous system, endocrine system, and immune system.

Psychological factors have the following four characteristics:

(1) Duality

Healthy psychological factors and negative psychological factors are mutually exclusive.

(2) Uniqueness

Individual psychological factors are influenced by growth, education level, and life experience.

(3) Easily Affected by External Factors

The more severe, varied, and longer the external stimulation on the psychological factors, the greater the role plays.

(4) Variance

Individual psychological tolerance is constantly changing. The interaction between subjective factors and objective factors is multi-level and dynamic.

6.2.1.1   Personality and Health

Personality refers to the psychological traits an individual consistently expresses. Heredity and environment both determine personality traits, which are closely related to health. Personality has three central components: trait, state, and action. The psychological characteristics of personality include temperament, personality, and ability. Character refers to an individual's enduring attitude toward reality and the habituated behavior corresponding to it. At present, human personality can be roughly divided into three types: A, C, and B. Individuals with a type A personality tend to be competitive, ambitious, hardworking, and irritable, with a sense of urgency and competitive aggression. Experiments have shown that blood stress hormones, such as catecholamine, pituitary vasopressin, and adrenocortical hormone are higher in people with type A personality compared to people with type B personalities. A study also found that individuals with type A personality have a higher incidence, recurrence, and mortality rate of coronary heart disease. Today, the type A personality has been identified as a risk factor for coronary heart disease and is itself a major risk factor, independent of other risk factors. Individuals with type B personality tend to be uncompetitive, calm, stable, meek, easy-going, less ambitious, thoughtful, generous, and indecisive. People with this personality type seldom argue and communicate through low-key speech. Some people with type B personality may resemble type A or type C personalities, and they may change, to a certain extent, through environmental influence or changes in their self-belief. People with type C personality are very cautious, careful, and tolerant. Individuals with type C personality tend to be perfectionists, exhibit emotional instability, and are not adept in dealing with negative emotions. This kind of individual tends to pursue a life in a familiar environment and perpetuate disappointment, sadness, depression, and other emotional experience when unfortunate events occur. Domestic studies have shown that people with type C personalities experience a higher incidence of cervical cancer, and they are at a higher risk of stomach cancer, liver cancer, and other cancers of the digestive system.

6.2.1.2 Emotion and Health

Emotions are related to people's specific desires. They are people's subjective and conscious experiences and feelings related to external stimuli. Emotion and affect are caused by objective stimulation, which is the fountainhead for mood. Emotion is closely related to individual cognition and directly related to human needs. In China, since ancient times, there have been such sayings as "happy and sad", "anger hurts the liver", "thinking hurts the spleen", "sadness about the lungs", and "fear of hurting the kidney", which show that traditional Chinese medicine has attached great importance to the relationship between human emotions and health. When a person's mood changes, there is often a corresponding physiological change. For example, when a person is frightened, the pupils might appear to dilate, the person might be thirsty and perspire, and the face might become white through a series of pathological changes. Under normal circumstances, these physiological changes have a positive role because they can mobilize all parts of the body to adapt to changes in the external environment. But excessive negative emotions, such as long-term unhappiness, fear, disappointment, worry, and sadness, will inhibit gastrointestinal movement, thereby affecting digestive function. People who are emotionally negative, depressed, or overly stressed tend to suffer from a variety of diseases. Only by maintaining an optimistic mood can people truly maintain their health.

The following three points summarize the functions of emotions:

(1) Motivational Function

Emotions are accompanied by motivational actions—positive emotions can promote behaviors and negative emotions can inhibit behaviors.

(2) Organizational Function

Positive emotions promote behavioral activities, while negative emotions discourage or play a destructive role in behavioral activities.

(3) Adaptive Function

Emotions mobilize the body's energy to adapt to changes in the external environment through physiological reactions. At the same time, individuals understand their surroundings through experience, and individuals can exert certain influences on others.

6.2.2 Psychological Stress and Health

6.2.2.1 Definitions of Stress

Stress is a physiological change and emotional fluctuation caused by changes in the external environment and internal state of the body. It is simply defined as the result of failing to adapt to changes.

Stress can be simply divided into eustress (good stress) and distress (bad stress). Eustress can be beneficial, because it can help with motivation, focus, energy, and performance. By contrast, distress can cause anxiety, worry, and a decrease in performance. Distress can negatively impact human health and can lead to serious issues if not addressed. For example, distress can cause physical conditions, such as headaches, digestive issues, and sleep disturbances as well as psychological and emotional strains, such as confusion, anxiety, and depression. According to the American Psychological Association, untreated chronic stress can result in high blood pressure or a weakened immune system. Chronic stress can also contribute to the development of obesity and heart disease.

Stressors refer to factors that direct stress reactions, including biological stressors, mental stressors, and social stressors. The distinction between a stressor and actual stress is as follows: a stressor can be a person, place, or situation that causes stress, whereas stress is the biological response to one or a combination of those stressors. The vast majority of stressors causing psychological problems are integrated. Examples of common stressors include relationship conflicts at home or at work, increasing work responsibilities, financial strain, loss of a loved one, and health problems. Examples of common chronic stressors include fatigue, difficulty sleeping, and poor problem-solving.

6. 2. 2. 2 Basic Theories of Stress

(1) Biological Stress Theory

The physiologist Claude Bernard defined stress as the collective adaptive response to external stimuli. Stress is the body's attempt to return to equilibrium.

Stress refers to a person's reaction in the face of difficulties or adversity. It is a dynamic process, including three basic links: feeling stimulus, stress response, and coping style (behavior).

Stressors can be divided into the following three categorie.

① Life events stressors: Life events refer to the major changes encountered in life, which can disturb people's psychological and physiological homeostasis.

② Environmental stressors: Environmental stressors refer to some major or sudden changes in the natural and social environment that destroy the individual's physiological and psychological homeostasis.

③ Work stressors: Negative stressors from work mainly include unsafe working conditions, high-pressure work environments and expectations, conflict within the occupational role, and interpersonal tension among colleagues.

The body's response to stress and its impact on health are as follows.

① Psychosomatic response. This is the initial test stage of physiological changes caused by stress. It is a series of short physiological reactions that occur when the body is under stress, such as increased heart rate, shortness of breath, increased blood pressure, increased muscle tension, facial flushing or paleness.

② Psychosomatic disorder: When stress occurs for a long time, repeatedly acting on the individual, the psychosomatic reaction continues to exist. The body adapts to the difficulties and will eventually initiate pathological reactions, such as neurosis.

③ Psychosomatic diseases: The above situation will lead to sustained deviation of body function, tissue damage, and structural changes of organic diseases. This kind of affliction, called psychosomatic disease because of the continuous existence of psychosocial stress, plays an important role in the occurrence of the disease.

(2) Social Event Stimulus Theory

Social event stimulus theory targets negative and positive life events. Life events refer to occurrences that cause mental imbalance in people's daily life. Psychological stress caused by life events has superimposed effect within a certain time range (usually one year), and has a certain relationship with physical health. The nature, intensity, and frequency of stressful life events can have varying effects on health, which may be caused by problems in learning, love and marriage, health, family, work and economics, interpersonal relationships, environment, law and politics, etc.

(3) Psychological Cognitive Theory

According to the theory of psychological cognition, stress is not only the external stimulus, nor the body's response to the external stimulus, but the transformation process between the two. Stress source, stress response, and stress management are the basic elements of psychological stress. Stress source refers to internal and external stimuli and situations; stress response refers to the body's response to stimulus, which is manifested in physiological, behavioral, emotional, cognitive, and other symptoms; and stress management refers to controlling and changing stress source and stress response.

Prolonged excessive stress can result in adverse health consequences. People often struggle to control their emotions when they are under high pressure for a long time and exhibit inexplicable irritability, anxiety, anger, fear, and even depression. The persistence of these negative emotions is likely to cause a series of physiological changes and behavioral abnormalities mentioned above. Excessive stress can also affect cognition, such as memory decline, inability to concentrate, impaired thinking, and so on. Too much pressure for too long will easily lead to low self-esteem or the individual thinking he or she is incompetent and helpless. In terms of behavior, people who are chronically stressed tend to be indifferent to others, have conflicts with others, or close themselves off. These manifestations can lead to delayed resolution of stress and create new problems in relationships. Some people resort to unhealthy habits, such as smoking, drinking, and drug use. When people are not in control of their emotions, they are more likely to engage in self-harm, suicide, and other impulsive behaviors.

6.2.3   Psychological Interventions

6.2.3.1   Individual Interventions

(1) Relaxation Training

Relaxation training enables an individual to consciously control or adjust his or her own psychological and physiological activities, so that the body and mind are in a broad state of relaxation and develop a sense of euphoria. Relaxation training can normalize the activities of the terminal organs of the central nervous system, inhibit brain excitement, reduce tension, and calm the psychological response to effectively improve anxiety, depression, and other adverse emotions. Several studies found that emotional therapy based on relaxation training can effectively relieve the anxiety, depression, and other adverse emotions of patients with ischemic stroke and enhance their confidence to participate in exercise. In addition, combinations of relaxation training methods, such as imagination relaxation, muscle relaxation, and breathing relaxation, can assist patients to cope with psychological disorders, improve anxiety, depression and other adverse emotions, help improve patients' compliance with exercise, and promote rehabilitation of limb motor function.

(2) Positive Reinforcement

Operant conditioning theory was first proposed by American psychologist and behaviorist B. F. Skinner. The theory holds that human behavior is regulated and controlled by external conditions, so changing stimuli can change behavior. People or animals act on their environment to achieve a certain goal. When the consequences of the action are favorable, the action is repeated. When unfavorable, the behavior can abate or disappear. This process is called environmental reinforcement of behavior. Although first used to train animals, the method was later developed and applied to human learning, and is now widely used to motivate and reform human behavior.

6.2.3.2   Group Interventions

(1) Health Education

Health education is an organized, planned, and implemented activity designed to help individuals and groups master health care knowledge, establish health concepts, and voluntarily adopt healthy behaviors and lifestyles. Health education includes information dissemination and behavioral intervention. Proper health education theories, targeted content, and appetency of means should all be emphasized when implementing behavioral intervention.

(2) Group Counseling and Psychotherapy

Group counseling provides psychological help and guidance in the context of a group. In other words, the counselor forms a task group based on the similarity of the participants' questions or the participants' initiative to solve the common issues of the members through joint discussion, training, and guidance. Group psychological counseling is a process of helping others through observation, learning, experience, self-understanding, self-exploration, self-acceptance, adjustment and improvement of interpersonal relationships, learning new attitudes and behavior patterns, and developing sound life adjustment through interpersonal interactions within the group.

(3) Social Engineering Intervention

Social engineering intervention refers to applying social measures, such as social facility intervention and social policy intervention, to influence behavior. For instance, a scale might be placed in snack bars, computerized nutrition systems might be added to supermarkets, and mental and behavioral health ads might be broadcast in public places.

6.2.3.3　Place Interventions

(1) Family Interventions

In family interventions, behavior modification takes place within a family unit and home. Applying intervention strategies at this level enables the family to take responsibility for the members' health.

(2) Community Interventions

Community interventions refers to the use of psychological theories and principles to maintain and promote the mental health of people living within a certain community. Community interventions encourage people to pay attention to and improve their mental health as a way of preventing physiological and mental disease.

(3) School Interventions

An increasing number of interventionists are finding value in fostering the sustainable development of adolescent mental health education through the combined actions of the school, family, and community toward promoting psychological education. In this scenario, the family serves as the foundation, with the school operating as the primary influence and the community serving as a strong supplemental influence. By instituting communication platforms, strong cooperation among the school, family, and community can be established to use these resources most effectively.

(4) Workplace Interventions

Workplace intervention includes improving the working site, the health of employees, and the comprehensive quality of enterprise management. Workplace health promotion (WHP) refers to using a multidisciplinary approach that incorporates multiple departments and intervention measures to improve operating conditions; promote healthy lifestyles; control health risk factors; reduce the rates of illness, injury, and absenteeism; promote the health of workers, families, and community residents; and improve the overall quality of life. The main WHP factors include a supportive environment, continuous community engagement, enterprises' sense of social responsibility, and the workers' participation and enthusiasm.

6.3   Behavioral Factors and Health

According to WHO, 40% of human health and longevity depends on heredity and objective conditions, among which 15% are genetic, 10% are social factors, 8% are medical conditions, 7% are climatic conditions, and 60% are lifestyle and behavioral habits established by the individual. Healthy behaviors include a consistent routine of balanced nutrition, regular physical exercise, and healthy mental outlook. About 80% of chronic diseases are caused by poor lifestyle choices and behavior patterns. The report identifies the following top ten risks, globally and regionally, in terms of the burden of disease they cause: underweight; unsafe sex; high blood pressure; tobacco consumption; alcohol consumption; unsafe water, sanitation, and hygiene; iron deficiency; indoor smoke from solid fuels; high cholesterol; and obesity.

In the most industrialized countries of North America, Europe, and the Asian Pacific, at least one-third of all disease burden is caused by tobacco, alcohol, blood pressure, cholesterol, and obesity. Furthermore, more than three-quarters of cardiovascular disease— the world's leading cause of death—results from tobacco use, high blood pressure, or high cholesterol, or a combination of these elements.

6.3.1   Smoking and Health

The custom of smoking dried tobacco leaves spread from America to the rest of the world after European colonization began in the sixteenth century. Given that smoking harms nearly every organ of the body, coupled with its addictive properties and widespread use, it is a dangerous psychoactive drug. Severe withdrawal symptoms and a craving for tobacco make this among the most refractory of addictions.

Nicotine is the psychoactive compound in tobacco. Nicotine is absorbed quickly and reaches the brain within seconds. Tolerance, the need for increasing amounts to achieve the same physiological response, develops to some but not all effects of nicotine. Many tobacco users who abruptly quit experience a withdrawal syndrome of irritability, aggressiveness, hostility, depression, and difficulty concentrating. These symptoms may last several days or even weeks and are accompanied by electroencephalographic changes. Many tobacco users relapse, often within days of attempting to quit.

6.3.1.1   Toll of Smoking

(1) High Mortality Rates

Cigarette smoking has been identified as the leading cause of preventable and premature death. Coronary heart disease (CHD), multiple cancers, and various respiratory diseases account for the majority of deaths related to cigarette smoking. As many as two-thirds of life-long smokers will die of a smoking-related disease. According to China's reported health hazards of smoking (2012), the number of deaths globally attributed to tobacco is as high as

6 million each year, accounting for one-tenth of the total number of annual deaths. The average life span of smokers is 10 years shorter than that of nonsmokers. In China, more than 1 million people die each year from smoking, with more than 100,000 deaths due to exposure to second-hand smoke.

(2) Economic Costs

Health care expenditures due to smoking-attributable diseases totaled a purchasing power parity (PPP) of $467 billion in 2012, or 5.7% of global health expenditures. The total economic cost of smoking (from health expenditures and productivity losses together) totals PPP $1852 billion in 2012, equivalent to 1.8% of the world's annual gross domestic product (GDP). Almost 40% of this cost occurred in developing countries, highlighting the substantial burden these countries suffer. Smoking imposes a heavy economic burden throughout the world, particularly in Europe and North America, where the tobacco epidemic is most advanced.

6.3.1.2 Smoking-Related Disease

(1) Cardiovascular Disease

Despite encouraging advances in prevention and treatment of atherothrombosis, cardiovascular disease (CVD) remains a major cause of death and disability worldwide and will continue to grow mainly due to the increase in incidence in low-and middle-income countries (LMIC). In Europe and the USA, CHD mortality rates have decreased since the mid-1990s due to improvements in acute care; however, the prevalence of CHD is increasing, largely due to the overall aging of the population, increased prevalence of cardiovascular (CV) risk factors, and improved survival of patients after a CV event. In China in 2010, the total deaths due to cardiovascular and circulatory diseases reached 3.1362 million, the mortality rate reached 233.70 deaths per 100,000 people, and the age-standardized mortality rate was 256.90 deaths per 100,000 people. Atherosclerosis is characterized by the deposition of lipids in the inner layers of the arteries, by fibrosis, and by thickening of the arterial wall. Atherosclerotic plaques develop over time, slowly progressing from early lipid deposition (fatty streaks) to more advanced raised fibrous lesions that decrease the arterial lumen, ultimately resulting in clinical events. The process of plaque destabilization is thought to be associated with inflammatory changes and thrombotic events that obstruct the blood flow and result in clinical manifestations of disease, such as myocardial infarction (MI) or stroke. The highly regulated physiologic interface between the blood and the arterial wall components is strongly and adversely affected by the toxic products from cigarette smoke that are added to the blood-stream. The smoking-related development of CHD includes at least five interrelated processes: atherosclerosis, thrombosis, coronary artery spasm, cardiac arrhythmia, and reduced oxygen-carrying capacity of the blood.

① Ischemic heart disease and cerebrovascular disease: From 2011 to 2015, mortality due to chronic ischemia cardio-cerebrovascular disease in Xuzhou residents was 261.2 deaths per 100,000 residents, 269.9 deaths per 100,000 for male residents, 252.0 deaths per 100,000 for female residents; the mortality rate in men was significantly higher than that in women. For urban residents, the mortality rate due to chronic ischemic cardio-cerebrovascular disease was 243.8 deaths per 100,000, which was lower than the rate of rural residents.

Both ischemic and hemorrhagic cerebrovascular diseases are major causes of death in the United States. Although stroke deaths have declined substantially during the past two decades, ischemic and hemorrhagic strokes accounted for approximately 158,000 deaths (6%) in the United States in 2003. Each year more than 500,000 new and 200,000 recurrent strokes occur. The risk of stroke increases with age. Smoking has been well demonstrated as a major cause of stroke. The 2004 Surgeon General's report noted that only hypertension is as consistently related to stroke risk as smoking. Smoking increases both the incidence and mortality from stroke.

② Peripheral vascular disease: The strongest risk factor predisposing persons to atherosclerotic peripheral arterial occlusive disease is cigarette smoking, which has been shown to be directly related to lower extremity atherosclerotic disease of both large and small arteries. Smoking prevalence is high among victims of aortoiliac (98%) and femoropopliteal (91%) disease. Intermittent claudication is more frequent among smokers than nonsmokers.

A recent cohort study found that, when compared to people who have never smoked, people who currently smoke experienced a 50% increase in the progression of atherosclerosis over 3 years, and people who currently are nonsmokers but who used to smoke experienced a 25% increase. Complications of peripheral vascular disease are consistently reduced, and performance and overall survival is improved among patients who quit smoking. Five cohort studies that analyzed the risk of death due to aortic aneurysm for current, former, and never smokers found that among men, risk among former smokers is two-to-three times higher than never smokers and about 50% lower among former smokers than current smokers. Patterns are similar for women. Multiple cross-sectional and cohort studies have shown that smokers have a higher abdominal aortic aneurysm mortality rate than nonsmokers.

The strong association between smoking and peripheral vascular disease is likely mediated by the mechanisms that promote atherosclerosis, as described earlier. The peripheral vasoconstrictive effects of smoking probably also play an important role. The association of smoking with ischemic stroke is likely mediated by the mechanisms that promote atherosclerosis and thrombus formation. Cigarette smoking appears to increase the risk of stroke by decreasing cerebral blood flow.

③ Coronary heart disease: Smokers have a higher death rate due to CHD at all ages. However, since the incidence of CHD increases sharply with age for both smokers and nonsmokers, the relative risk for smoking-related CHD peaks for men at age 40—44 years and for women at age 45—49 years. The percentage of CHD deaths attributable to smoking is 84% for men aged 40—44 years and 26% for men aged 75—79 years. The smoking attributable percentage of CHD deaths is 85% for women aged 45—49 years and 23% for women aged 80 years and older.

Results from cohort studies clearly demonstrate that the risk of death from CHD is increased by smoking early in life, the number of cigarettes smoked per day, and the depth of smoke inhalation. For example, data from the Nurses' Health Study show that, although the risk of CHD is increased for all smokers regardless of the age at which they begin smoking, the risk is higher for women who started smoking before age 15. The positive effect of smoking cessation on both primary and secondary prevention of CHD has been extensively studied and validated. The 1990 Surgeon General's report evaluated this research and concluded that, compared with continued smoking, cessation substantially reduces the risk of CHD among men and women of all ages.

④ Endothelial injury or dysfunction: Data from animal studies suggest that nicotine causes endothelial damage, and data from humans indicate that smoking increases the number of damaged endothelial cells and the endothelial cell count in circulating blood. Young and middle-aged smokers without disease had a significant reduction in endothelium-dependent vasodilatation compared with nonsmokers. Smoking also appears to stimulate smooth muscle cell proliferation and to increase the adherence of platelets to arterial endothelium. Animal studies have demonstrated that exposure of rat endothelium to blood from a person who had recently smoked two cigarettes resulted in the deposition of a large number of platelets on the endothelial surface. Cigarette smoke exposure in dogs resulted in increased endothelial permeability to fibrinogen.

⑤ Thrombosis/Fibrinolysis: Smoking may also increase thrombus formation. Fibrinogen levels are elevated in smokers, as is platelet-fibrinogen binding and other clotting abnormalities that tend to promote thrombus formation. Compared to plaques from nonsmokers, plaques from smokers more frequently have thrombosis along the artery walls. Smoking also increases the expression of tissue factor, a glycoprotein that initiates the extrinsic clotting cascade. The prothrombotic effect of smoking is thought to be the main underlying factor that links smoking to sudden cardiac death.

⑥ Inflammation: Current ideas about the pathogenesis of atherosclerosis increasingly emphasize inflammation as having a central role. Smoking induces a systemic inflammatory response, as demonstrated by increases in inflammatory markers, such as blood leukocyte count. Smoking is also associated with elevated levels of C-reactive protein, which is another measure of inflammatory activity. High C-reactive protein levels are associated with risk of CHD, stroke, and peripheral artery disease.

⑦ Increased oxygen demand: Cigarette smoking increases myocardial oxygen demand by increasing peripheral resistance, blood pressure, and heart rate—effects which are probably attributable to nicotine. In addition, the capacity of the blood to deliver oxygen is reduced by increased carboxyhemoglobin, greater viscosity, and higher coronary vascular resistance due to vasoconstrictor effects on the coronary arteries. Reduced oxygen-carrying capacity may contribute to infarction in the presence of significant atherosclerotic narrowing of the vessels. Coronary artery spasm can cause acute myocardial ischemia and may promote thrombus formation. Arrhythmias can precipitate heart attacks and can increase the case fatality rate of myocardial ischemia; smoking has been shown to lower the threshold for ventricular fibrillation.

(2) Chronic Obstructive Pulmonary Disease

In the 40-year follow-up of the British Physicians' Study, the risk of chronic obstructive pulmonary disease (COPD) among smokers was found to be almost as high as the risk of lung cancer. Dose-response relationships have been consistently observed, with the risk of death from COPD influenced by the number of cigarettes smoked per day, the depth of smoke inhalation, and the age of smoking initiation. The 2004 Surgeon General's report concluded that smoking causes COPD. The report also concluded that the evidence was suggestive but not sufficient to infer a causal relationship between smoking and acute respiratory infections among persons with preexisting COPD.

Studies have identified the likely mechanisms by which cigarette smoking induces COPD. The current model suggests that after a long latency period, COPD develops because of a more rapid decline in lung function during adulthood or because of a reduction in maximal lung growth in childhood and adolescence. Atopy and increased airway responsiveness are associated with a more rapid decrease in pulmonary function, and cigarette smoking is a cause of exaggerated airway responsiveness. Smoking also causes injurious biologic processes (oxidant stress, inflammation, and a protease/anti-protease imbalance) that result in airway and alveolar injury. If sustained, such injury results in COPD.

After smoking cessation, prior smoking patterns (duration and daily consumption) and the number of years since cessation are used to determine the rate at which the risk of COPD is reduced. Smoking cessation reduces respiratory symptoms and respiratory infections. Smokers who quit have better pulmonary function than those who continue to smoke. For persons without overt COPD, pulmonary function improves about 5% within a few months of quitting. Cigarette smoking accelerates age-related decline in lung function; with cessation, the rate of decline is comparable to those who never smoked. With sustained abstinence, the risk of developing COPD and the COPD mortality rate are lower than in continuing smokers, but these risks do not return to the level found in nonsmokers, probably because smoking has resulted in irreversible injury to the airways and parenchyma.

The 2004 Surgeon General's report concluded that a causal relationship exists between active smoking and chronic respiratory symptoms (chronic cough, phlegm, wheezing, and dyspnea) among adults. These symptoms have a dose-response relationship with the number of cigarettes smoked per day, and they decrease with cessation. Smoking contributes to these symptoms by decreasing tracheal mucous velocity, increasing mucous secretion, causing chronic airway inflammation, increasing epithelial permeability, and damaging parenchymal cells. The Surgeon General also concluded that there was inadequate evidence to determine a causal relationship between active smoking and asthma in adults, that the evidence was suggestive but not sufficient to infer a causal relationship between active smoking and increased nonspecific bronchial hyperresponsiveness, and that active smoking was a cause of poor asthma control.

(3) Mouth Diseases

Epidemiological studies from several countries have shown that cigarette smokers have more periodontal disease than do nonsmokers, and the 2004 Surgeon General's report concluded that smoking causes periodontitis. A strong association has been noted between both the duration of smoking and the number of cigarettes smoked per day and the level of periodontal disease. The likely mechanism for smoking-related periodontal disease is reduction in immune response, possibly making the smoker more susceptible to bacterial infection. Smoking also impairs the regeneration and repair of periodontal tissue. Leukoplakia or gum recession occurs in 44%—79% of smokeless tobacco users and can occur even among young people. Gum recession commonly occurs in the area of the mouth adjacent to where the smokeless tobacco is held. Among adult users of smokeless tobacco or snuff, the risk of oral disease has been well documented, and changes in the hard and soft tissues of the mouth, discoloration of teeth, decreased ability to taste and smell, and oral pain have been reported.

(4) Gastrointestinal Disease

Smokers of both sexes have a high prevalence of peptic ulcer disease, with a clear dose-response relationship. Up to 100 percent of duodenal ulcers and 70%—90% of gastric ulcers are associated with *H. pylori* infection. Duodenal ulcers heal more slowly among smokers than nonsmokers, even with therapy. Both gastric and duodenal ulcers are also more likely to recur among smokers. Likely mechanisms by which smoking promotes peptic ulcer disease include the potential for tobacco smoke or nicotine to increase maximal gastric acid output and duodenogastric reflux, and to decrease alkaline pancreatic secretion and prostaglandin synthesis. Bicarbonate secretion from the pancreas is reduced immediately after smoking, leading to a decrease in duodenal bulb pH. The pH level appears to be the most important determinant for the development of gastric metaplasia in the duodenum, which allows colonization by *H. pylori*. Smoking cessation is associated with fewer duodenal ulcers, improved short-term healing of gastric ulcers, and reduced recurrence of gastric ulcers.

(5) Other Diseases

The 2004 Surgeon General's report noted several other causal relationships between smoking and disease. The report concluded that smoking diminishes health, which could manifest as increased absenteeism from work and increased use of medical care, adverse surgical outcomes related to wound healing and respiratory complications, low bone density in postmenopausal women (in men, the evidence was suggestive but not sufficient to infer causality), and hip fracture. The report also concluded that smoking causes nuclear cataracts.

6.3.1.3　Cancer

(1) Lung Cancer

Among malignant lung tumors, 90% belong to four major cell types, which are commonly designated as bronchogenic carcinoma: squamous cell, small cell, large cell, and adenocarcinoma. Smoking induces all four major histologic types of lung cancer. Initially, squamous cell carcinoma was seen most often in smokers, followed by small cell carcinoma. However, since the late 1970s, adenocarcinoma has been increasing, and is now the most common histologic type. It has been suggested that the increasing incidence of adenocarcinoma may be related to the switch to low-tar, filtered cigarettes, which may allow increased puff volume with increased deposition of smoke in the peripheral airways. Low-tar cigarettes also contain increased levels of tobacco-specific nitrosamine, a carcinogen shown to induce adenocarcinoma. Lung cancer has a propensity to metastasize early and widely. Five-year survival in lung cancer patients is 15%. The survival rate is 49% for localized disease, but only 16% of lung cancer is diagnosed at this early stage.

Smokers who report slight or no inhalation have a relative risk of cancer up to eightfold higher than nonsmokers. The 2004 Surgeon General's report and 2004 International Agency for Research on Cancer (IARC) report confirmed and expanded the evidence base supporting the conclusion that smoking causes lung cancer. The number of years smoking and lung cancer mortality are also directly related. Lung cancer incidence appears to increase with the square of the amount smoked daily, but with the duration of smoking raised to a power of four or five. Smoking mechanics, such as the degree of inhalation, also affect lung cancer mortality. Both case-control and cohort studies have demonstrated some reduction in lung cancer risk in smokers who switched from non-filtered to filtered cigarettes. For those who have always smoked filtered cigarettes, the risk of lung cancer is still very high, but may be 10%—30% percent lower compared to lifelong smokers of non-filtered cigarettes.

For persons who stop smoking cigarettes, the decrease in lung cancer mortality is relative to smoking history (e.g. dose, duration, type of cigarette, and depth of inhalation) as well as the number of years since cessation. Risk reduction is gradual; after 10 years the risk is about 30%—50% of that for continuing smokers. However, even with the longest duration of quitting, the risk remains greater than for lifetime nonsmokers. It is hypothesized that the absolute risk of lung cancer does not decline after cessation, but the additional risk that comes with continued smoking is avoided.

Components of tobacco smoke are potent mutagens and carcinogens. Tobacco smoke contains more than 60 known carcinogens that have both cancer-initiating and cancer-promoting activity. The 2004 Surgeon General's report concluded that smoking causes genetic changes in lung cells that lead to the development of lung cancer. Although research during the past 25 years has led to a greatly expanded knowledge of the major factors contributing to the toxicity and carcinogenicity of cigarette smoke, the mechanisms responsible for initiating lung tumors from tobacco smoke constituents are complex and not yet completely understood. The bronchial epithelia of smokers show progressive abnormal changes; the frequency and intensity of these changes increase with the amount smoked. The number of cells with atypical nuclei decreases with an increased number of years since smoking cessation. An association between smoking and the presence of DNA adducts has also been reported.

(2) Oral, Laryngeal, and Esophageal Cancer

Smokeless tobacco causes oral cancer. Long-term use of snuff is associated with cancers of the cheek and gum. The death rates from oral and pharyngeal cancer vary more than 100-fold across countries, with the highest rates among men in Sri Lanka and the western Pacific region, where tobacco is chewed in combination with betel. All forms of tobacco use, such as cigarettes, pipes, cigars, chewing tobacco, snuff, reverse smoking (in which the lit end is placed inside the mouth), and "pan" (tobacco, areca nuts, slaked lime and betel leaf) chewing increase the development of premalignant lesions and cancer of the oral cavity and pharynx. Cigar smoking causes oral, laryngeal, and esophageal cancer.

A large number of cohort and case-control studies from many countries support the conclusion drawn by the U. S. Surgeon General and IARC that smoking is a cause of oral and laryngeal cancer, adenocarcinoma, and squamous cell carcinoma of the esophagus. Pipe smoking causes lip cancer and is also associated with oral, laryngeal, and esophageal cancers.

(3) Pancreatic Cancer

The 1-year survival rate for pancreatic cancer is 24%, and the 5-year survival rate is 4%. Even for those diagnosed with local disease, the 5-year survival rate is 17%. The 2004 Surgeon General's report concluded that smoking causes pancreatic cancer.

(4) Cervical Cancer

Epidemiological studies have consistently shown an increased risk of cervical cancer in cigarette smokers. There is a dose-response relationship with duration of smoking and number of cigarettes smoked per day. It is postulated that smoking may increase the rate at which cancer develops in women with persistent infection or possibly increase the risk of persistent infection. Both the Surgeon General and IARC have concluded that smoking causes cervical cancer. In most studies, former smokers at one year after cessation are at lower risk for cervical cancer than are continuing smokers. Human papillomavirus (HPV) is causally related to cervical cancer and appears to be necessary to its development. Components of tobacco smoke (including NNK and nicotine) have been found in the cervical mucus, and the mucus is mutagenic in smokers. In addition, tobacco-related DNA adducts were higher in cervical biopsies of smokers compared with nonsmokers.

6. 3. 1. 4   Health Risks of Secondhand Smoke

The International Agency for Research on Cancer identified secondhand smoke (SHS) as a human carcinogen. The number of deaths due to exposure to SHS is estimated to be approximately 600, 000 each year worldwide. SHS exposure can cause cardiovascular disease, lung cancer, numerous health problems in infants and children, and adverse reproductive outcomes. Globally, about 35% of female nonsmokers are involuntary smokers and are exposed to secondhand tobacco smoke. Smoking is prevalent among men in China. One result is that a large number of nonsmoking Chinese women may be exposed daily to SHS.

(1) Constituents of Secondhand Smoke

SHS is a serious health hazard. SHS is a diluted mixture of "mainstream" smoke exhaled by smokers and "sidestream" smoke from the burning end of a cigarette or other tobacco product. It is chemically similar to the smoke inhaled by smokers and contains a complex mix of more than 4,000 chemicals, including more than 50 cancer-causing chemicals and other toxic substances, such as benzene, cadmium, arsenic, nicotine, carbon monoxide, and nitrogen. Sidestream smoke is the major component of SHS, providing nearly all of the vapor-phase constituents and more than half the particulate matter. Sidestream and mainstream smoke differ in the tobacco combustion temperature, pH, and the degree of dilution in air. Five known human carcinogens, nine probable human carcinogens, three animal carcinogens, and several toxic compounds such as ammonia and carbon monoxide are emitted at higher levels in sidestream smoke than in mainstream smoke. Vapor-phase nicotine and respirable suspended particulate matter have been identified as markers for the presence and concentration of SHS in the environment; cotinine (a metabolite of nicotine) and, to a lesser degree, nicotine are widely used biomarkers of SHS exposure and uptake in people.

(2) Secondhand Smoke and Sudden Infant Death Syndrome

The China Report on the Health Hazards of Smoking concluded that SHS causes a particularly serious risk to the health of pregnant women and children. Ample evidence suggests that SHS can lead to sudden infant death syndrome and lower fetal birth weight. In addition, there is evidence that exposure to SHS in pregnant women can also lead to preterm birth, neonatal neural tube deformities, and cleft lip and palate.

(3) Secondhand Smoke and Children's Health

According to the China Report on the Health Hazards of Smoking, ample evidence suggests that SHS causes respiratory infections, bronchial asthma, decreased lung function, acute otitis media, recurrent otitis media and chronic middle ear effusion, and other diseases in children. In addition, there is evidence that SHS can also lead to a variety of childhood cancers, aggravate the condition of children with asthma, and reduce the effectiveness of asthma treatment. Mothers who quit smoking may reduce the risk of respiratory diseases in their children.

(4) Secondhand Smoke and Adults

China is the world's largest producer, consumer, and victim of tobacco, accounting for about 40% of global cigarette production and sales. The smoking rate of the population is high (especially the adult smoking rate), and SHS exposure is very common. According to the China Report on the Health Hazards of Smoking, 40% of adolescents worldwide, 33% of adult males, and 35% of adult female nonsmokers are exposed to SHS. About 740 million nonsmokers in China are exposed to SHS, making SHS an important risk factor affecting the health of our residents, especially women and children. Public places, workplaces, and families are the main places of exposure of SHS in China. Among adults, exposure to SHS primarily occurs in the workplace and in the home. Among healthy adults, the most common complaints after exposure to SHS are irritation in the eye conjunctiva and mucous membranes of the nose, throat, and lower respiratory tract.

(5) Secondhand Smoke and Diseases

① Cardiovascular disease: SHS increases the risk of coronary heart disease by around 30%, which is larger than might be expected based on the risks associated with active smoking and the relative doses of tobacco smoke delivered to smokers and nonsmokers. Protection of nonsmokers through smoke-free environments leads to a decrease in heart disease mortality through a combination of reduced exposure to SHS and an environment that encourages smoking cessation.

More than 20 studies have examined the association between heart disease and exposure to SHS in nonsmokers. In 2006, the Surgeon General concluded that SHS causes morbidity and mortality from coronary heart disease among both men and women, with an estimated 10%—30% increase in risk. Various experimental and clinical studies suggest mechanisms for the cardiovascular effects of SHS. In 2006, the Surgeon General concluded that SHS has a prothrombotic effect, causes endothelial cell dysfunctions, and causes atherosclerosis in animal models. It was also noted that these acute cardiovascular effects occur with short duration of exposure. Others have noted that SHS appears to cause decreased oxygen supply and increased oxygen demand—all effects consistent with the mechanisms found for active smoking.

② Respiratory disease: The effect of SHS on chronic respiratory symptoms or disease in adult nonsmokers is difficult to measure. Exposure to SHS has been estimated to increase the symptoms and severity of existing bronchitis, sinusitis, and emphysema by 44% and respiratory work-related disability by 80 percent (from exposure to SHS at work).

(6) Secondhand Smoke and Cancer

① Lung cancer: The 2006 Surgeon General's report concluded that smoking causes lung cancer among lifetime nonsmokers and that the risk of lung cancer increases 20%—30% from SHS exposure associated with living with a smoker. The report also concluded that the mechanisms by which SHS causes lung cancer are probably similar to those observed in smokers. For example, exposure to SHS causes a significant increase in urinary metabolites of the tobacco-specific lung carcinogen NNK.

The report also specifically looked at workplace exposure and noted that indoor air nicotine and/or respirable suspended particulate concentrations levels were comparable between work and residential environments, and that SHS exposures in homes and workplaces were qualitatively similar in chemical composition and concentration. Studies showed a trend of increased risk with increased duration of exposure, and a threefold increased risk among persons with the highest level of workplace exposure (based on both years and intensity of exposure). As a result, the Surgeon General concluded that the risk of lung cancer applies to all SHS exposure, regardless of location.

② Sinus Cancer: IARC noted that four cohort studies and one case-control study that looked at the relationship between exposure to SHS and upper respiratory track cancers. A positive association was found in most of the studies. According to the China Report on the Health Hazards of Smoking, evidence exists that SHS can cause sinus cancer.

6.3.1.5   Tobacco Interventions

(1) Preventing Tobacco Use

Evidence shows that knowledge of adverse and long-term health effects does not translate into reduced smoking among youth. Therefore, efforts are focused on developing valid theoretical models of smoking initiation and prevention programs. Smoking initiation among children and adolescents occurs in five stages: ① A preparatory stage in which attitudes and beliefs about the utility of smoking develop. Even before it is initiated, smoking may be viewed as having positive benefits. ② Trying stage, which includes the first two or three times an adolescent tries smoking (usually in a situation involving peers). ③ An experimentation stage with repeated but irregular smoking, in which smoking is usually a response to a particular situation. ④ Regular use: at least weekly smoking across a variety of situations. ⑤ Nicotine dependence, the physiological need for nicotine. Community-based interventions (tobacco price increases, countermarketing campaigns, minors' access restrictions, and school programs) have been the primary modalities used to prevent initiation.

Increasing price: In 1993, a consensus panel from the National Cancer Institute (NCI) concluded that an increase in cigarette excise taxes may be the single most effective intervention for reducing tobacco use by youth. A robust body of evidence supports the effectiveness of price increases on youth initiation. One study concluded that youth consumption may be three times more sensitive to price increases than adult consumption. Another analysis of cigarette excise taxes concluded that increasing the federal cigarette excise tax would encourage an additional 3.5 million Americans to forgo smoking, including more than 800,000 teenagers and almost 2 million young adults aged 20—35. Other studies have reported that for every 10% increase in price, total cigarette consumption among youth decreases 7%.

Countermarketing campaigns: Media campaigns, when combined with other interventions, are an effective strategy to reduce youth initiation. The 2,000 Surgeon General's report noted that multicomponent youth-directed programs with a strong media presence have shown long-term success in reducing or postponing youth tobacco use.

(2) Increasing Cessation

Ex-smokers report the following reasons as contributing to their cessation attempts and continued abstinence: health problems; strong family pressures, both from spouses and children; peer pressure from friends and coworkers; cost of cigarettes, especially for lower-income individuals; fear of potential adverse effects on personal health or on the health of their children; the likelihood of their children starting to smoke; and concern for cleanliness and social acceptance.

① Increasing the price of tobacco products: Price increases are one of the most effective interventions to increase adult cessation, as shown by a substantial body of evidence. For every 10% increase in price, cessation increased 1.5%.

② Countermarketing: Evidence for the effectiveness of counter-advertising comes from both national and international data. An econometric analysis of the U. S. Fairness Doctrine (which required one antismoking message for every three to five tobacco advertising messages) concluded that counter-advertising substantially deterred smoking. An evaluation of a Greek media campaign showed that the annual increase in tobacco consumption was reduced to nearly zero as a result of the campaign. When the campaign stopped, consumption again rose to the precampaign rate. In all studies, the campaign was concurrent or coordinated with other interventions such as tax increases, community education programs, self-help cessation materials, individual counseling, or other mass media efforts. Various endpoints were measured in the various studies. The campaigns increased cessation by a median of 2.2% points, reduced tobacco consumption by a median 17.5%, and reduced prevalence by a median of 3.4% points.

③ Advertising bans: Evidence for the effectiveness of advertising bans is mixed. One study used multiple regression analyses to evaluate the effectiveness of advertising restrictions, price, and income on tobacco consumption in 22 countries from 1960 to 1986. Above threshold levels, both advertising restrictions and higher prices were effective in decreasing tobacco consumption. Similarly, other studies have suggested that partial bans are not effective, but that complete bans can decrease consumption.

④ Quitlines: Quitlines (telephone-based support programs for people who want to quit smoking) can increase cessation rates. The Guide to Community Preventive Services found 32 high-quality studies of the effectiveness of quitlines. In all studies, telephone support was coordinated with other interventions, such as patient education, provider-delivered counseling, nicotine replacement therapies (NRT), a cessation clinic, or a televised cessation series. Cessation rates were increased by a median of 2.6% points. Six studies that examined the effect of quitlines plus patient education materials, compared with patient education materials alone, had a similar magnitude of effect.

6.3.1.6　Challenges in Tobacco Use Prevention and Control

Tobacco companies invest huge sums to advertise and promote cigarettes. Although the effect of this activity on overall cigarette consumption is difficult to assess, advertising and promotion likely make smoking more attractive to youth, make continuing smokers less motivated to attempt cessation, and perhaps increase recidivism by providing omnipresent cues that smoking is fun and relaxing and contributes to conviviality.

Public health agencies and preventive medicine practitioners can help accelerate social pressure to not smoke by supporting strict clean indoor air legislation and its enforcement.

Economic incentives are one of the most effective strategies to reduce cigarette consumption, prevent initiation, and increase cessation. Health and public health professionals can support initiatives to raise tobacco taxes. Health care professionals should routinely assess tobacco use and advise users to quit. New and innovative strategies are also needed, especially those that address tobacco use among youth.

6.3.2　Drinking and Health

6.3.2.1　Introduction

Alcohol is the most commonly abused drug in the world, and the consequences of alcohol use are pervasive in society. From a public health perspective, alcohol use presents a unique dilemma, referred to as the "prevention paradox". This paradox stems from the observation that health and economic consequences resulting from alcohol use are far greater due to hazardous drinking than drinking patterns that constitute a formal diagnosis of alcohol dependence. This paradox is further complicated by findings that suggest low to moderate levels of alcohol use may play a role in reducing mortality for certain disorders, such as cardiovascular disease. To better understand this paradox and the risk of alcohol use, it is helpful to stratify alcohol use and risk along a continuum stretching from abstinence to dependence.

6.3.2.2　Categories of Alcohol Use Along the Drinking Continuum

(1) Safe (Low-Risk) Drinking

Based on the concept of a continuum of risk, some organizations have proposed guidelines for "safe (low-risk)" drinking, some of which include both the characteristics and circumstances of the drinker as well as levels of consumption. Chinese guidelines for safe drinking generally recommend no more than 25 grams of absolute alcohol per day for men, and 15 grams of absolute alcohol per day for non-pregnant females. Meanwhile, the report of the Australian National Health and Medical Research Council (NHMRC) recommends that men should not exceed 4 units or 40 g of absolute alcohol per day on a regular basis; and that women should not exceed 2 units or 20 g of absolute alcohol per day on a regular basis.

In essence, no level of alcohol consumption will always be safe for all individuals under all conditions. Rather, increasing levels of consumption hold a progressively increasing risk of causing either acute or chronic damage. Moreover, the level at which risk occurs and its significance are influenced by a combination of personal and environmental factors that render the individual more or less vulnerable to damage from alcohol.

(2) Hazardous Drinking

The term "hazardous drinking" has been used to describe levels of alcohol consumption that expose the drinker to a high risk of physical complications. Under certain circumstances, relatively low levels of consumption on isolated occasions may result in damage to the individual drinker. Evidence suggests that levels of consumption far below those found in people diagnosed as alcohol dependent are linked with increased risks of adverse health consequences. A special case involves the survival and normal development of the fetus of a pregnant woman who drinks. In this instance, some authorities would assert that no level of consumption is safe, or that such a level may be impossible to define. As information grows on the health hazards of alcohol it becomes increasingly difficult to define what is safe. Rather, alcohol use involves a continuum of risk, defined by host and environmental factors as well as by the levels of alcohol consumption.

6.3.2.3 Alcohol Abuse and Alcohol Dependency

(1) Definitions

The definitions of alcohol abuse and dependency have evolved over time and differ somewhat among various organizations [e. g. WHO, American Psychiatric Association (APA), Chinese Association of Drug Abuse Prevention and Treatment (CADAPT), Asia-Pacific Society for Alcohol and Addiction Research (APSAAR)]. WHO has recently published its 10th edition of the International Classification of Diseases (ICD-10), while the APA recently published its fourth edition, text revision, of the Diagnostic and Statistical Manual of Mental Disorders (DSM-IV-TR). The definitions differ primarily in the number and definition of symptoms required before a diagnosis of alcohol abuse or dependency are met.

(2) Epidemiology

① Epidemiology of alcohol consumption in China: More than half of the adult Chinese population regularly consume alcohol. In the 2017 white paper Moderate Drinking Condition of Chinese Drinkers, the prevalence of current alcohol consumption was much higher for men (84.1%) than for women (29.3%), with 65% of consumers displaying unhealthy drinking patterns. The prevailing problem is overdrinking. In 2016, the consumption of alcoholic products in China was 45.5 liters per capita, equivalent to 5.7 liters of absolute alcohol, which was a 2.0% increase over previous year (2015). In a study by Xu using data from the 2010—2012 National Survey on Nutrition and Health Status of Chinese Residents, 34.3% of those surveyed consume alcohol, the drinking rate in males (54.6%) was significantly higher than that in females (13.3%; 38.5 g); in the 45—59 year age bracket, the drinking rate and alcohol intake were the highest among all groups (38.6%); more beer

(64. 6%) is consumed than hard liquor (38. 7%) and low spirits (29. 7%); the average daily alcohol intake was higher in males than (32. 8 g) in females (8. 0 g); the rates of hazardous drinking were 30. 4%, 34. 8% and 11. 7% for all, men and women, respectively.

② Epidemiology of alcohol abuse and dependency worldwide: Large population-based studies have demonstrated that the lifetime prevalence of alcohol use disorders (abuse and dependence) is even more common. Study demonstrated that, among community-dwelling, non-treatment seeking individuals, the lifetime prevalence of alcohol dependency was 13. 7% in United States. Surveys done in health care settings present a startling example of alcohol-related costs. In a primary care outpatient setting, problem drinking rates of 8%—20% are seen, and between 20%—40% percent of patients admitted to general medical hospitals have a history of alcohol use disorders. Medical morbidity of this extent obviously translates into significant mortality. According to WHO, over 3. 3 million people in 2012 died because of drinking. These summary statistics can be further broken down into risk indicators, which are more useful for preventive health purposes, such as targeting screening and prevention efforts. Alcohol use disorders are more common in males than females, with the ratio of affected males to females being approximately 2 : 1—3 : 1. While rates of females affected with alcohol use disorders are lower, health-related consequences of alcohol use in females who do not meet diagnostic criteria for alcoholism are more severe than in males.

• Age: Age can be used to characterize risk. Alcohol use disorders typically are most common in individuals under 59 years of age. According to the China Alcoholic Drinks Association (CADA), the age group between 18—35 drinks more alcohol than people in any other age brackets. Health-related morbidity varies across the age span, with more unnatural deaths (e. g. accidents, suicides, homicides) observed in younger age groups and more chronic disorders seen in the older age groups. Screening tools and definitions of alcohol use disorders in the elderly are less satisfactory than in middle age, and thus rates of alcohol use disorders in the elderly may be underestimated.

• Socioeconomic groups: Alcohol use disorders are present across all socioeconomic groups. Alcohol use disorders cluster weakly in lower socioeconomic groups, but this may simply be secondary to alcohol's contribution to poor school and job performance. Persons of Asian descent have lower rates of alcohol related disorders, presumably related to decreased levels of alcohol-metabolizing enzymes, which lead to effects such as flush reactions, tachycardia, and headache that serve to encourage limited alcohol consumption. The differences between blacks and non-blacks are significant, and generally show lower rates of alcohol use disorders among non-black populations, in both males and females.

• Comorbidity: Comorbidity of alcohol use disorders and other psychiatric disorders is very common. Study found that about half of individuals with alcohol use disorders had a concomitant psychiatric disorder. The most commonly observed psychiatric comorbidities include antisocial personality disorder, mood disorders, and anxiety disorders.

6. 3. 2. 4　Alcohol-Related Dysfunction and Damage

(1) Morbidity and Mortality

① Overall situation: WHO and several institutions reviewed the major health problems related to alcohol, including alcohol withdrawal syndrome, psychosis, hepatitis, cirrhosis, pancreatitis, thiamine deficiency, neuropathy, dementia, and cardiomyopathy. Alcohol use also plays a key role in injury and accidents, suicide, and homicide. An important concern is also the range of adverse pregnancy outcomes and fetal abnormalities caused by alcohol's embryotoxic and teratogenic effects. In men, the most common medical problems, in terms of decrease one's overall lifetime among the alcohol dependent and heavy drinkers, are trauma, acute alcoholic liver disease, peptic ulceration, chronic obstructive lung disease, pneumonia, hypertension, gastritis, epileptiform disorders, acute brain syndromes, peripheral neuritis, ischemic heart disease, and cirrhosis.

This pattern of lifetime morbidity contrasts greatly with the ranking in terms of excess mortality, namely, cardiovascular disease, suicide, accidents, cirrhosis, malignant neoplasms, pneumonia, and cerebrovascular disease. The differences in these patterns of morbidity and mortality are related to the lethality of the conditions, the risk of this population dying from these disorders compared with the community-at-large, and the frequency of the conditions in the general adult population.

② Sexual difference: Alcohol use in females results in exposure to all the risks reviewed for men. Several consequences of drinking are more common in females and they often manifest with a lower quantity of alcohol compared to males. In adolescent and young adult females, accidents and suicide mortality predominate as health consequences of drinking. In middle age, breast cancer and osteoporosis become issues of concern. Drinking appears to be more detrimental to women than men with respect to liver disease. Cirrhosis rates are higher among female alcoholics as compared to male alcoholics, with females having lower consumption rates, as observed in a variety of studies. Alcohol is also the most widely used substance associated with domestic violence. Females are most commonly the victims of domestic violence, and both their use of alcohol and their partner's use of alcohol appear to increase risk. The risk of HIV/AIDS and alcohol use presents similar concerns in both females and males. Use of alcohol may influence the risk of acquiring HIV infection, both through direct effects on the immune system, as well as increased likelihood of unsafe sexual behavior during periods of intoxication.

(2) General Mechanisms of Alcohol-Related Dysfunction and Damage

Besides its direct toxic effects on target tissue, alcohol also may act indirectly through a variety of mechanisms. Other alcohol-associated behaviors involving tobacco, risky sexual behavior, illicit drugs, and other chemicals as well as nonalcohol-related disease processes, may contribute as cofactors to the development, course, and outcome of alcohol-induced primary damage. In addition, alcohol may influence the development, course, and outcome of coincidental diseases.

Much of the tissue damage that occurs in association with alcohol use has been attributed, at least in part, to direct toxic effects; examples include alcoholic hepatitis, cardiomyopathy, and neuronal degeneration. However, new findings suggest that excitotoxicity mediated through alterations in glutamate neurotransmission may be responsible for many of the central nervous system (CNS) degenerative processes associated with alcoholism (e. g. Wernike-Korsakoff syndrome, cerebellar degeneration, dementia associated with alcoholism). The effects on the CNS are also of great importance in the development of various alcohol-related problems associated with acute intoxication and withdrawal from alcohol, as well as alcohol dependence. Acute effects are particularly important in circumstances under which drinkers may injure themselves or others.

Alcohol also may act indirectly by producing metabolic disturbances, endocrine changes, immune system changes, aggravation of obstructive sleep apnea, and displacement of dietary nutrients or impairment of their absorption or use, as well as through the effects of diseases caused by alcohol. Obstructive sleep apnea, a complication of alcohol use that occurs as a result of acute intoxication, is potentially important as a direct cause of morbidity and mortality. It may contribute also to the course and outcome of other alcohol-and nonalcohol-related diseases. This disturbance and its precipitation and aggravation by alcohol have been recognized only recently. When an alcohol-related health problem does occur, its course and outcome may be influenced by the affected individual's continued exposure to alcohol and alcohol-related hazards. Furthermore, course and outcome may be influenced by whether or not the affected individual seeks, has access to, receives, and adheres to effective treatment, not only for the complications of alcohol use but also for the drinking behavior itself.

6. 3. 2. 5   Estimating the Public Health Importance of Alcohol-Related Problems

Alcohol-consuming nations usually consider the public health importance of alcohol-related health problems to be significant, although the impact of alcohol-related health problems on the total burden of ill health varies from country to country. Many different groups experience the effects of alcohol-related health problems. This includes those with alcohol-related health problems, their families, other individuals or groups who may suffer injury or loss due to others' use of alcohol, those who provide services for the prevention and treatment of alcohol-related problems, and the community at large.

Many of the effects are tangible but immeasurable, such as the pain and suffering of the alcohol-damaged individual and his or her family. However, other manifestations of alcohol-related problems are suitable for empirical study; examples include the incidence and prevalence of alcohol-related health problems, the costs of health and social services attributable to these problems, the number of people who are disabled or die from alcohol-related problems, and the economic costs of illness, disability, and death. It may be possible to make reasonably good estimates for specific aspects of mortality and morbidity, for example, the burden of alcoholic psychoses in specialized institutions.

(1) Epidemiology of Alcohol-Related Problems

WHO reported that, in 2014, alcohol consumption contributed 5.1% of the burden of global disease and injury, as evaluated by disability adjusted life year (DALY). According to report on alcohol-related deaths in Canada in 1980, of the almost 18,000 such deaths (10.5% of all deaths), the vast majority (88.0%) were classified as indirectly related; that is, they were due to accidents, cancers, and circulatory and respiratory diseases in which alcohol was a contributing factor. This problem is further exemplified by U.S. studies and also epidemiological studies in China.

(2) A New Measurement Model for Alcohol-Related Problems

A different approach to quantifying the effects of alcohol-related health problems is to express them in monetary terms. Such an approach is useful because it provides an estimate of the relative distribution of the costs, for example, across organ systems or various health and social services, as well as a measure of total costs. Thus, these figures can be used to compare the costs of alcohol-related problems with other health problems as a basis for focusing the attention of the community or making policy decisions regarding the funding of prevention, treatment, and research.

(3) Universal Prevention Efforts

① Per capital consumption: A substantial body of evidence now supports the view that increases in overall or per capita consumption are associated with higher rates of heavy drinking and, consequently, with increased frequencies of alcohol-related health problems. Studies of relationships between per capita alcohol consumption and alcohol-related morbidity and mortality have focused on cirrhosis, where a strong positive correlation has been established. Per capita consumption also has been correlated positively with total mortality in men, international variations in deaths from diabetes mellitus, deaths from alcohol-related disease, alcoholism death rates, and hospital admission for alcohol dependence, alcoholic psychosis, liver cirrhosis, pancreatitis, Wernicke's encephalopathy, and Korsakoff's psychosis.

Recognition of the relationships among per capita alcohol consumption, rates of heavy use, and the incidence of alcohol-related health problems has focused attention on universal prevention strategies aimed at the drinking population, generally with the principal objective of reducing per capita alcohol consumption. Critical reviews suggest that measures addressing the economic and physical accessibility of alcohol are among the most effective in this regard.

② Community-based programs: Beyond the individual, broader community context factors are also strong predictors of alcohol use and problems. Community use patterns, availability of alcohol (including legal drinking age, cost, and enforcement), and peer group behavior affect the use and abuse of alcohol. Universal prevention efforts have been attempted in various forms, but community-based programs for the prevention of alcohol abuse and alcohol-related problems are difficult to design, implement, and complete. A more direct universal prevention strategy involves limiting availability, increasing enforcement of laws pertaining to alcohol use, legislating stricter laws, improving community standards, and increasing the cost of alcoholic beverages through taxation.

③ Prevention strategies: The public health approach to disease prevention was first classified in 1957 as proposed by the Commission on Chronic Illness. Primary, secondary, and tertiary prevention techniques were defined. In this model, primary prevention is geared toward efforts to decrease new cases of a disorder (incident cases), secondary prevention is designed to lower the rate of established cases (prevalent cases), and tertiary prevention seeks to decrease the amount of disability associated with existing disorder or illness.

Gordon later proposed an alternative classification system that incorporated a concept stating risks and benefits measures are desirable only for a select population who are at above-average risk for developing a disorder. Preventive measures are applied, as indicated, to individuals who, upon screening examination, demonstrate a high risk of developing a disorder.

The Institute of Medicine (IOM) noted that both classification systems were designed and optimized for traditional medical disorders, but that their application to mental disorders was not straightforward. The IOM proposed an alternative system, which is referred to as the Mental Health Intervention Spectrum for Mental Illness. This system incorporates the whole spectrum of interventions for mental disorders, from prevention, through treatment, to maintenance. The term prevention is reserved for those interventions that occur before the initial onset of the disorder, and it incorporates many of Gordon's concepts such as universal, selective, and indicated measures.

(4) Accessibility

① Economic accessibility: Numerous studies, reviews, and reports have examined the use of price control via taxation in reducing alcohol consumption and alcohol-related problems. The accumulated evidence indicates that price control could be effective and, in some instances, powerful, both in relation to other measures and in combination with them.

Based on an analysis of the price of beer and spirits, other economic and sociodemographic factors, and various regulatory control variables, Ornstein concluded that price was the most important policy tool available to regulators in the United States. Others, however, have been more guarded in their support for price manipulation as a control measure, pointing out the methodological limitations in econometric analyses, the modest or conflicting implications of some findings, and the possible role of countervailing forces.

Price control via taxation has been recommended repeatedly as a strategy for stabilizing or reducing per capita consumption and thereby preventing alcohol-related health problems.

② Legal accessibility: Age limitations represent a legal barrier to alcohol. Most countries have age restrictions on alcohol purchase and/or consumption. Although the data are neither unflawed nor entirely consistent, much evidence indicates that the lower the drinking age, the higher the consumption of alcohol and the higher the incidence of alcohol-related problems, particularly among teenagers.

An investigation by WHO on accidents in 2008 showed that approximately 50%—60% of traffic accidents are related to drunk driving, and drunk driving has been listed as the main cause of death from traffic accidents. In China, tens of thousands of traffic accidents are caused by drunk driving and more than 50% of fatal accidents are related to drunk driving each year. Therefore, drunk driving was officially codified into the Criminal Law of the People's Republic of China on August 23, 2010. Recently, in the United States, most states instituted lowered blood alcohol content limits for legal driving. The effect of such measures on automobile crashes and automobile fatalities will be an important outcome measure.

(5) Screening

① Screening for alcohol dependence: The most commonly used tools for screening alcohol dependence are questionnaires and laboratory values. The most common screening questionnaires include the Michigan Alcoholism Screening Test (MAST), the abbreviated Brief-MAST, and the CAGE instrument. Several newer instruments include the Alcohol Use Disorders Identification Test (AUDIT) and the TWEAK instrument. Laboratory screening tests include blood alcohol levels, liver enzyme elevations, erythrocyte mean corpuscular volume, lipid profiles, and carbohydrate-deficient transferrin.

② Screening questionnaires: Allen et al. offer guidelines for selection of screening tests in primary care. Based upon their review of the literature, use of the AUDIT, CAGE, or MAST was recommended. Because of time constraints in primary care, the AUDIT or CAGE were first choice recommendations, and the TWEAK was recommended for pregnant women. For adolescents, the adolescent drinking index (ADI) was suggested as a good option. In the elderly, two studies point to deficiencies in the CAGE as a screening tool and suggest the need for more sensitive and specific tools in this population.

③ Laboratory screening tools: Unfortunately, to date, laboratory tests for screening have not been as sensitive nor as specific for alcohol use disorders when compared to the screening questionnaires reviewed above. Liver enzymes, including gamma glutamyltransferase (GGT), aspartate aminotransferase (AST), alanine aminotransferase (ALT), and alkaline phosphatase have all been used as screening tests. The GGT is the most useful of the liver tests, demonstrating a sensitivity of 50%—90% for ingestion of 40—60 g of alcohol daily (3—4 standard drinks). The GGT rises most rapidly in response to heavy alcohol use, and with abstinence it returns to normal most rapidly. Other liver enzyme tests such as the AST, ALT, and alkaline phosphatase are less specific and sensitive than the GGT.

In a general medical setting, liver enzymes and mean corpuscular erythrocyte volume (MCV) are often ordered as part of the medical work-up for individuals who present for care. Laboratory studies in combination with screening questionnaires can be useful in discussions with patients regarding the health consequences of their alcohol use.

(6) Effective Intervention

Recent evidence strongly suggests that brief interventions in the early stages of heavy drinking are both feasible and effective. Some studies have shown the effectiveness of brief intervention in socially stable, healthy, problem drinkers who do not have a high degree of alcohol dependence and whose histories of problem drinking are short. In confirmed heavy drinkers, a careful assessment of alcohol dependence is required to determine if brief intervention is appropriate.

The degree of alcohol dependence is also crucial in determining whether the treatment goal should be moderation (i. e. controlled drinking) or abstinence. Moderation appears to be a realistic alternative in problem drinkers who are not heavily alcohol dependent, as is often the case in early-stage heavy drinkers. Moderation may be a more acceptable treatment goal particularly in environments where alcohol use is especially diffuse and among young drinkers, who may perceive the penalty of abstinence to outweigh the risks from continued drinking.

In summary, most heavy drinkers do not seek treatment for their alcohol problems, but socially stable persons at early stages of problem drinking have a better prognosis. Health professionals in primary care settings are in an excellent position to identify problem drinkers, and brief intervention by health professionals can be effective in reducing heavy alcohol use.

Alcohol use problems are not restricted to those with alcohol abuse or dependency. Recognizing that hazardous drinking is linked to many health-related and societal burdens is a first step toward a rational public health policy. Primary care providers are asked to screen for and be able to treat many different disorders. Alcohol use problems have, for too long, been viewed as either untreatable or requiring specialty management in all cases. However, evidence suggests that office screening tools, combined with relatively brief interventions, can be powerful methods to help assist a large population at risk. While alcohol screening must compete with many disorders for primary care providers' attention, it is hoped that the data presented in this chapter will raise the priority of alcohol use disorder in the minds of those caregivers.

(Dai Yue, Yan Zhao, Zhang Qiao, Zhao Jinshun, Jenny Bowman)

Exercises

图书在版编目(CIP)数据

预防医学＝ Preventive Medicine：英文 / 赵进顺,倪春辉,
孟晓静主编. —杭州:浙江大学出版社,2020.7
ISBN 978-7-308-20295-4

Ⅰ.①预… Ⅱ.①赵…②倪…③孟… Ⅲ.①预防医学－
教材－英文 Ⅳ.①R1

中国版本图书馆 CIP 数据核字(2020)第 103987 号

预防医学

赵进顺　　倪春辉　　孟晓静　　主编

丛书策划	朱　玲	
责任编辑	李　晨	
责任校对	陈丽勋	
封面设计	春天书装	
出版发行	浙江大学出版社	
	(杭州市天目山路 148 号　邮政编码 310007)	
	(网址:http://www.zjupress.com)	
排　　版	浙江时代出版服务有限公司	
印　　刷	杭州高腾印务有限公司	
开　　本	787mm×1092mm　1/16	
印　　张	29.5	
字　　数	935 千	
版 印 次	2020 年 7 月第 1 版　2020 年 7 月第 1 次印刷	
书　　号	ISBN 978-7-308-20295-4	
定　　价	75.00 元	